A Physician's Journey

Yoga & Meditation
to
Holistic Medicine

Dennis K. Chernin, MD, MPH

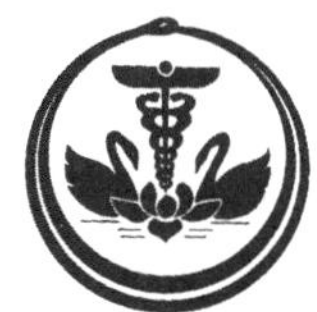

Himalayan Institute Hospital Trust
Swami Ram Nagar, P.O. Jolly Grant
Dehradun 248016 Uttarakhand, India

Editing: Dr. Barbara Bova
Cover design: Connie Gage
Cover chakra illustration: Tabi Walters
Dantian flow chart: Tom Rosenbaum

© 2021 Himalayan Institute Hospital Trust
ISBN 978-81-88157-99-0
Library of Congress Control Number 2020951763

Published by:
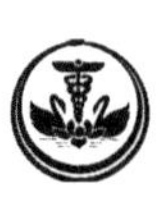
Himalayan Institute Hospital Trust
Swami Ram Nagar, P.O. Jolly Grant,
Dehradun 248016, Uttarakhand, India
Tel: 91-135-247-1233, Fax: 91-135-247-1612
src@hihtindia.org; www.hihtindia.org

Distributed by Lotus Press, P.O. Box 325, Twin Lakes, WI 53181 U.S.A.,
www.lotuspress.com, 1-262-889-8561, lotuspress@lotuspress.com.

Contents

Preface

After many years on the path of meditation and holistic health, I'm delighted to finally tell the story of my professional and spiritual journey. I am using the singular *journey* because my spiritual and professional lives have melded into one. I began writing the first edition of this book by chance. While doing research for a meditation class that I was to teach in my children's school in the year 2000, I found that books on meditation often used a lot of Sanskrit terminology or were not systematic in their description of the practice, leaving the reader with some theory but without the practical tools to establish a practice. To fill this gap, I decided to write the book, *How to Meditate Using Chakras, Mantras and Breath*, describing the meditation practice that I had been initiated into by Swami Rama and that I have used in my holistic medical practice.

For the last seven years I had been thinking of updating and expanding the book on meditation by adding some important concepts the original book had not included, such as how a holistic medical practice could be understood within the paradigms of meditation and yoga philosophy. However, every time I attempted to take up this task, I would develop a severe case of writer's block. I tried to use mantras, various concentration techniques and meditation on the fifth chakra, the center of communication and creativity, but to no avail.

Understanding my angst about writing a memoir and wanting to release me from this quagmire, Ruma wisely suggested that I expand *How to Meditate Using Chakras, Mantras and Breath* by incorporating more about my personal spiritual and professional medical journey. As we had often talked about my early experiences in a yoga ashram, she encouraged me to incorporate these reminiscences into a personal memoir of my lifelong experiment of integrating meditation and holistic medicine, and to illuminate it with personal anecdotes and case histories. Initially, I was uncomfortable with this idea as I wondered whether it would be an egotistical exercise. I also wondered if anyone would really be interested in my story. Then, a few months later, I received an email from my friend Kamal (Patrice Hafford), who had been Swami Rama's long-time personal secretary. As the director of Swami Rama Center (SRC) at the Himalayan Institute Hospital Trust in northern India, she asked if I would consider being a contributing author in a book called *At the Feet of a Himalayan Master: Swami Rama, Volume 6*, which was part of a series of the personal experiences of those who had lived and interacted with Swami Rama. Although I decided with some hesitation to accept this offer, when I sat down to begin this project, to my astonishment the words came flowing out.

A Physician's Journey: Yoga & Meditation to Holistic Medicine combines my previous book on meditation with some of the material from the above-mentioned biographical chapter. In addition, I explain how all this relates to my medical practice. In a sense, this book is a personal memoir.

In Part I, I share stories and anecdotes of my life journey, including my childhood years, my family, medical school, meeting Swami Rama, the birth of my children and my life in Ann Arbor.

Part II delves into my study of yoga philosophy, the foundation of my meditation practice. It includes summaries of three major paradigms from yoga and meditation philosophy, the koshas, the chakras and raja yoga, which I have used in both my medical practice and my personal spiritual practice for many years and which I feel offer clear and comprehensive models to understand human health and interpret disease. I also touch upon my foray into other forms of meditation such as tai chi, kirtan, Jewish Kabbalistic and the microcosmic Taoist meditation practices and compare them to the yogic meditation path.

Part III presents the theory and practical application of raja yoga, the royal path of meditation, which integrates all the other paths of yoga.

Part IV is a practical guide to the meditation system taught to me by my teachers from the Himalayan Mountain tradition, which uses chakras, mantras and the breath as a focus of concentration. These techniques make up the basis of my own personal meditation practice and what I teach my students and patients on their own spiritual and healing journeys.

Part V, the final section of the book, provides a detailed description of the therapeutic modalities I use in my medical practice, including nutrition, Ayurveda, exercise, breathing techniques, meditation, psychotherapy and homeopathy. To illuminate how I integrate the above modalities within the paradigms of the chakras and the koshas I have included several case histories.

In addition, I have briefly introduced a number of other topics that are complementary to a holistic medical practice. However, I cannot claim to be a scholar on some of the subjects that I have ambitiously touched upon in this book. To sum it all up, I am a generalist and enjoy integrating the yogic concept of the interconnectedness of body, mind and spirit and multi-dimensional healing into modern medicine while also offering the reader a practical guide to yoga and meditation.

Acknowledgments:
My Spiritual Family

I am a relationship-centric person and my family and friends are most important to me. These relationships form the very backbone of my existence both emotionally and spiritually. So I begin by acknowledging the people who have inspired and supported me on my path of meditation and medicine.

My life partner, Ruma Banerjee, PhD, has been very important in my personal journey. Not only do we share a deep interest in the practice of meditation and hatha yoga, we also enjoy discussions of the underlying philosophy. She is a professor in biochemistry at the University of Michigan Medical School, and we often share ideas on the relationship between meditation and medicine. I also want to acknowledge Ruma's wonderful editorial skills, which were important in polishing this book, as well as her elegant postures that appear in the section on hatha yoga.

Central to my spiritual approach to life is my relationship with my children, Abe, Ethan and Ari. My kids are wonderful people whom I love dearly. They inspire me to be the best man I can be. Abe was born in 1978 and my second son, Nathaniel, was born in 1980. During the sad, dark days after Nathaniel's death from SIDS in 1981 at the age of fourteen months, meditation was my refuge and afforded me moments of peace. Ethan and my daughter Ari were born in 1982 and 1984. I experienced the wonders of their homebirths and I'm so grateful to have actively guided and watched their growth, academically, creatively and athletically. I was very fortunate to have been able to coach my kids' sports teams for thirteen years. We have always been very close, and my children lovingly tease me about my unusual interests in the metaphysical world and medicine.

My kids are now married with Abe living in Chicago, Ethan in Tampa and Ari in the Denver area. Our family is still growing, and I am now a grandfather to nine little ones. Abe and Sarah have three children (Phoebe, Owen and Penelope) and Ethan and Leah have four children (Noah, Madeline, Oliver and Jacob). Ari and Michael have two sweet baby girls, Ives Ever and Lyon Lilly. Ives Ever and are about to be blessed with another child. Being a grandfather is a very spiritual experience for me. Without the worry of managing the stresses of life and schedules, it affords me the opportunity to love, help, watch, listen and guide. They are constantly in my dreams and I know we will continue to be in each other's lives through time and space.

My father, Jack, who passed away in 2002, and his wife, Jackie, had always loved and supported me, even when my earlier ashram life seemed a bit strange to them. My sister, Donna Chernin Kurit, and I were extremely close. We shared the joys and struggles of our lives from our childhood, and with her passing two years ago, I am deeply missing her loving presence in my life. As a child growing up, my mother, Berneice, exposed me to many cultural, academic and athletic pursuits and encouraged me to be sensitive and respectful of others.

Swami Rama was my first teacher of meditation and homeopathy and taught me how to incorporate the art and science of raja yoga and meditation into a medical practice. I also appreciate Alan Ajaya, PhD, who not only introduced me to the Himalayan Mountain meditation tradition but also encouraged me to meet Swami Rama. Rudolph Ballentine, MD was my first homeopathic mentor and his rigorous training helped me to be the curious and careful homeopathic physician I have become.

My childhood friend, Rick Frires, MD, continues to be a close confidant and we enjoy comparing notes from our long and intersecting spiritual paths. We are both involved with kirtan and he and his wife Char often join my kirtan chanting group. My lawyer, friend and fellow tai chi practitioner, Marty Kriegel, and I have shared many books, laughs and abstract late-night discussions on the theory and practice of meditation.

Glenn Burdick, MA has been a rock of a friend and we often share stories about personal spiritual experiences and the spiritual teachers with whom we've studied. Rosanne Emanuele, is a close and valued friend from the Himalayan Institute, as is Jerry Gore, MD, whose dedication to Judaism and holistic medicine is a source of inspiration. I also appreciate the many discussions on the link between meditation and biology that I have shared with James Arond-Thomas, MD, a holistically oriented behavioral oncologist. I also thank my good friend and homeopathic colleague, Greg Manteuffel, MD, with whom I coauthored *Health: A Holistic Approach.*

I'd be remiss if I did not mention my old medical school friend Rick Goodman, MD, JD, MPH. Our public health practices have intersected over forty-nine years, and although he doesn't share my interest in meditation and its place in holistic medicine, he has always supported me while also ribbing me on occasion about these interests. My Ann Arbor physician friend, Jack Scheerer, MD, and I enjoy our monthly lunch chats and I appreciate his continual coverage for my medical practice, which allows me to travel internationally as much as I do. I also want to acknowledge Cinda Hocking, my long-time office manager, friend and fellow tai chi practitioner.

In 1998, I traveled to northern India where I taught meditation and holistic approaches to physicians and nurses at the Himalayan Institute Hospital Trust, a huge medical, education and research institute that was founded by Swami Rama. This was my first time in India and I found the experience both inspiring and exhilarating. While I was there, I enjoyed reconnecting with Barb Bova, a homeopath and old friend from the Himalayan Institute in Glenview, whose devotion to yoga and healing closely parallels my own. Barb, Ruma and I stay in close touch and Barb has worked tirelessly to edit this book and has done a wonderful job. I can't thank her enough for her dedication in reorganizing this book and making it ready for publication. As my old friend, Wesley Van Linda, who along with Kamal Hafford, Prakash Keshaviah, and Vijay Dhasmana, has been involved with publishing this book, wisely said, "Every writer needs a reader." Also, Wesley was very helpful in clarifying concepts related to yoga philosophy.

My practice of kirtan, the ancient meditative form of call-and-response chanting, finds expression in my Ann Arbor Kirtan group. I acknowledge fellow members including, John Churchville, Matthew Pancone and Alice Greminger. We chant with the community monthly. Jai Uttal is both a good friend and kirtan teacher, and I've learned about Indian music theory from him by participating in his kirtan camps.

From 2008 to 2018 I taught meditation and shared my kirtan practice at the Sivananda ashram in the Bahamas, Grass Valley, CA, Woodbourne, NY and in Kerala, India. With their emphasis on raja yoga and the many similarities with Swami Rama's teachings, the Sivananda organization felt familiar to me. Also, Ruma and I completed the yoga teacher training program in the Bahamas.

Very recently I reconnected with an old childhood friend who lives in Israel, Rabbi Avraham Trugman. He and I shared stories of middle and high school and how our lives turned out similarly with respect to closeness to family and spiritual journeying. We exchanged books we've written, and I appreciate his edits in the section on Jewish mysticism and the tree of life in this book.

I also appreciate Ruma's daughter, Maya Ragsdale, for demonstrating the meditation and relaxation poses in this book. Ahmed Mori did a great job photographing Ruma and Maya and doing the necessary editing to bring the postures to life.

Tabi Walters did a very nice job redrawing the chakras on the front cover of this book. To me, they look like little jewels. Connie Gage also did a beautiful job designing the cover. I also want to thank Tom Rosenbaum for drawing the picture of the flow of the chi through the dantian as part of the Taoist microcosmic orbit meditation. Tom is a friend and very gifted artist who in the last six months has encouraged me to learn to draw and paint (with his tutelage), something that had been totally outside my comfort zone and inherent talent level. Stick figures have always been a major challenge for me, so it was with much trepidation that I have ventured out to dabble with sketching with pencil, pastels and charcoal as well as painting very abstract pieces in acrylics and watercolor. Perhaps I've made a bit of progress. Ruma is a very good artist in her own right and we enjoy giving each other helpful hints. With her encouragement she helps me be the best person (and fledgling artist) I can be. What fun!

All of the above people have not only made it possible for me to practice medicine in a way that is compatible with my lifestyle and philosophical approach to living, but also have given me the necessary love and support to live fully and with gratitude. For this, I thank all of them from the depth of my heart.

PART I:

Becoming a Holistic Physician

A JEWISH KID FROM CLEVELAND

I was an ordinary middle-class Jewish kid from Cleveland, minding my own business but also a bit of a know-it-all. I spent quite a bit of time in my youth dealing with the sadness and confusion that followed my parent's breakup and studying hard in school so that I could get into a good college and eventually go to medical school. I also spent a lot of time enjoying being a jock, playing high school basketball and baseball. I was raised along with my older sister Donna. We were fortunate to have been very close friends throughout our lives. We were also close to my mother's parents with whom we lived when I was a young child. Many people who knew us, have said my demeanor reminded them of my grandfather. He tended to be a quiet man, especially in groups, and was patient and hard working. In fact, he worked well into his nineties as a landscaper and died peacefully as he was approaching 102 years.

I was a fast-food junky in my earlier years, having been raised on McDonald's and plenty of candy, which my mother enthusiastically gave us. White bread was a staple, and I especially liked it slathered with sugary red jelly.

Even when I was a little kid, I knew that I wanted to be a doctor. The World Book Encyclopedias tucked under my bed after late night reading, with pictures of human anatomy, famous scientists and doctors and weird bacteria attested to this desire. I felt an inner drive to help individuals who were ailing, not only physically but also emotionally and mentally. I have always enjoyed talking to and being around people, and serving others in a healing capacity is simply a part of my DNA.

Along with this inner drive to become a physician, for as long as I can remember there has been a deep desire to fathom the unknown. Throughout junior high and high school my close friends and I would often talk about the infinite nature of the cosmos and whether we believed in God as a person or something more expansive. Those were fun discussions and I guess I'm still asking the same questions today.

COLLEGE AND MEDICAL SCHOOL

As a pre-med student I majored in cultural anthropology at Northwestern University. It was fascinating to discover how people from different cultures looked at their lives in vastly different ways, especially in indigenous societies. Likewise, their approach to healthcare and disease treatment varied widely.

I was fairly straight-laced in college and studied diligently for long hours so I could get the grades necessary to get into a good medical school. I seldom drank alcohol and didn't touch pot while at Northwestern. It was the late '60s and early '70s, so this seems surprising in retrospect. However, it was the era of the Vietnam War and I did my share of campus protesting.

Having completed my studies at Northwestern, I attended the University of Michigan Medical School at Ann Arbor where I let my hair down, so to speak, but I still played it pretty safe. I did actually grow my hair very long, so that by the time I graduated from medical college it was down to the middle of my back, while my bushy beard extended to the middle of my chest. In fact, when I did my surgery rotation, the attending surgeons made me wear three surgical masks, one over my mouth and nose and two over my beard. I was quite a sight!

As I thought about specialization, I realized I wasn't particularly fond of aggressive medical procedures, so internal medicine specialties didn't really appeal to me. Also, the patient's mind and spirit were often left out in the analysis of medical problems. Surgery was out of the question, since I did not have good fine motor skills due to my poor eyesight. I was born with cataracts, which slowly matured as I moved through college and medical school, leaving me blind at various times in my life. I've had five eye surgeries over the years and I am forever grateful to modern medicine for helping me to regain and retain my sight.

Ultimately, I decided to enter psychiatry as my medical specialty. Medical anthropology and transcultural psychiatry were also of particular interest. I considered going to the University of Vermont for its beauty or to Syracuse University for its expertise in my area of interest, but eventually I picked the University of Wisconsin Madison. This decision turned out to greatly influence my spiritual journey.

I chose Wisconsin because I had discovered there was a strong spiritual community in the city, and two of my close friends from medical school were also going there for residency. It was a very good program with emphasis on classical Freudian analysis, Rogerian empathic approaches, family systems and group therapy. Initially I enjoyed the psychiatry program and learned a great deal about human behavior and psychopathology, but I was disappointed they hadn't developed an orientation on the integration of body and mind. Other aspects that interested me that were not part of the Wisconsin program were Jungian analysis and medical anthropology. I was also deeply immersed in yoga and Buddhist philosophy and was most interested in the interface between Eastern thought, meditation and Western psychology. My final decision to leave the program occurred when I met Swami Rama and he asked me to study meditation, homeopathy and psychotherapy with him in Glenview, Illinois at his ashram.

MY SPIRITUAL BIRTH

My journey into the world of spirit, meditation and healing actually began without conscious awareness years before I met Swami Rama, my primary meditation teacher. As a young child I used to have terrible dizzy spells, especially at school. When this happened the school nurse would have to call my mother to come and pick me up early from classes. These episodes became especially frequent during the time my parents were going through their divorce. The stress and sadness I was experiencing were very intense in those days. Then one night I somehow discovered that by slowing down and smoothing out my breath, I was able to stop the dizziness. I was very happy about this discovery.

Many years later, while I was reading about breathing exercises in yoga, I was surprised and delighted to find out that I had spontaneously started to practice breathing exercises as a child and that I had discovered the power inherent in these techniques. Then as I reached my early twenties an intense craving arose in me not only to study various spiritual paths but also to experience more altered and expansive states of consciousness. My early exploration of different spiritual traditions ultimately proved to be an important influence on my spiritual path.

During the holocaust, many of the great Jewish spiritual leaders lost their lives. We post-war children were looking to move away from the relative conformity of Reformed and Conservative Judaism. We were seeking spiritual guidance, but often our rabbis were not able to captivate us. Even though great Jewish spiritual souls were undoubtedly there, the information and teachings we sought seemed hidden and inaccessible. To exacerbate the problem, religious discrimination in many European countries prompted mystically oriented Jewish spiritual teachers who had survived the Holocaust to go underground in order to avoid further persecution. In addition, they tended to make their teachings available only to very serious Orthodox students over the age of forty. All of these facts contributed to the lack of teachers and teachings that were available to us young and less religious spiritual seekers.

While there had been much interest in Eastern philosophy for hundreds of years in the West, along with a substantial body of scholarship in the 19th century, it wasn't until the 1960s and '70s that popularity of these subjects really took off. Yoga arrived from India, Buddhism came from Japan and Tibet and Taoism from China. This opened doors to new ways of holistic living, paths for dietary improvement through natural foods or vegetarianism and health through the practice of yoga, breath awareness and meditation. At the same time, the Beatles arrived. Their foray into the music and spirituality of India captivated me. My father Jack, whom I was very close to, had served in India during WWII. He was quite the amateur photographer and had taken lots of wonderful pictures in India. I became fascinated with India and wonder if his experiences there influenced me to explore India's great philosophies.

In addition, the ongoing traumas of the Vietnam War and the changing spiritual milieu in the US spurred many of us to look for higher meaning and truth. During this time, I explored several different approaches to meditation, including Zen and Tibetan Buddhism as well as Taoism and tai chi. Being Jewish, I also explored meditative approaches and more spiritually-based practices of Judaism. But mostly I absorbed myself in books about Eastern philosophy. Yogananda, Alan Watts, Suzuki Roshi, Ramana Maharishi, Sir John Woodruff, Gandhi and Lao Tsu were my earliest teachers. Like many people in the '60s and '70s, I was introduced to the theory and practice of meditation through books on Zen Buddhism and Eastern philosophy written by Alan Watts and the *Autobiography of a Yogi* by Paramahansa Yogananda. I found that the great philosophies and traditions of India had particular appeal for me and inspired me. They presented the techniques of meditation in a concise, systematic and thorough way.

In the midst of this avalanche of spiritual books, I read about a yogi from India, Swami Rama, whom I also refer to as Swamiji in this book. In laboratory experiments he had shown that he could control involuntary body functions and brainwave patterns. This included voluntarily putting his heart in ventricular tachycardia, changing the temperature by ten degrees on opposite sides of the same palm and maintaining active awareness in the delta EEG wave pattern, usually associated with deep sleep. In my quest to understand his amazing abilities and explore different states of consciousness, I continued to read voraciously. One book that especially caught my attention was *Yoga Psychology*, written by Swami Ajaya, who was teaching in Madison at that time. He was an American trained psychologist and meditation teacher, having studied with Swami Rama. In his book he did a wonderful job explaining the theory of meditation and its practical applications in Western psychological terms.

SWAMI RAMA COMES INTO MY LIFE

Meeting my spiritual teacher Swami Rama was part of a most unexpected adventure. As I had begun my psychiatry residency in Madison, I had also started to study meditation with Swami Ajaya and had received my first initiation with a personal mantra from him. My first actual exposure to homeopathy came in 1975 when Swami Ajaya introduced me to the work of his teacher, Swami Rama, and to one of his fellow students, Rudolph Ballentine, MD. At that time, they were living and practicing holistic medicine in the Chicago area, combining alternative approaches of nutrition, yoga therapies, meditation, psychotherapy, Ayurveda and homeopathy with conventional medicine. He said their work was brilliant, unique and inspiring and he strongly encouraged me to meet Swami Rama the next time he came to Madison. He said he was a most unusual man and he didn't know how long Swami Rama would be staying in the US.

And so I met Swami Rama after a lecture he gave in Madison in March 1976. After his talk, he walked up to me in the audience and said, "I've been waiting for you to come back to study with me. Come visit me in Chicago and we will discuss how best to arrange for you to learn deeper meditation practices." Needless to say, I was quite surprised. Did he mean I was destined to study with him? Did I know him from a previous life? Yet, while I questioned what he had meant, I also recognized within myself that what he said made sense.

I continued my studies until one day I had an epiphany: why not integrate my burning desire for spiritual growth and keen interest in meditation with my passionate desire to serve as a physician? And so I decided to accept Swami Rama's invitation to intensively study meditation as well as alternative and holistic medicine with him at his ashram near Chicago. I often ponder if that first meeting with Swami Rama was destiny or happenstance. He certainly changed my life. It is said in the yogic tradition that when the student is ready, the teacher will appear. So there he was, and I felt ready. Swami Rama was my first spiritual guide and continues to be my most important teacher through time and space.

It is also said that the teacher-student relationship continues even after the teacher leaves his body. Life and death are two states that the individual soul repeatedly passes through on its long journey towards enlightenment. Swamiji taught us that consciousness is not dependent on physical form and that as conscious beings we exist on many levels both in life and in death.

MOVING TO THE ASHRAM

In 1976 I left Madison and my psychiatric residency to move to the Himalayan Institute, Swami Rama's ashram in Glenview, Illinois, a suburb just north of Chicago. My ex-wife Jan and I lived there for four and a half years. While we were there, I meditated, learned homeopathy, taught classes, ran a holistic medical center, discovered how to care for and love my patients and helped manage a spiritual center. During my early years at the Himalayan Institute, I was immersed in attaining knowledge of the philosophy and practice of meditation, yoga and breathing. Raja yoga, the eight-fold path of yogic meditation, was the basis of my practice, and jnana yoga, the path of knowledge, was also an important focus. I studied the Bhagavad Gita, the Vedas and the Upanishads and also practiced karma yoga. We were encouraged to do our work with skill and thoughtfulness so as not to create new unhealthy karma.

When I first arrived at the Himalayan Institute, I had been studying meditation and yoga philosophy for several years but still felt like I was a beginner on the path. Within a few months, Swamiji asked me to teach classes on the science of breath, nutrition, homeopathy and various aspects of meditation. When I told him I felt uncomfortable starting to teach already, he just smiled and said not to worry, that he was going to take me to the top and I would be a great teacher. At the time, I wasn't sure what he meant but I now realize that teaching others is one of the best ways to immerse oneself in a subject and learn more quickly.

A LESSON IN EGO

I had kept my hair and beard very long during medical school and residency and they were still very long when I arrived at the Himalayan Institute. Swamiji immediately told me to cut my hair. Of course I was strongly resistant to this idea and so I cut my hair just a bit, still retaining the hippie look. After weeks of gentle scolding and my lack of responsiveness, he said loudly and sternly in front of a group of people, "Leave the ashram and don't come back."

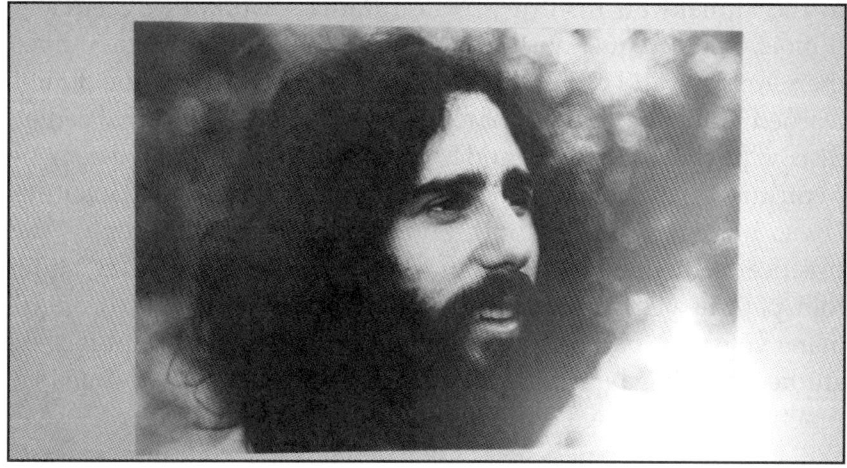

Dennis during his ashram days

After some tears and regret over my stubbornness, I talked to my homeopathy mentor, Rudolph Ballentine. He said that cutting my hair was like changing clothes and that I should change and be unattached to outward appearances. So, I finally cut my hair short. But was it too late? With some trepidation, I walked over to Swamiji's room and knocked on his door. He opened the door, looked at me sternly, cocked his head, but then said with a smile, "Sonny, I love you, now get to work." He mostly called me Sonny, and sometimes Dr. Chernin. Only once did he call me Dennis.

While I was happy that he had accepted me back into the fold, he surprised me again the next day when he said, "You look so good now, so to even improve on this appearance, I'd like you to also start wearing a short white coat, like the ones doctors wear in hospitals." I gently explained to him that doctors have long white coats and the short ones are for medical students. He smiled, seemed amused and said that he thought the shorter one would be better.

Since I had spent years as a medical student and young physician cultivating the image of a rebellious doctor with holistic leanings, I felt embarrassed that I had to appear like a traditional student in training. But I had learned my lesson. Quietly though begrudgingly, I started to wear a short coat.

To add to my embarrassment, a few months later my very close childhood friend from Cleveland, Rick Frires, also a young doctor and whom I hadn't seen in a few years, tapped me on the shoulder and said, "Denny Chernin, it's really good to see you in the ashram. I had no idea you lived at the Himalayan Institute. I saw your picture on the wall and was looking around for you." He then chuckled and said, "Nice short white coat!" We hugged, and then shared a big laugh when I told him about the hair and coat incidents.

What I learned from those incidents was the need to keep my ego in check. I had become very attached to my hair and to my general appearance. It reflected my need to separate myself from traditional doctors who I felt didn't have a holistic approach to healing and medicine. Swamiji taught me a very valuable lesson. He would say that one needs a strong ego for self-development, self-respect, identity and personal power, but that one should not get attached to it. He often said to use the ego like a good shoe. You should take good care of it and wear it well but toss it aside when it is worn out. Like the shoe, it is important to let the ego protect you as you walk through life, but when it is no longer useful as your consciousness expands to greater realities, toss it aside.

Swamiji would tell us to be free of all attachments and to identify with the real Self, the divinity within. He said all reality is Brahman or pure consciousness, and all else is illusion or maya. He emphasized the importance of identification with the all-encompassing inner Self, not the temporary sense of ego and its inherent separateness from the universal truth.

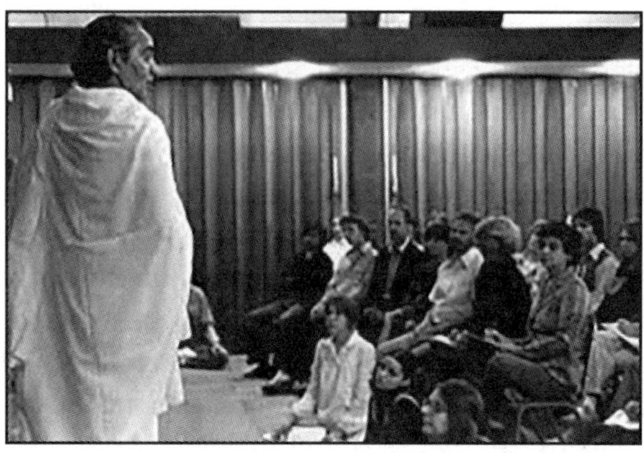

Swami Rama lecturing at Himalayan Institute, Glenview, Il

TRAINING IN HOMEOPATHY

Looking back at my medical school experience at the University of Michigan, I remember hearing the word *homeopathic* once. I believe it was when one of my internal medicine professors talked about the small amount of replacement thyroid hormone needed for someone who had had their thyroid irradiated (and destroyed) as a treatment for Graves' disease, a form of hyperthyroidism. He called this minute quantity a "homeopathic dosage." Despite using this term, I'm virtually certain he had no idea what homeopathy really was. At the time I wondered what he meant by this statement but quickly moved on as I was trying to absorb the voluminous amounts of information coming my way. Little did I know that I would later spend a lifetime studying, contemplating, absorbing and practicing this absolutely fascinating therapeutic system of medicine.

As stated earlier, Swami Rama had invited me to study with him at the Himalayan Institute and to work in Dr. Ballentine's medical clinic, the Center for Holistic Medicine. Our one-year commitment turned into a four and a half-year stay that included the birth of two of our four children, two years of supervised training in homeopathy and two years of helping train many other young physicians in the art and science of homeopathy. In the mid

'70s, there were only a few living homeopaths in the States and those people were bridges to the great physicians of homeopathy's golden years. We were fortunate to study and learn from these elder statesmen, including Drs. Rood, Panos, Sutherland, White, Williams and Rodgers.

During this period, the doctors and staff would have weekly clinics to discuss difficult cases with Swami Rama, himself an experienced Indian trained homeopath, seeing many patients in a short time. We would have two-hour long huge Indian lunches together with our staff and other doctors and teach classes and meditate in the evening together. Sometimes there would be three or four physicians training with us, and besides being stimulating, it was very enjoyable to share so much of our lives. We were a community brought together with a common goal of healing, study and meditation. This was a time of tremendous growth and learning, sometimes challenging, and generally a lot of fun.

A NEW HOME

After having lived off-site from the Himalayan Institute campus without a salary for six months, Swamiji called me at 9 a.m. one Sunday morning and said he was going to teach me and that we should move into his house on the Himalayan Institute campus, as he would be moving to an apartment nearby. Needless to say, again I was stunned by this offer. I thought he had already been teaching me, but then I supposed that he was withholding the real teachings until I showed him I was committed to the path and was ready for deeper initiations. Moving into his house felt like an unbelievable gift at the time. As it turns out, living in an ashram setting was an amazing communal experience but also at times quite stressful, a bit like living in a glass house. There was little privacy!

The Center for Holistic Medicine occupied one side of our house, and the waiting room for patients during the day was our living room at night. There was a swinging door between the communal space and our kitchen area. One day, after a heavy lunch (causing me to have my usual post-meal fatigue crash), I fell asleep with my head on the waiting room side of the door and my legs

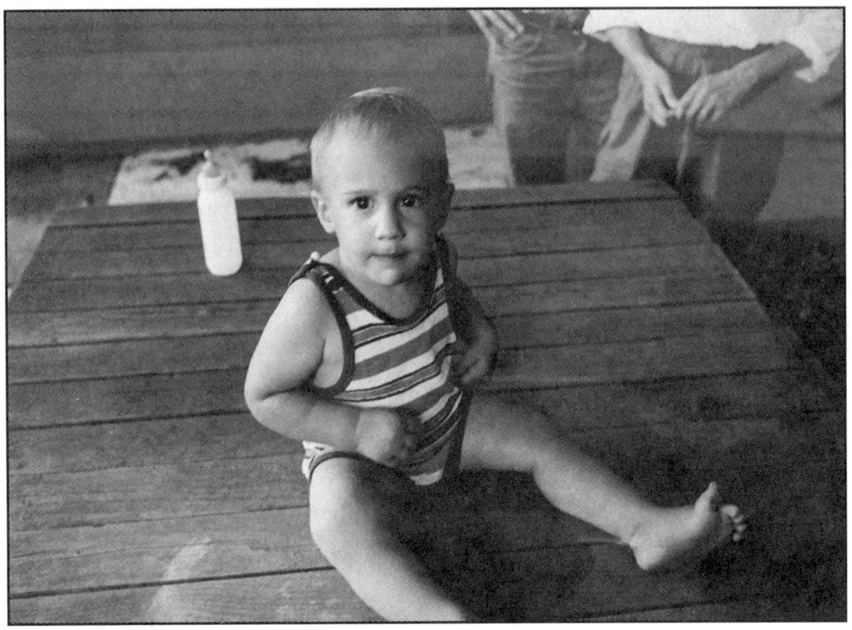

Abe

on the kitchen side. Although the afternoon patients had begun to come in, my doctor friends, amused at the sight of me, just let me lie there in full view of the patients! I woke up startled and looked around with embarrassment, while everyone chuckled.

My first two children were born in that house. Having two children in the communal setting of the ashram was enjoyable for me. My eldest child, Abe, would sit in my lap when I meditated and would pull on my beard when he got bored or wanted my attention. He used to walk right up to me while I was teaching my evening classes and start to imitate me and attempt to teach. Sometimes when Swamiji would be lecturing in the evenings, Abe would strut up to the stage, grab the eraser and wipe out Swamiji's notes. He would begin talking and babbling to the audience (he was two at the time), mimicking Swamiji, who would actually encourage him, start laughing and tell him and the students that Abe was a very good boy. At other times, Swamiji would enjoy giving Abe ladoos (a sugary Indian sweet). My second son, Nathaniel, was born 27 months after Abe. He was a sweet little boy and his stay at the

Glenview Center was short, since we ended up moving away six months after his birth.

WAS HE READING MY MIND?

Sometimes it seemed like Swamiji knew what I was thinking. Once, I was walking down the hall and I heard his booming voice behind me say, "Sonny, you should stop worrying about finances, you will be taken care of. The universe will provide." At that very moment, I had been fretting that we had such a small bank balance. Then there was the time when I was sitting with several other people having lunch in his room and we were chatting about the excellent tasting Indian food in front of us. My mind wandered and I began to think of a patient's mysterious illness. Swamiji turned to me and asked that I please give this very same patient a specific homeopathic remedy. I witnessed this type of thing several other times with myself and with other people.

SPIRITUAL TEACHERS I'VE MET
ON THE WAY

One of the great opportunities of living and teaching at the Himalayan Institute back in the late '70s was participating in the yearly international conferences that we organized, which brought together thousands of spiritual seekers. I met many of the spiritual teachers who came from the East as well as many religious leaders trained in the West. These included Swami Satchidananda (student of Swami Sivananda), Pir Vilayat Khan (leader of the American Sufis), Yogi Bhajan (founder of the Kundalini Yoga organization), Pramodaji Chitrabhanu (Jain leader), Roy Eugene Davis (student of Yogananda), Ravi Shankar (renowned sitarist) and Rabbi Joseph Gelberman (leading Jewish Kabbalist). It was a great privilege to interact with, learn from and sometimes attend to these great teachers as a physician. I was a moderator in the first year that I participated in this conference. The next several years, I gave lectures on such topics as the science of breath and how the chakra system could be used as a healing paradigm.

Later, on one of my visits to India I rediscovered an important spiritual connection to one of Swami Rama's most erudite students, Dr. Usharbudh Arya, who was now Swami Veda Bharati. Until the time of his passing, he continued to be one of the foremost scholars of meditation, mantra and Vedic knowledge in the world. Ruma and I had the great pleasure of meeting with him in 2012 in his ashram in Rishikesh. Luckily, our visit preceded his vow of five years of silence, and I felt very privileged to be able to renew our friendship over a cup of tea. He invited me back to his ashram and to teach whenever possible. Sadly, Swami Veda passed away in 2015. My meeting with him was helpful in getting me reconnected with the Himalayan Institute tradition.

More recently, Ruma and I had the privilege to spend time with a Tibetan Buddhist nun, Jetsunma Tenzin Palmo. She was one of the first women ordained into the Tibetan monastic tradition and had spent twelve years living alone in a cave high in the Himalayan Mountains. We visited her at the Sivananda Ashram in India. She was a very focused, pleasant and humorous person, noticeably at peace with herself. Currently, she is running a Buddhist monastery for young women in the Himalayas.

WE MOVE TO ANN ARBOR

In 1981, we felt it was time to leave the Glenview ashram. We were getting a little tired of being in a big city and wanted to be closer to family in the Detroit area and in Cleveland, Ohio. Earlier we had briefly discussed moving to another spiritual community, The Abode, located in upstate New York. They were oriented towards the Sufi tradition and had just started the Omega Institute. I would have been involved in building Omega into a spiritual retreat center as well as starting a private medical practice. We decided instead to move to Ann Arbor, a decision that Swamiji supported. He encouraged me to start a branch of the Himalayan Institute, if and when I was ready, and promised to visit often to help the center grow and thrive. I had also decided it was time to finish my psychiatry residency and get board certified in a specialty. I had previously been accepted to the University of Michigan's

Department of Psychiatry and had two years left to finish the program.

Unfortunately, when I got to Ann Arbor I discovered the Psychiatry Department's program had become very medication-oriented and less psychotherapeutic in scope. I was no longer moving in this direction as I was intent on trying to integrate Eastern forms of meditation into traditional forms of psychotherapy, especially Jungian approaches to dream analysis. Since this seemed incompatible with the emphasis on medication in the traditional psychiatry program, I decided for a second time not to finish the psychiatry residency.

The first time I had left the psychiatry program was at Madison so I could study with Swami Rama and learn holistic medicine and meditation. Having learned to treat the whole person, I found the traditional approaches to treating the mind with medication too narrow for my liking. In my work at the Himalayan Institute I had learned that the treatment of suffering individuals must ultimately focus on the mind, where, according to ancient medical systems, disease largely originates. Although Western psychology has undoubtedly played an integral role in how we understand mental illness, the split between man's psyche and soma has been widened by increased sub-specialization in medicine and psychiatry. If the patient's problems are not viewed in totality, treatment can only be fragmentary, and the patient may not really understand how to interrelate emotional problems with specific physical ills.

MY SON PASSES AWAY

Our second son, Nathaniel, was five months old when we moved to Ann Arbor. He had been a happy and sweet baby and was a gift to us, albeit for a very short time. When he was almost fourteen months old he passed away from sudden infant death syndrome. I experienced more grief than I thought was possible. He was full of life, was crawling and had begun to communicate with words. When he didn't wake up at his usual time one morning, I went to check on him and discovered that he had died quietly in his sleep. We were devastated.

Swamiji called us soon after Nathaniel's passing and, with great love, said that Nathaniel's life was short because he only needed a short amount of time in this physical world to complete his work. He said that he was now free of body consciousness and could easily move to other realms. He also said that he was closely connected to us karmically and we were very important to him in this and other incarnations. Swamiji's words were very comforting at a time of great sorrow. We received this card from Swamiji and the residents of the Himalayan International Institute, Honesdale, Pennsylvania, after Nathaniel's death.

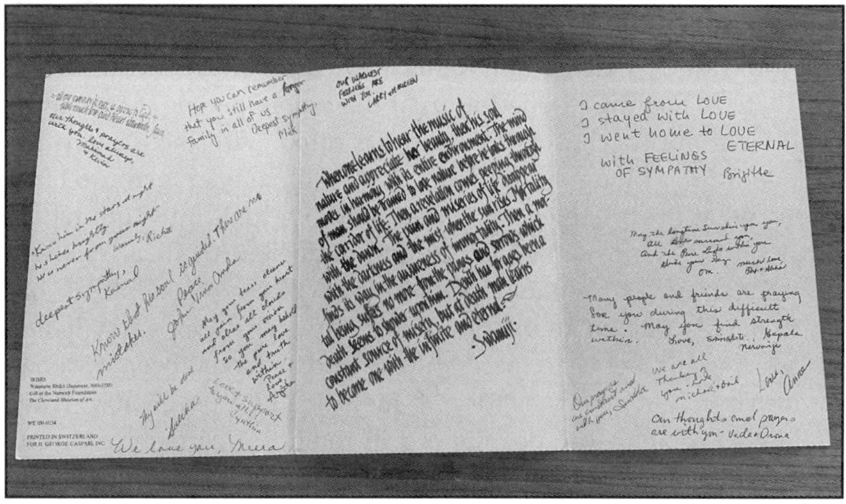

Card sent from Swamiji and Himalayan Institute residents
after Nathaniel's death

I often feel that Nathaniel has been my angelic guide. He made me a better, more sensitive and compassionate physician. His passing helped me feel others' pain more deeply. His sudden death caused me to move into inner spaces of sadness and emotional survival daily. Those were long and heavy days, and just getting up in the morning was sometimes a challenge. As we had no savings, I had to go back to work three days after his passing. The community of friends, colleagues and patients rallied around us, which helped comfort us. I have many beautiful letters that people sent at that time, which I rediscovered recently. I have now reread them and realize there was great love surrounding us. After losing Nathaniel, we never again thought of leaving Ann Arbor. Establishing roots and raising my children here felt right and I do not regret that decision. Ann Arbor is a safe and intellectual community, full of interesting people, arts and music.

A NEW BEGINNING

Shortly after we had moved, I set up a solo medical practice using and refining the same methods and modalities I had learned at the Himalayan Institute. Fortunately, I had begun to see patients privately before my psychiatry program was to begin, and I already had a long waiting list. In exchange for teaching homeopathy to my colleague, Lev Linkner, MD, he sent patients my way to help build my practice. It was a mutually beneficial exchange and my practice grew quite quickly. In 1987, Lev and I purchased two beautiful Victorian homes and moved those buildings three miles from downtown Ann Arbor, restoring and connecting them together to create a truly complementary and holistic medical center. Presently, I continue to treat patients there and to teach interested doctors, health care practitioners, medical students and lay people about homeopathy.

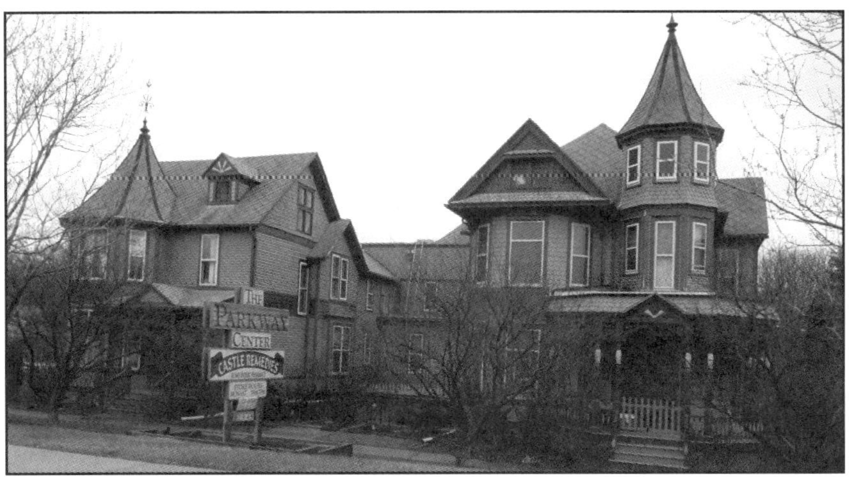

Our holistic health center in Ann Arbor, Michigan

In 1983, I decided to start a residency in preventive medicine and public health and to obtain a masters in public health (MPH). I finished in 1987 and remain board certified in this specialty. I still continue to work two days a week in two county public health departments where I function as the medical director and chief epidemiology officer for these counties. Both counties are rural, one being mostly poor and white and the other being mostly poor and white but with a sizable immigrant community of Mexican workers. My many years of working in rural Michigan have opened my eyes to the grinding poverty, health inequalities, poor housing and education that plague rural communities like those I work in.

I'm happy that I have had an opportunity to work in public health and help people in underserved communities. Public health measures (e.g. clean water, milk free from tuberculosis and other bacterial infections, better sanitation methodology and immunization) have accounted for ninety percent of health improvement and increased life expectancy in the last century and I am privileged to have contributed to implementation of these changes in local communities.

When I look back on my career, I am very grateful to have practiced preventive medicine on multiple levels besides the individual. My public health work has had innumerable community and global implications. During my public health career I have worked with such important public health issues as AIDS, bioterrorism, Lyme disease, measles, hepatitis A, the H1N1 influenza and West Nile outbreaks as well as enabling children to receive necessary immunizations and food stamps (WIC).

As I'm editing this book now, we are in the midst of the COVID-19 pandemic. I am helping with local public health activities, hospital testing procedures, coordinating local quarantining and working at ending the current lockdown. I have been in constant dialogue with state reps, sheriffs, judges, nursing home owners, hospital administrators, ER physicians, county commissioners, other medical directors and county health officers and often discuss important issues on radio and TV. During the current lockdown, we as a nation have learned how important public health planning, disaster preparedness and epidemiological investigation are in the prevention of disease and maintenance of community and world health.

I'm very proud to be part of the US public health infrastructure and really hope that those afflicted with the virus and those whose jobs have ended due to the sequestration and lockdown are able to recover quickly. And to those doctors, nurses and staff on the front line treating the very sick, I send my sincerest thanks.

FEELING GRATITUDE

Swamiji had always been kind and loving to me and my family. Looking back, I feel grateful for my time with him at the ashram and have few regrets about those remarkable years. There was a great amount of excitement during most of my time there and the learning was constant. While I have studied with several other teachers over the years, my meditation practice continues to be that which Swamiji taught me through face-to-face instruction and by his communication through my meditation.

I continued to visit Swamiji in Honesdale in the early '80s, usually organizing my trip around a meditation conference or homeopathy workshop. Occasionally we would visit or write to Swamiji. Here is one letter (next page) he lovingly wrote to us.

My involvement, however, with Swamiji and the Himalayan Institute slowly diminished in the late '80s and early '90s. I was immersed in building a medical practice and a holistic center in Ann Arbor and now had three children to care for. Also during that time, controversies about some of Swamiji's actions troubled me and I needed some distance from the organization. I spoke to Swamiji about my concerns and he was respectful of my feelings. He encouraged me to continue my practice and to use the teachings and my meditation as my ultimate guides. This was extremely important to me because I realized that if my inner self were part of the universal consciousness, then all the answers were within me.

I sometimes regret the lapse in my contact with Swamiji. I didn't know that he was very ill and felt sad when I got word of his passing in 1996. I would have liked to say goodbye and tell him how he had helped me grow in so many ways. I have talked to

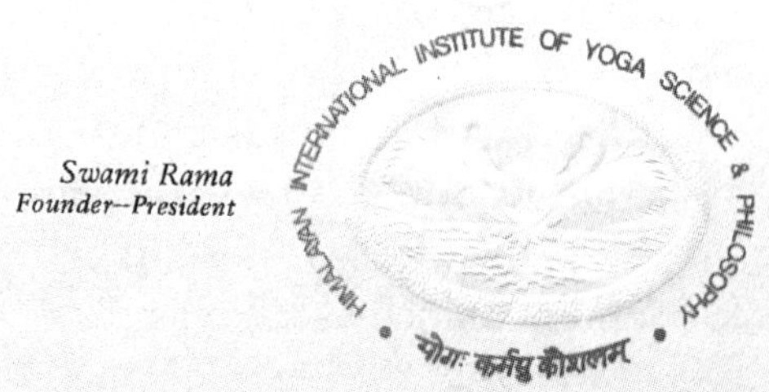

Swami Rama
Founder--President

INTERNATIONAL INSTITUTE OF YOGA SCIENCE & PHILOSOPHY

Himalayan International Institute
RD 1, Box 88, Honesdale, PA 18431
717/253-5551

July 19,1985

Dr. Dennis Chernin
2225 Packard, Suite 1
Ann Arbor Michigan

Dear Dennis and Jan:

God Bless you. I was delighted to meet you both at the Congress. I was very
happy that Abraham remembered me. I love him very much. The children are
all very dear to me. You know that I love you both very much.

I am very glad to know that your work is going well. You should both definitely
finish your degree programs. It is a temporary sacrifice but it will help
you both to do some useful work in the world.

You should definitely start a branch of the Himalayan Institute when you are
able to do it comfortably without too much stress. Whether you do it now or
after your degree is completed is up to you. Whatever you can do, whether
you continue to teach students on your own, or open a center, you know
that I will help you in any way that I can. You are both in my thoughts
and I pray for you often. If you do decide to open a center, you should
make sure that you can continue to provide well for your family.

At present I am very busy and do not feel much like traveling. I am
most interested in writing and staying quietly to rest for awhile. You should
see the Institute grounds even since Congress. We have built a bridge by the
Red Dot trail for the children to play on. Give my love and blessings to
the children. God Bless you.

Yours in the Service of the Lord,

Swami Rama

Copy of a letter Swami Rama wrote to Dennis in Ann Arbor

Ruma about my times and remarkable experiences with Swamiji. Interestingly, even before I met Ruma, she and her family had read Swami Rama's book, *Living with the Himalayan Masters*. Over the last ten years Ruma and her children, Maya and Rishi, and I have often meditated together, and we have used the practices, mantras and techniques Swamiji had taught me years ago.

Swamiji said to love others as yourself because we are all one. It was essential to sit in meditation but to apply meditation to daily life and activity was also of great importance. None of us is free until all beings are free to experience enlightenment, which is the great Buddhist concept of the bodhisattva principle. It is our duty to help ourselves as well as others on the path.

When I look back on my years with Swamiji, I remember the excitement of his presence. He was gentle at times but could be harsh and critical at others. He was an enigmatic and charismatic man who had great depth of knowledge and experience with meditation, which he readily shared with serious students. He transmitted energy *(shaktipat)* through his gaze, through touch and through meditation as a vehicle for teaching those students who were prepared. Through my association with him I learned that the knowledge and power gained from meditation needed to be harnessed and directed carefully. I also learned that it is essential to trust one's inner meditation practice rather than depend too heavily on a teacher for spiritual guidance. I continue to feel Swamiji's presence especially during the quiet of meditation. While I miss seeing him in person, I know that he continues to guide me in subtler realms.

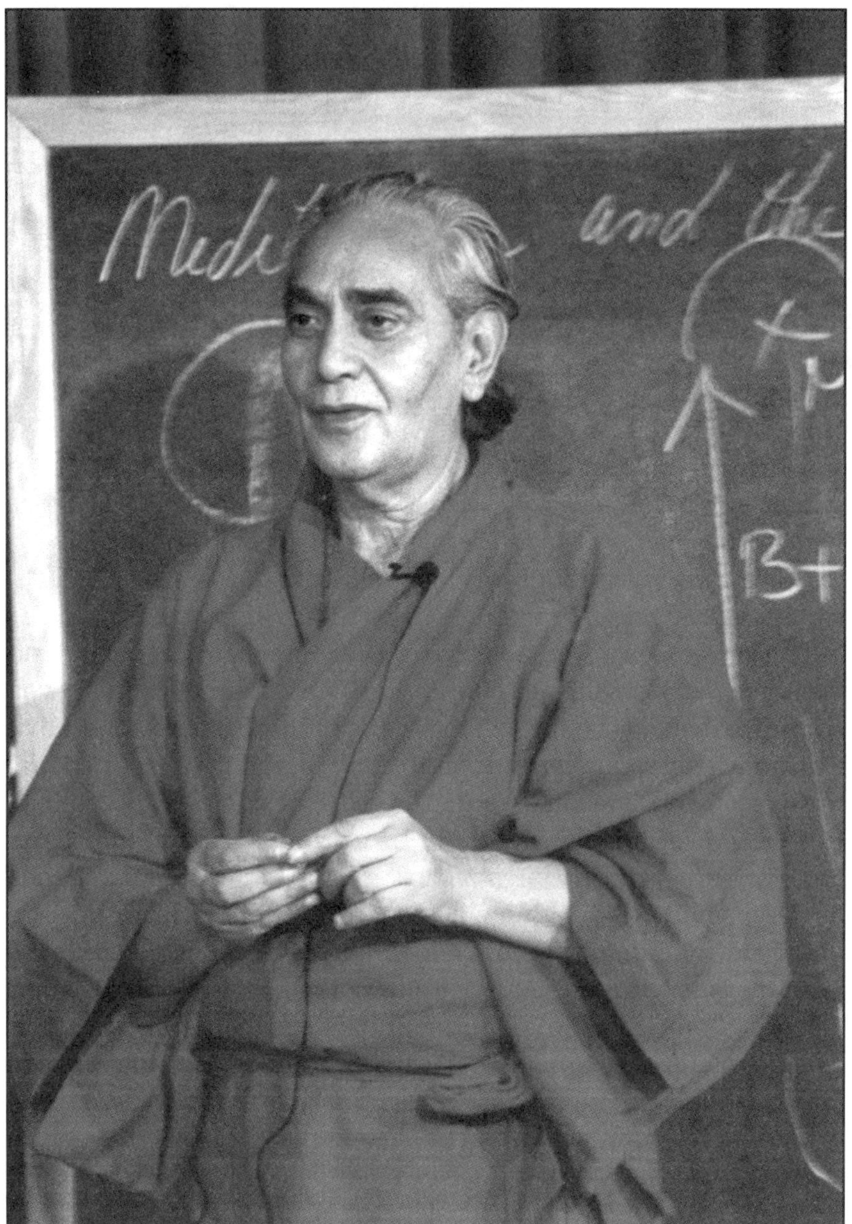

Swami Rama

PART II:
Yoga Philosophy, the Foundation

Before discussing the principles of yoga and meditation in relation to holistic medicine, it is necessary to establish a basic understanding of yoga philosophy. As yoga is a vast subject, we will only be touching on its various aspects. The bibliography at the end of the book will guide you to further studies in yoga and meditation and holistic medicine.

THE TEACHINGS

The Origins of the Universe

One of the greatest advantages of living at the Himalayan Institute was having the opportunity to receive teachings in yoga philosophy directly from Swami Rama, particularly those of Advaita Vedanta, the great Indian monistic philosophy. According to Vedantic philosophy, the all-encompassing pure consciousness, the undifferentiated Oneness, is called Brahman. Brahman never changes or ceases to exist; therefore only Brahman is real. Inherent within Brahman is the desire to know itself. It was this desire that led to manifestation. Thus, Brahman is the underlying substrate of the entire cosmos and the ultimate source from which all energy and matter have manifested.

Brahman cannot be defined, but the state of Self-realization or the experience of the Oneness of consciousness has several names and has been described in several ways: Atman merging with Brahman, the merger of I and Thou, cosmic consciousness, God consciousness, pure consciousness without an object, the Tao, and samadhi or nirvana. It should be understood that these words merely approximate Brahman as they are but limited descriptions of the Absolute. True knowledge of the ultimate nature of

Brahman can be experienced within Brahman alone. The closest verbal description of this indescribable state of true awakening is *satchidananda,* which can be broken down as: *sat* (existence, reality, or that which is), *chit* (pure consciousness) and *ananda* (absolute bliss).

This idea of Brahman being the absolute reality comes from the nondualistic philosophy of Advaita Vedanta, which was codified by Adi Shankaracharya, a spiritual teacher who lived around 800 AD. The truths he described are: 1. Brahman alone is real *(Brahma satyam),* 2. The world *(jiva)* is an illusion *(jagan mithya),* and 3. Brahman and the world are essentially not different *(Jiva Brahmaiva na aparah).*

Advaita Vedanta

Vedanta means "the end of the Vedas." The philosophical system of Advaita Vedanta is found in the concluding section of the Vedas in the Upanishads, which explains in detail the nature of Brahman. The Vedas are not of human origin but instead were revealed to the rishis, the great saints of ancient times, while they were in the deepest states of meditation. The rishis were seers of truth who had the ability to awaken others, so they were perfect agents for transmitting this knowledge.

Vedanta is an intellectual system of knowledge based on the ancient texts, the Upanishads and the Vedas. At the heart of this philosophy is the idea that consciousness, mind, energy and matter are not separate entities. All that exists is ultimate, unified and singular consciousness. Separation of body and spirit and all changes in the universe are only illusory. The changeless underlying substructure of pure consciousness is the only truth. This differs in a fundamental way from Samkhya philosophy, which maintains that consciousness and matter coexist simultaneously.

According to Vedanta and Tantric philosophy, pure consciousness (Brahman) is single, unified and complete. It is the intelligent life force that underlies and encompasses all existence, inclusive of all forms of subtle energy and all animate and inanimate objects from the most rudimentary particle to DNA and the entire universe. Inherent within pure consciousness is the desire and the ability to know and experience itself. Thus, consciousness needs to become differentiated from the One into many so that the many can know the One. For this creative urge to manifest, consciousness must take action and does so through will or intent.

Maya Shakti is the energy that initiates manifestation and is also the illusory power responsible for the manifestation of the universe in all its names and forms. Maya has two aspects or powers: the veiling power *(Avarana Shakti)* and the projecting power *(Vikshepa Shakti)*. Brahman, along with the power of manifestation of Maya Shakti, is Ishwara. Ishwara is similar to the idea of God in the religions of the world. Ishwara's creative aspect is Brahma; Vishnu is the sustaining and preserving power of Ishwara; and Shiva is the destructive and transformative aspect of Ishwara.

In Advaita Vedanta only Brahman is real; the apparent world is considered to be merely an illusion. Relative reality *(mithya)* is characterized by names, forms and constant change, and although it appears to be real, it is not. To say that matter and mind are not real does not mean they don't exist; they simply cease to exist in the state of enlightenment. To believe the apparent world is real is comparable to a person who identifies with the dream world and thus believes the dream is reality. Just as dreams seem real to us in the sleeping state but not in the waking state, our waking lives seem real to us in the waking state but not in the enlightened state or transcendental consciousness of Brahman.

In other words, although mind and matter are experienced as real during the state of maya, they disappear in the light of pure knowledge. Life is not simply a hallucination, nor is it arbitrary or meaningless. Identification with body and mind, however, is similar to seeing the temporary formation of a cloud as permanent. The body does indeed have form but it is impermanent and eventually disappears, just as the mind merges into a more universal awareness in deep meditation. From this perspective, the only reality that is absolute is the all-encompassing, underlying whole. Maya involves mistaking parts of the whole for the whole itself. The paradox is that maya exists only in the phenomenological world of names and forms. Brahman is not transformed into the physical universe but only appears to be part of the illusion of the universe because of our lack of deep spiritual awareness and insight *(avidya)*. Human beings, in their illusion, superimpose the apparent world upon Brahman.

Avidya is individual ignorance that hides one's true nature and causes the aspirant to identify with the individual sense of self/ego. Attachment to the experience of life generates avidya, the veil that covers the truth of Brahman and the ocean of bliss. Avidya causes identification with *upadhis,* the limiting factors that create a false sense of identification with body and mind and a false sense of jiva, the individual soul. Because of the mind's distortions, our experience remains limited to the mere manifestations of Brahman.

From the standpoint of mind and individual consciousness, it is said that Brahman and Atman (the inner individual Self) are one and the same. Atman, the innermost Self within the individual, is a reflection of the universal consciousness of all beings. It is the same as Brahman, but Atman as experienced by the individual is also considered to be pure absolute consciousness. When the veil of ignorance is removed, the individual soul (Atman) realizes that he or she is actually one and the same as Brahman. This is the real goal of yoga—the union and complete identification and absorption in Brahman, one's true nature.

The Big Bang

The Vedantic theory of consciousness having differentiated from one into many may be thought of as similar to the Big Bang theory of the origin of the universe described in modern cosmology. According to this theory, if one were to travel back to the beginning of time, they would find the universe becoming smaller, hotter and denser the farther back they were to go. In the very beginning, all forces, matter and energy were unified in one singular, undifferentiated point of infinite mass and potentiality. Expansion from this single infinitesimally small point resulted in differentiation into the universe as it is known today. This explosion, called the Big Bang, occurred billions of years ago and continues to echo all around the universe. It can still be heard today by giant earth-based radio telescopes and orbiting satellites.

As the expansion phase of the Big Bang continues and the distances between the objects of the universe increase, the gravitational forces holding the objects of the universe become weaker. This process will eventually lead to the universe collapsing in upon itself, the Big Crunch, in which the universe will return to a single infinitely concentrated point. The continual cycle of expansion and contraction of the cosmos is described in Vedantic philosophy as the universal inhalation (expansion phase) and exhalation (contraction phase), or the eternal breath of Brahman.

The first manifestation of the differentiation from the Oneness to the many was a vibration. A similar vibration to this infinite vibration can be experienced in deep meditation, when the senses and the mind have been quieted. What one is actually hearing are the faint echoes of the underlying universal undifferentiated consciousness before it manifested into form. Human beings experience similar vibrations in the form of subtle sounds called mantras.

Tantra

In Tantra, the human being is considered to be a microcosm that is a doorway to the macrocosm. According to Tantra, there are thirty-six levels of reality, reflecting a complex description of manifestation from the singular universal consciousness to the multiplicity of the seen and unseen universe.

In Tantric thought, Shiva represents pure consciousness, which is called Brahman in Vedantic philosophy. Shiva begins his evolution from the Oneness to the multiplicity of time, space and form. At the beginning of the process, the three gunas—*sattva* (harmony, balance, joy), *rajas* (activity, energy, passion), and *tamas* (inertia, inactivity, dullness)—are not yet manifest and are considered to be in a potential state of manifestation. The process of manifestation unfolds through the energy of Shakti, who is considered to be the dynamic feminine force of manifestation, equivalent to Maya Shakti in Vedanta. Shiva is similar to the

Vedantic concept of Brahman and is the holder of all potential manifestation and knowledge, but his knowledge belongs to Shakti, which includes the human mind and the knower of the mind. In the beginning before manifestation, Shiva and Shakti are in complete union and are indistinguishable. Shiva, who manifests from the One, simultaneously remains the One. This is similar to the Vedantic idea in the Upanishads where Brahman remains as One, but at the same time also has the possibility of becoming the many through the force of manifestation of Maya Shakti.

Tantric philosophy also believes in a singular consciousness but differs from Vedanta in that from the Tantric viewpoint the multidimensional universe actually exists, as it evolves out of the Oneness and is not merely an illusion. In other words, Vedanta teaches that the world has only apparently been created, while in Tantra the world is inherently existent in the absolute unity of consciousness. Tantra believes that the world already existed as a potentiality in the Oneness and therefore is as real as the underlying Oneness. Likewise, the ultimate reality of Shiva includes the principle of creation and therefore it too is real. Thus, the Shiva and Shakti principles co-exist in the cosmic play called life.

In Tantric philosophy, the chakras (the chakras are discussed below and in greater detail in Part V) are directly related to the concept of how consciousness manifests into form, going from the One to the many. The creative process of manifestation into the various names and forms of the universe is called *vikriti*. This state is also called grossification, where consciousness goes from the subtlest (Shiva) to the grossest manifestation, (Shakti and her world of thought and activity). The chakras emerge in the process of manifestation as the elements associated with the chakras begin to take form, beginning with pure consciousness, devolving into mind and then to space, air, fire, water and earth. In an analogous way to the Big Bang theory, first there was space in which different energies and forms established themselves. This space was filled with a gaseous substance, air, which consolidated and condensed from intense nuclear reactions to form fire. Fire became liquid (lava). As lava cooled and solidified, it became solid earth. Here the process of vikriti ends.

Samkhya

Swamiji also introduced us to Samkhya, one of the great Indian philosophical systems that deals with the universe of mind/matter and consciousness. In Samkhya, the all-existent principle of consciousness is called Purusha. The goal of meditation is to purify the mind and realize that one's true nature is pure consciousness/Purusha. Purusha is unchanging and represents the true Self. Purusha is similar to Brahman in Vedantic thought and Shiva in Tantric philosophy.

In this system, Prakriti represents the power of undifferentiated consciousness and the potential for the formation of mind/matter. Prakriti is also described as an unconscious principle, the ultimate underlying cause of nature, the essence of matter and the supreme cause of the cosmos. Prakriti manifests into the material universe through the forces of the three gunas. Mind/matter manifests through evolution when the three gunas are out of balance.

An important goal of meditation is to create a clear mind to be able to differentiate mind/matter from consciousness. Buddhi or *mahat,* the intellect and first evolute of Prakriti, is the quality of the individual mind that is primarily sattvic. In this state, one can see clearly and can recognize truth from unreality. It is like looking at a mirror and knowing that the person staring back is not really you but merely a reflection of you.

The three philosophical systems, Vedanta, Tantra and Samkhya, differ in the way they describe how the universe manifests and unfolds through the *tattvas.* Prakriti, the energy of manifestation of the phenomenological universe and the ever-changing world of nature, is similar to the concepts of Maya Shakti in Vedanta and Shakti in Tantra. But while Vedanta says that the world with all its names and forms is merely an illusion, both Tantra and Samkhya proclaim that the world is not unreal but is a manifestation of Shiva through the power of Shakti, and Purusha through the evolution of Prakriti, respectively.

While Samkhya doesn't really mention the *koshas,* the Taittiriya Upanishad, an ancient Vedic text does describe them as a further manifestation of the gunas and representation of the different levels of consciousness as experienced by humans. A more detailed discussion of the koshas is found below in the section, "Consciousness and the Five Koshas."

The Tattvas

There is an important concept in Vedanta and Samkhya that describes the three worlds/realms of existence. These realms obscure the underlying reality of the pure consciousness of Brahman and Purusha. The subtle astral and physical worlds originate from the subtle causal world and also exist on the plane of potentiality. The causal, astral and physical worlds break down further into the twenty-four tattvas to manifest the world as it is known today. (See below for a more detailed description of these three worlds, also called the three bodies, in relation to the koshas).

According to Samkyha, evolution develops from the undifferentiated consciousness of Prakriti into the following tattvas:

- The four aspects of mind: *buddhi,* also called mahat (intellect or intuition); *chitta* (unconscious and reservoir of samskaras, the subtle impressions of all experiences past and present); *ahamkara* (ego); and, *manas* (lower mind or sensory mind).
- The five *jnanendiryas* (sense organs): hearing, touch, sight, taste and smell.
- The five *karmendriyas* (the organs of action): grasping, locomotion, evacuation, speech and procreation.
- The five *tanmantras* (subtle elements): the underlying essence of the physical elements.
- The five *mahabhutas* (physical elements): space (ether), air, fire, water and earth.

The Five Elements (the Five Mahabhutas)

All that we call life is composed of combinations of the five basic elements: ether (space), air, fire, water and earth. It must be remembered that these elements are not in any way similar to the elements of modern physics and chemistry and Mendeleyev's Periodic Table. The five ancient elements represent a system for classifying phenomena. The element of fire, for instance, is not only associated with heat and flames, such as the sun, but is also the primary element involved with the digestion of food in the body and in the generation of body temperature. It is furthermore associated with anger, a short-tempered or choleric personality as well as various types of food. A detailed discussion of the five elements is included in the section on the chakras.

The Doshas

The doshas, vata, pitta and kapha, represent a further refinement of the five elements as follows: Air and space become vata, fire becomes pitta and earth and water combine to form the kaphic state. These forces create the body/mind complex and their imbalances are reflected as disease, growth and aging as well as mental and emotional states. The Indian system of Ayurveda uses the three doshas as the basis for diagnosis and treatment and also uses dosha analysis as a window into the deeper aspects of the human organism.

Prana, tejas and *ojas* represent the subtler and deeper counterparts of the three doshas and are responsible for well-being, creativity and health. In Vedantic thought, when the body and mind function in equilibrium, prana, tejas and ojas are in a steady state. These underlying principles are the healthy and positive forms of the three doshas, vata, pitta and kapha. When this balance is disturbed, the doshas lead to a loss of energy, ill health and disease.

Prana

In Vedantic philosophy, all aspects of creative manifestation have an underlying subtle essence. The entire universe is made of different forms of energy at different states of manifestation and levels of vibration. Prana is the underlying dynamic energy that provides the integrating link between the physical, mental and spiritual realms of creation. Since mankind's physical and mental being is a microcosm, a reflection of nature's macrocosm, all vibrations and forces within the human organism also exist in the outer world. In a sense, the universe is an ocean of prana and each person a small pranic wave in this vast sea, individual yet part of the whole. Thus, by identifying, controlling and thoroughly knowing one's pranic essence, one can better understand the subtle forms underlying the greater universe.

Prana manifests as both the inherent life force and the subtle energy present in the atmospheric air. This subtle force underlies all physical, emotional, mental and spiritual functioning. For example, it is responsible for governing coordination of the breath, for sensory experiences and for mental functioning. In addition, prana governs the unfoldment and integration of all states of consciousness. Yogic breathing exercises, meditation and raja yoga practices serve to increase and balance prana.

The concept of prana is not unique to yoga. Prana is the same as libido, the psychic energy referred to in Freudian psychology, the vital force of homeopathy and chi in Chinese medicine and martial arts. These names all characterize the life force that animates the human organism. The breath and food are vehicles for the intake of prana.

Prana enters the body with the inspired air and flows into the nadis that have their origin in the nose. If the flow of pranic energy through the inspired air is regulated, smooth and consistent, this is usually associated with good physical and emotional health. Abnormal rhythms often indicate illness. Other portals of entry also exist, and as one learns to follow its movement, prana can be consciously drawn inwards at various locations such as the chakras.

Once in the body, prana flows to different locations and controls specific functions as the five pranas: *Udana* is located in the area of the throat and is responsible for speech and control of the sensory nerves. *Samana* is located around the center of the abdomen and is responsible for digestion, metabolism and assimilation. *Apana* is located in the area of the anus and bladder and is responsible for elimination, excretion and urination as well as the exhalation part of breathing. *Prana* is located in the cardiac and lung region and is responsible for inhalation. *Vyana* circulates throughout the entire body and is responsible for circulation of blood, lymph and nerve impulses.

Type of Prana	Location of Prana	Function of Prana
Udana	Throat area	Speech, senses
Samana	Naval area	Digestion, metabolism
Apana	Anal area	Elimination, excretion, urination, exhalation
Prana	Chest area	Inhalation
Vyana	Entire body	Circulation of blood, lymph, nerve impulses

Tejas

Tejas is called the inner radiance and represents the subtle essence of fire. It is described as the active force that gives us will power, fortitude and courage, and provides the inner heat and power that allow for efficient digestion, assimilation, metabolism and reproduction. Tejas is increased by herbs, a balanced diet, yogic practices and meditation, all of which help to improve metabolism, destroy toxicity and improve digestion.

Ojas

Ojas represents the subtle essence of water and fluids in the body and of energy reserves, often described as the end product of perfect digestion that allows for balanced immunological, endocrine, nervous, reproductive, cardio-pulmonary and musculoskeletal system function. It is the subtle force that underlies the biological fluids of the body that support immunity, vigor and longevity. Ojas is the power that underlies one's endurance and all forms of exertion of both the body and mind. It is like the glue that holds the body, mind and spirit into a functional whole. Ojas is built up by living a balanced, sattvic life with nutritional food, exercise and meditation.1

To summarize, on the level of pranic functioning, prana is the energy that flows along the nadis and is used by the body and mind; tejas is the heat moving along the nadis that directs prana through metabolism, and ojas is the subtle lubricating fluid that lines the nadis and makes prana operational.

Consciousness and the Five Koshas

Vedanta, Center of Consciousness and the Koshas

Consciousness is the underlying substrate of the entire cosmos from which all energy and matter have manifested. Yoga and Vedanta philosophy teach us that consciousness is not dependent on the physical form. All conscious beings exist on many levels both in life and in death, the two states that the individual soul passes through on its long journey towards enlightenment. Thus, consciousness is described as being multidimensional with awareness existing on several levels.

According to Vedanta and the Upanishads, there are five levels of consciousness that surround and obscure the true Self, the center of consciousness. These are known as the five koshas or sheaths and are called *anandamaya kosha, vijnanamaya kosha, manomaya kosha, pranamaya kosha* and *annamaya kosha*. In the context of the koshas, the word maya means "made of" and not "illusion or underlying power of creation." These five levels of consciousness are called sheaths because of their concentric arrangement, although they all interpenetrate and overlap each other. These sheaths form a continuum, and all levels are interdependent, interconnected and closely coordinated. The denser, gross external levels obscure the finer, less material inner layers. These five levels of consciousness span a much larger spectrum of human experience than described in Western thought. Associated with each level is a specific type of awareness. Humans exist simultaneously on all these levels.

The center of consciousness is often compared to a light source and the different sheaths to lampshades that obscure to different degrees the clarity and brilliance of the underlying light. The outermost sheaths are the densest, allowing the least amount of light to penetrate. Therefore, those who identify only with the most external sheaths, such as the body, remain oblivious to the more inner levels of consciousness and the center of consciousness. They experience life only on a mundane physical level and cannot feel the deeper, more subtle and spiritual aspects of their existence. On the other hand, those who practice meditation can learn to penetrate the sheaths so they can experience the complexity and subtleness of life and more clearly see the source of the inner light.2

The Three Gunas

As we have discussed earlier, according to Vedantic philosophy, Brahman is the ultimate reality and is unmanfest as pure consciousness and pure existence. Inherent in Brahman is Maya Shakti, the energy behind manifestation as well as the three gunas (sattva, rajas and tamas). The three gunas are the primordial expressions of Maya Shakti and constitute the three inherent qualities of nature. The movement of the three gunas, as instigated by Maya Shakti, from static balance and potentiality to dynamic activity, results in creation of the infinite law of karma of cause and effect, all energy exhanges, all mental activity as well as all physical structures. In other words, the gunas are the fundamental building blocks of all that has manifested from pure consciousness. The quality sattva is characterized as purity and balance; rajas represents kinetic energy, change, movement and action; and, tamas is described as inertia and represents matter, solidity, decay, destruction and death.

The Three Stages of Manifestation (Causal, Astral, Physical Bodies) and the Five Koshas

In the following section, when referring to the terms causal, astral and physical, there are various descriptors that can be used: *realm, plane, world, form, state of being* and *body*. When describing a state or level of consciousness, *world, realm* or *plane* is used, whereas when referring to an individual's personal existence, the term *body* or *form* is used. In this discussion, we are referring to the manifestation of the human body and so will use the term *body*.

Maya Shakti's energy of manifestation proceeds from the undifferentiated Oneness to the manifest universe in three stages: the causal body *(karana sharira,)* the astral body *(sukshma sharira)* and the physical body *(sthula sharira). Sharira* means "body." The three subtle gunas precede the formation of the causal, astral and physical bodies (the three stages of manifestation), and provide the subtle substrate for the progressively denser levels up to the state of physical matter.

In the first stage of manifestation, the causal body, the world of potentiality, includes the three gunas, which exist in a state of balance. When the gunas are no longer in balance, this leads to the formation of the next stages of manifestation — the astral body and the physical body. Thus, the causal body underlies the individual's astral body. The five koshas can be understood as evolving in association with the causal, astral and physical bodies as follows. From the innermost center of consciousness to the outermost kosha are the following levels of consciousness: anandamaya kosha, the blissful or superconscious/transcendental sheath; vijnanamaya kosha, the intuitive or intellectual/unconscious sheath; manomaya kosha, the mental sheath; pranamaya kosha, the energy sheath; and annamaya kosha, the physical sheath. With respect to the three stages of manifestation, anandamaya kosha is associated with the causal body; vijnanamaya kosha, manomaya kosha and pranamaya kosha are associated with the astral body; and, annamaya kosha is associated with the physical body.

The Causal Body and Anandamaya Kosha

The causal body (karana sharira) underlies the individual's astral body and dense physical body. Anandamaya kosha, also called the blissful superconscious, is associated with the causal body. *Ananda* means "bliss" and this sheath, being the innermost sheath closest to the Self, corresponds with the most subtle states of mind, characterized by joy, equanimity, truth, knowledge and bliss. The emotions associated with this sheath are pure bliss and the experience of universal truths. In Samkhya, this sheath represents pure sattva, which in its essence is blissful. The qualities of anandamaya kosha are: *priya* (happiness from looking at an object),

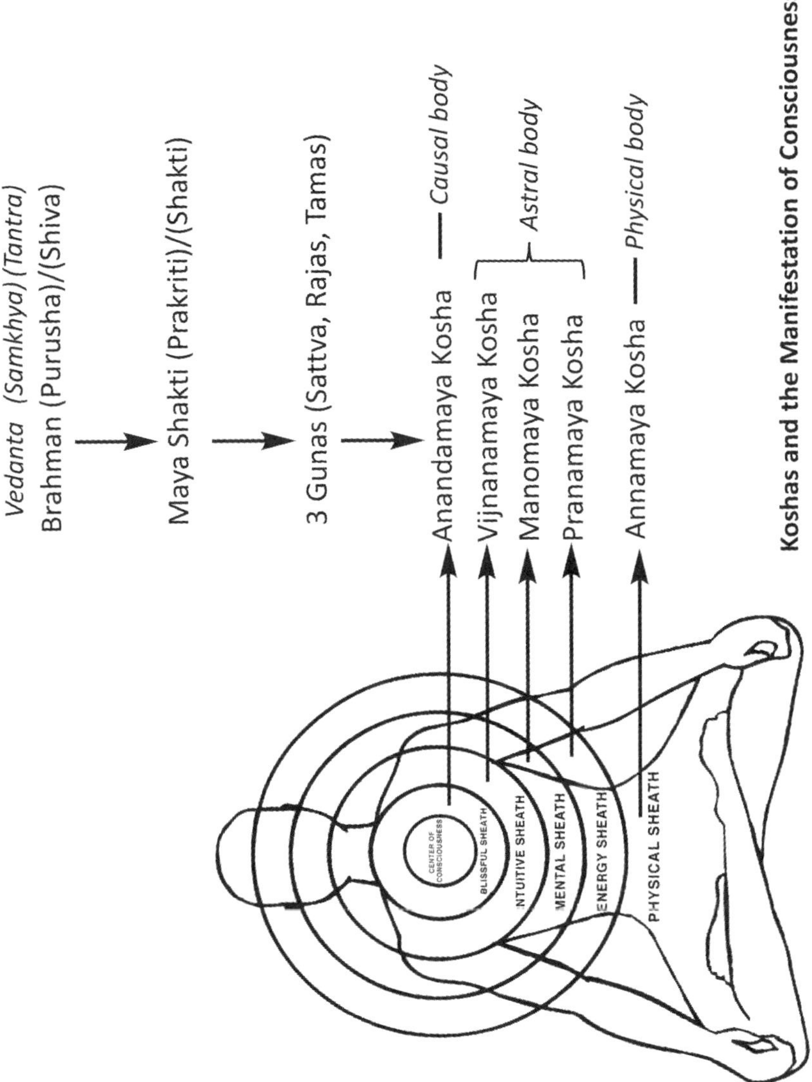

Koshas and the Manifestation of Consciousness

moda (happiness from owning an object) and *pramoda* (happiness from experiencing an object).

The Astral Body and Vijnanamaya Kosha, Manomaya Kosha and Pranamaya Kosha

The astral body (sukshma sharira) is associated with three koshas: vijnanamaya kosha, manomaya kosha and pranamaya kosha. There are five components of the mind — buddhi, ahamkara, chitta, manas and the vrittis — and these five dimensions of the mind can be understood in the context of the astral body.

Vijnanamaya Kosha

Vijnanamaya kosha is also called the intellectual or unconscious sheath. *Vijnana* refers to the intuitive knowledge of consciousness and this level corresponds to some degree with the Western idea of the unconscious mind. Here a refining of the intuitive nonverbal faculties is found, allowing deeper unexplored levels of the human psyche to be integrated within the individual. Vijnanamaya kosha is associated with two aspects of the mind — buddhi (intellect and intuition) and ahamkara (sense of self and ego--and thus is characterized by the qualities of I-ness, clarity, discrimination and wisdom.

Buddhi guides action on the core of information received by manas, the sensory part of the mind, resulting in how one responds to an urge, thought, emotion, or desire and what course of action to take. Buddhi is responsible for our ability to clearly discriminate right from wrong as well as intuition. According to Samkhya philosophy, within the vijnanamaya kosha, prakriti begins manifesting from the pure consciousness of Purusha. Buddhi, spiritual awareness, which is the first evolute of Prakriti, is considered pure in this refined state of consciousness.

Ahamkara is the function of the mind that gives humans self-awareness. It is the sense of *I* that separates awareness of oneself from other people. It is similar to the idea of the ego in Western psychology. Associated emotions are those that manifest in dreams, archetypes and symbols. Awareness of spiritual truths comes at this level.

Manomaya Kosha

Manomaya kosha, the third sheath, is the mental body. *Mano* means "mind." Qualities of manomaya kosha are: thinking, doubting, anger, lust and various other emotions. Manomaya kosha is made up of the other two aspects of mind—manas (the lower, sensory mind) and chitta (subconscious thoughts and memories)--and the five jnanendriya (organs of knowledge): hearing, touch, vision, taste and smell.

Manas is the mental screen that registers impressions as it is most directly in contact with incoming data from the senses. The mind has the capacity to look both inwards and outwards as it identifies with the five senses. Manas receives, collects, selects and synthesizes data from the five senses (hearing, touch, vision, taste and smell). It also receives input from the memory and the unconscious. Following collection and organization of the sensory and memory data, thoughts (vrittis) arise. The manas component of the mind coordinates the incoming sensory information and associated thoughts with active motor responses. Manas responds to this information by force of habit or through primitive instincts or emotions. This function of the mind is under the influence of the basic urges, including the need for food, shelter, sleep and sex.

When functioning alone, manas reacts instinctively and directs a mechanical response. However, it cannot make decisions on its own. Intelligent use of all the information available to manas depends on the activity of two other components of the mind, ahamkara and buddhi. Impressions first appear on the mental screen of manas, thoughts are created (vrittis), impressions and thoughts become integrated to the person's sense of self (ahamkara) and lead to the ability to make decisions (buddhi).

Chitta is similar to the unconscious in modern psychology, acting as a passive reservoir that receives and stores information from the senses. Chitta also corresponds to the memory, containing impressions *(samskaras)* of past thoughts and experiences from this lifetime and previous lifetimes. Emotions often get activated and stimulated from memories contained in chitta.

According to Vedanta philosophy, the human mind manifests from the unfoldment of the tattvas and gunas. Sattva is the essential nature of the mind and represents purity of perception, intelligence and the laws of nature and truth, without distortion of the thinking processes. When the mind is sattvic, it perceives its own true nature, which is love and infinite bliss. Its manifestations in the mind are purity, clarity, tranquility, peace, bliss, harmony, balance and the one-pointed concentration of meditation.

Rajas is characteristic of the desire-filled mind. Human beings suffer because of desires for external objects and consider this to be the normal state of the mind. Rajas can be compared to the stormy waves of a lake that create agitation and obscure the vision of the lake's bottom, which in this analogy is like Brahman. Because the experience of inner bliss and harmony is covered by rajas, the individual is disconnected from the ultimate reality of Brahman. They do not perceive the state of rajas as pain because they have lost awareness of the bliss of Brahman and the reference point of sattva. In the mind, rajas manifests as scattered thinking, desire, restlessness, agitation, anger, attachment and feelings of liking or disliking something or someone. Under the influence of rajas the mind becomes distorted by the ego, the sense of I and mine and takes on exaggerated importance. This causes the ego to create disagreements, wars and conflicts with other people, differing religions and within families.

Tamas is the quality of mind characterized by inertia, dullness, laziness, sloth and depression. It is like a muddy lake, dark and heavy. The light of Brahman cannot shine through it. One becomes totally disconnected when dominated by tamas. It is vital to the aspirant to not allow the mind or body to sink into tamas. One should try to stay in rajas to keep up practices that lead to sattva and the ultimate realization of Brahman. A degree of tamas in normal daily living is necessary, however, as this quality helps one to rest and sleep. In essence, balance of all three gunas is important for healthy living in the world, but always with an emphasis on maintaining a sattvic attitude and lifestyle.

Components of the Mind	
Buddhi	Decision-making
Ahamkara	Sense of self, ego
Chitta	Memory, unconscious
Manas	Collects data, senses
Vrittis	Thought waves

Pranamaya Kosha

Pranayama kosha, the fourth sheath, is the pranic or energy body. It is sustained and nourished by the intake of prana through the breath. This kosha consists of the nadis and the subtle forces of prana and the chakras, which are discussed below after annamaya kosha and in subsequent sections. Yoga psychology and physics state that energy exists in one of two forms: manifest/kinetic or potential. Higher states of consciousness can be understood within this concept as representing different stages of this latent or potential force. Yoga sees an endless interchange between the two: evolution is the process whereby potential energy transforms into manifest matter, and involution represents the reverse process. In yogic thought, potential energy functions at a higher and faster vibrational level than its manifested form. Within this concept, higher states of consciousness can be understood to represent the subtlest stages of this latent or potential force.

Pranayama kosha provides the energy behind the five karmendriya (organs of action: grasping, locomotion, speech, evacuation and procreation). Its qualities are hunger, thirst and the experience of heat and cold. Pranamaya kosha also controls the five pranas (udana, samana, vyana, apana, and prana; the latter, though having the same name, also represents one of the sub classifications). While not included in the Samkhya twenty-four tattvas discussed earlier, these five pranas are included in the Vedantic description of the formation of the cosmos.

The Physical body and Annamaya Kosha

The physical body (sthula sharira) is the subtle precursor to annamaya kosha, the dense material physical body, which is also

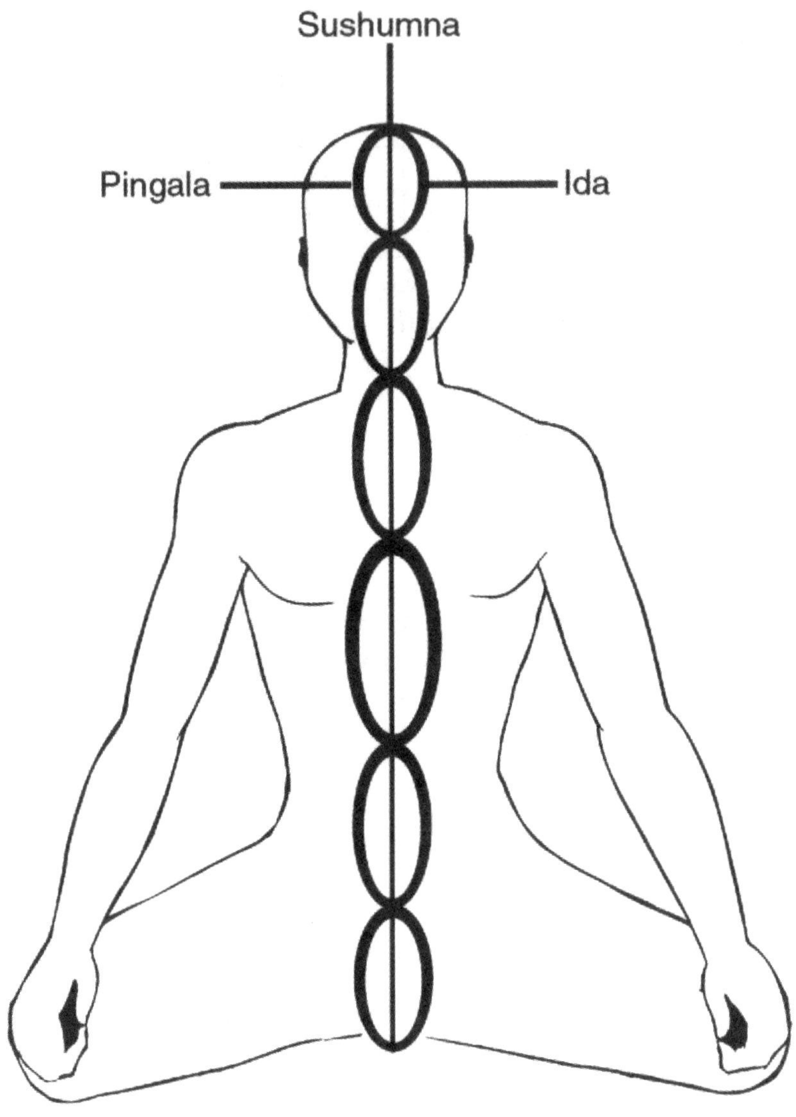

The Main Nadis

called the food sheath. *Anna* means "food." Thus, annamaya kosha refers to the physical body that is made of the elements derived from food and represents the densest level of illusion that obscures pure consciousness. Thus, the physical body is made up of the five elements of space, air, fire, water and earth, and its qualities include existence, birth, growth, death and decay. It includes the physical and anatomical structure of a human being such as the DNA, genome, molecules, cells, tissue and organs.

I will discuss some aspects of nutrition in Part V, as food represents the foundation of this sheath. Also, in Part V, I will present case histories based on the concept of the koshas.

Nadis

Nadis are energy pathways. Unlike the bronchial tubes that conduct air or the nerves that transmit electrochemical impulses, the nadis are not anatomical structures. They exist on a subtler level and cannot be seen by even the most powerful microscope, but can be perceived when the obstacles of body tension, breathing irregularities and rapidly changing thoughts are quieted and stilled through a regular practice of pranayama and meditation. Individuals deeply immersed in the practices of meditation have said there are approximately 72,000 nadis. While many nadis originate in the third chakra, located in the solar plexus area, fourteen of these nadis are considered to be of the greatest importance. These nadis flow from and merge into the concentrated energy areas known as the chakras. Two nadis, *ida* and *pingala,* travel upwards in a crisscrossed pattern through the major chakras along the spine, while *sushumna* travels upwards in a straight central path. Pingala is the nadi associated with the right side of the body. It corresponds to active metabolic processes and sympathetic nervous system activity. Yogic meditation symbolism describes pingala as being masculine and energizing, and its symbols are the sun and light. As air enters the right nostril, the prana is conveyed to pingala located within the right nostril. Ida is the nadi connected with the left nostril, the left side of the body, the parasympathetic nervous system, and the receptive and more feminine aspects of human nature. In meditative symbolism, ida is associated with darkness and the moon. Ida and pingala cross each other as they travel from the nose down and up the body, intersecting within the chakras. The sympathetic and parasympathetic nervous systems make up the autonomic (involuntary) nervous system, which is described in detail in Part V in the section, "The Science of Meditation."

Sushumna corresponds to the central axis of the human body and represents the uniting and integration of pingala and ida. It is said to be located within the spinal cord of the physical body. Prana flows through sushumna when both nostrils are open and directing the flow of air evenly.3

The Chakras

The subtle connections among the five koshas are maintained by the chakras, which integrate the physical, pranic, mental and spiritual energies from the various sheaths of consciousness. Each of the five koshas is expressed by each chakra, as each chakra is characterized by different and congruent aspects of human life, including the levels of body, energy, conscious, unconscious and superconscious minds. Thus, each kosha and chakra center offer a particular frame of reference through which the individual relates to and experiences the world.

There are seven major chakras that are interconnected, each center affecting and affected by the functioning of the other centers. In this way, body affects the breath, prana and the breath affect the mind, including the unconscious and the deeper spiritual levels, and vice versa. This is analogous to biochemical reactions where one activity affects another, creating an overall integrated reaction network and effect. The seven chakras are described in more detail in Part IV in "Objects of Concentration" and in relation to holistic medicine in Part V.

Chakra means "wheel or circle." The chakras are often described as whirling vortices of energy within the pranic body, where physical, psychological and spiritual forces interact and intersect. In a deep meditative state one can experience the chakras as an energy field.

Each chakra represents a force field that transforms energy from its source (consciousness) into various physical, mental and spiritual qualities. As the movement of spokes emanating from a central motionless hub characterizes the wheel, the chakras represent an area of energy surrounding a central point from

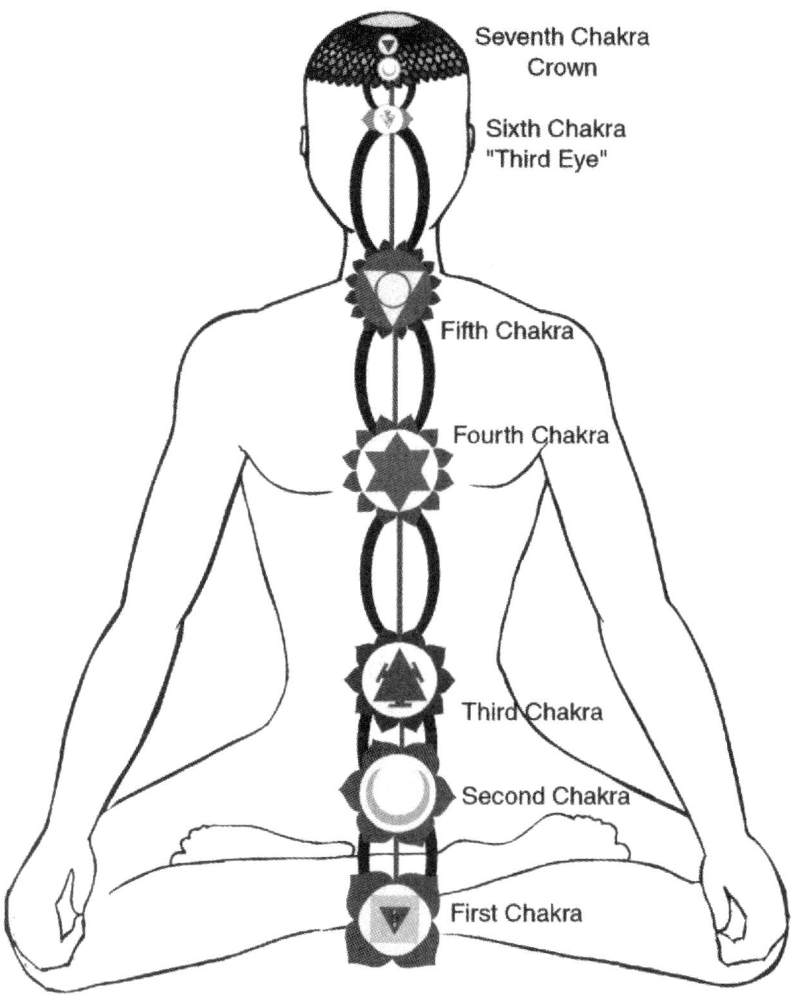

The Chakras and the Nadis

which motion and energy originate. The hub of each chakra is like a mini center of consciousness. The movement from the hub out through the spokes manifests as the various physical, emotional and spiritual experiences characteristic of that center.

There is also a constant exchange of energy between the inner and outer environments. As energy flows in and out of the pranic body, forces from the outside (light, sound, other people's emotions, constant worldly activity) affect the chakras, and the outer world is similarly responsive to the energies of the inner chakra world. Thus, there is a dynamic exchange of inner and outer forces creating a situation where the chakras are in constant change, flux and transformation.

As the chakras spin in a whirling fashion, they can do this in a rapid, smooth or erratic way. Yogis say that if a chakra is spinning in an efficient manner, it can absorb similarly congruent energy forces from the outside environment and use them positively to charge, energize and refresh. If the chakras are integrated but the rate of vibration is not similar to incoming disruptive vibratory frequencies of energy, a well-balanced chakra has the ability to cast off the influences of the incongruent forces. The opposite is also true. If the chakra is out of balance, then external forces can disrupt the inner chakra functioning and it can absorb some of the incoming negative forces.

Another concept about the chakras that is interesting is that as a person evolves emotionally and spiritually, they tend to focus their energy and life activities on the higher chakras and less on the lower three chakras. As one focuses on and identifies with the upper four chakras a shift in consciousness occurs, and one is drawn to the subtler vibrations and psychological and spiritual qualities of these higher centers.

The lower centers retain their importance as their activity supports all the qualities associated with the upper chakras. When this happens, the psychological and spiritual qualities of the lower chakras become balanced, and people turn to healthier behavior and activities. For example, one can become more connected to the positive attributes of the first chakra by caring for the earth, not overusing precious resources and by recycling. Issues associated with the second chakra become more focused such as directing one's sexual expression lovingly towards one's spouse or significant others. With respect to the third chakra, one learns to direct the ego and will power in positive ways such as helping others rather than primarily serving one's own needs.

Jewish Mysticism and the Tree of Life

I am not religious in the formal sense of the word, but I have explored my Jewish spiritual roots. While I identify myself as Jewish from a historical, familial and cultural perspective, I seldom go to synagogue or keep the Sabbath, although I do sometimes have a Passover Seder or break the fast with a Yom Kippur meal. I do, however, incorporate Jewish meditative practices in my daily spiritual disciplines, as there are some fascinating similarities between certain Jewish mystical practices and the yogic path.

I believe that similar spiritual teachings are the foundation of all religions and that all paths lead to the same goal: God-awareness, samadhi or enlightenment. Once in a lecture Swami Saroopananda of the Sivananda Ashram made a comment that provided me with an image of different spiritual paths. He talked of different paths as a tapestry, each having unique richness, beauty and patterns, while all reflect the one true goal of enlightenment and God identification.

An old childhood friend, Avraham Trugman, a rabbi in Israel who teaches and writes about kabbalistic concepts, wrote a very eloquent description of the *Shema*, the most important statement of faith in Judaism in relation to the notion of God. While there are at least seven different names for God in Judaism, it has always been clear that the Jewish people believe there is only one God. Rabbi Trugman's following statement is very similar to Vedanta's description of the unity and all-encompassing, undifferentiated oneness of Brahman. He says: ". . . the Jewish belief in one God does not merely mean that there are no other gods . . . rather, it expresses the belief that there is nothing other than God, and even though God surrounds all worlds and is beyond time, space and all description, He is paradoxically ever-present within every point of time and space."4

In the Kabbalah, the Jewish mystical philosophy, there is a system of subtle energy centers that are somewhat similar to the chakras. These spiritual centers, the *sefirot* (also spelled *sephiroth*) form what is called the tree of life, *etz chaim* in Hebrew. In Jewish thought, as stated in Genesis of the Old Testament, human beings are made in the image of God. The sefirot represent divine attributes through which God manifests Himself. The attributes of the sefirot allow humans to speak about and better understand God's immanence in creation. One of the manifestations of the sephirot is that they are expressed in humans as a series of energy spheres that are distributed along the energy body in accordance with the form of the physical body. Besides having emotional, mental and spiritual qualities, each *sefirah* (singular of sefirot) is associated

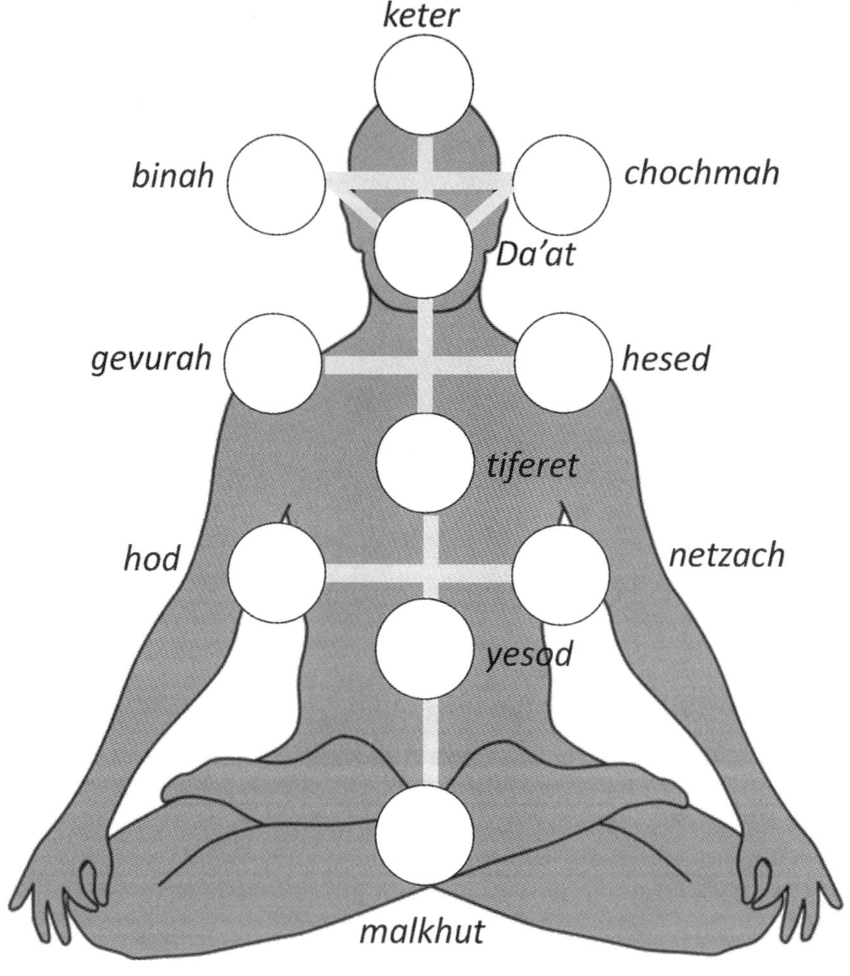

The Ten Sefirot of the Tree of Life

with a specific limb of the human body. These limbs look like the branches of a tree, hence the name, tree of life.

The sefirot are arranged along three axes, right, left and center, from the head to the legs and are connected by channels that provide a pathway for energy to travel from one to the other. As in the yoga chakras, since the sefirot are all interconnected, each center affects the functioning of the other energy centers of the tree of life accordingly. In this way they are like atoms that form complex molecules, each component interdependent for the overall functioning of the chemical or biological system.

While there are seven major chakras in yoga, there are ten sefirot. In the chakra system, all the chakras also have a left/right component, but they are considered as two halves of a single whole. Similar to the yoga chakra model, these sefirot have different associated physical, emotional, mental and spiritual qualities, and are arranged in a hierarchical yet holistic manner. Each sefirot of the tree of life has a name that reflects the different states of awareness and activity that characterize each center. Aspects of our consciousness, thoughts and actions are determined by the level of the sefirah to which we are attuned. In the chakra system, as we move through the various centers, we evolve emotionally and spiritually as we integrate and strengthen the qualities of each chakra. The lower chakra development is just as important as the higher centers, because a human being's health and well-being depend on a strong foundation. This is also true of the tree of life. Drawing down a higher sefirot's energy into a lower sefirot to help strengthen the qualities of the lower sefirot is just as important, and sometimes even more important than raising awareness into the higher centers. The sefirot are said to be formed in the individual at the moment of conception as the soul descends into the developing embryo.

There are rules of conduct and physical, breathing and spiritual practices that promote the movement through the tree of life. The ascension and descent occur within all levels of one's consciousness, but since the sefirot exist within every level of reality including the energy body and the etheric sphere, these centers can primarily be seen and experienced through one's subtle vision. In yoga, the

Microcosmic Orbit Meditation

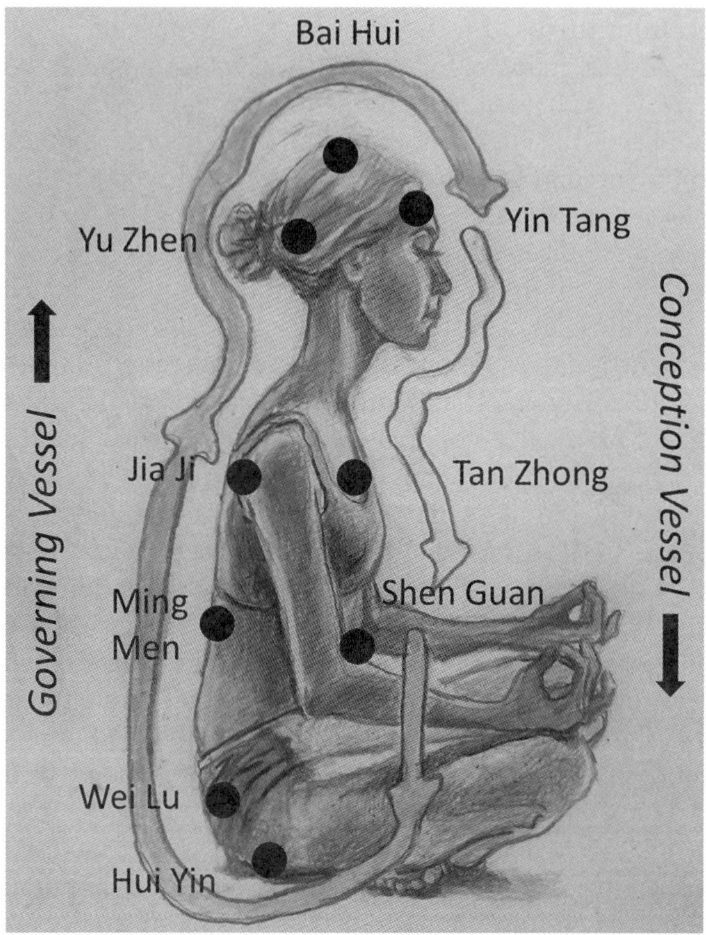

The Dantian and Correspondences with the Chakras

1. Hui Yin and muladhara (first) chakra)
2. Wei Lu and swadisthana (second chakra)
3. Ming Men & Sen Guan and manipura (third chakra)
4. Jai Ji & Tan Zhong and anahata (fourth chakra)
5. Yu Zhen and vishuddha (fifth chakra)
6. Yin Tang and ajna (sixth chakra)
7. Bai Hui and sahasrara (seventh chakra)

guru, live or deceased, can help an individual through this process of unfoldment; in Jewish mysticism it is the rabbi, called *rebbe* in the more spiritual sects, who can help in this evolutionary growth. Growth also takes place by following the precepts of the Torah historical messages of the Jewish prophets.

In Part III I will briefly discuss another interesting aspect of Kabbalistic thinking, the Shekinah, and in Part V I will discuss the physical, emotional and spiritual qualities of each sefirah as compared to the chakras.

Taoist Microcosmic Orbit and the Dantian

The Chinese Taoist system, the microcosmic orbit system, is quite similar to the chakra meditative systems of Tantra and yoga. The dantian are energy centers comparable to the chakras of yoga. Chi (energy) flows through the dantian in the microcosmic orbit in an analogous way that prana flows through the chakras in the system of yoga. I will discuss the theory of the microcosmic orbit a bit later in Part III under "The Taoist Idea of Chi."

In 2007 I met Liping Zhu, an acupuncturist from San Francisco at Tassajara, a Zen Buddhist monastery in Northern California. We became friends and colleagues and she and I subsequently taught a course together at Tassajara. She has been helpful in my understanding of the Chinese microcosmic orbit meditation system as well as introducing me to the swimming dragon form of tai chi.

Consciousness from the Western Perspective

In contrast to the philosophy of Vedanta and yoga, in the West it is believed that consciousness abides in and exists only in the mind, and thus is dependent on the synapses functioning in the brain. From this perspective, consciousness represents the totality of a person's thoughts, feelings and impressions. Self-consciousness represents the capacity of a sentient being to know itself, with humans having the greatest capacity to realize this.

Christof Koch, a prominent neuroscientist and biophysicist, has written about the neural bases of consciousness from a reductionist, biological perspective. His book, *Consciousness: Confessions of a Romantic Reductionist,* is a good introduction to the Western-based understanding of consciousness. Koch presents four facets of the phenomenon of consciousness: commonsense, behavioral, philosophical and neuronal. I have summarized these ideas and compared them with the yogic and Vedantic understanding of consciousness.

The *commonsense* definition of consciousness applies to what we are actually consciously aware of. We are aware that we dream at night and wake up in the morning and that we lose this awareness during deep sleep, under the experience of deep anesthesia or if we have an accident that affects critical brain functioning and we become unconscious.

The *behavioral* definition of consciousness refers to the awareness of sensory, mental and motor experiences. These actions and behaviors characterize all species, not just human beings.

The *philosophical* definition of consciousness asserts that a person knows they are alive because they can feel it. They feel they are conscious and therefore they are.

The *physiological* mechanisms that are needed for conscious experiences and sensations are described by the neuronal definition of consciousness. These include the synaptic and neuronal networks in the central and peripheral nervous systems, the neo-cortex, cerebellum and thalamic complex (thalamus, hypothalamus, basal ganglia and amygdala). If any one of these brain structures becomes dysfunctional or damaged, the experience of consciousness can be altered. Neurons that have intact and normal functioning connections between the sensory regions of the cortex with the pre-frontal cortex are particularly important for maintaining awareness and attention. Another area of the brain that plays a role in awareness is the hippocampus, which turns perceptions received from the outside into memories.

The nervous system passes an impulse of electrical charges along the membrane of nerve cells (action potential). These nerve impulses in the thalamic-cortical axis, in particular, allow for the human's unique capacity of self-consciousness and introspection to manifest. Thus, in this paradigm consciousness is dependent on coordinated neural networking that involves synergistic and integrating connections that are increasingly differentiated, especially as the organism becomes more self-aware and displays a higher degree of introspection, as in humans.5

Specific areas of the brain have differing functions and disruption or damage to these areas can lead to corresponding functional deficits. For example, the cerebral cortex has specific areas of neurons that recognize color, faces, forms of objects and memory for names, and when damaged accidentally or due to a stroke, these functions become impaired.

Altered conscious awareness is usually divided into two major categories: destructive and irritative. Destructive states of altered consciousness that affect the entire brain include, in ascending magnitude of order of disruption: confusion states (disoriented), delirium (more confusion), obtundation (difficulty staying awake but can respond), stupor (no response except for pain), coma (totally unresponsive though has the potential to recover) and persistent vegetative state (permanent coma). Dementias caused by Alzheimer's disease, Parkinson's disease, excessive alcohol intake, sleep disorders such as hypersomnia and problems related to paralysis, blindness and deafness are other destructive forms of altered consciousness.

Irritative forms of altered conscious awareness include extreme pain states, hallucinations caused by drugs, high fever and epileptic seizures. Psychogenic disorders that are more in the "mind" and that affect consciousness also fall into this category. The more serious disorders include: schizophrenia, other forms of psychosis, catatonia and more serious types of personality disorders. Less serious problems include depression, hysteria, phobias, panic disorder and obsessive-compulsive disorder.

On the other hand, certain areas of the brain can be conditioned to work in harmony even without conscious volition. Pre-frontal cortex activity is shifted to the cerebellum and basal ganglia through repetitive movement, action and continual practice. Since these parts of the brain are responsible for coordinated movements, the skill needed for these types of activities improves and becomes spontaneous, graceful and easy, even without conscious guidance. This can be seen when a person practices piano, dances, sings or plays basketball diligently. Over time, the action becomes "second nature."6 The same is true as one practices yoga, tai chi or meditates for lengthy periods of time.

To summarize, from a Vedantic perspective, consciousness reflects the manifestation of Maya Shakti in the physical world. In contrast, what Dr. Koch refers to as consciousness, is actually conscious awareness. Humans have self-awareness and animals also have awareness of themselves, although their self-awareness is generally only in relationship to their surroundings. From a yogic perspective, consciousness exists independently of the brain and nervous system, is singular in that all sentient beings share in the same ocean of consciousness and this continues on even after death. The brain only facilitates awareness in the physical and mental worlds. Science can answer important questions about the intricacies and patterns of conscious awareness and how it comes together in a neural networking way but cannot explain what the unconscious mind is or why consciousness even exists.

THE YOGA WAY

The path of action and manifestation from the One to the many is called *pravriti;* the path of dissolution, and the accompanied inner knowledge of unity gained from this process is called *nivriti.* In order to be liberated from pain, suffering and feelings of separation and aloneness, one must retrace the path from multiplicity back to the unity of consciousness.

The ultimate goal of this journey is to develop insight and discrimination *(viveka),* to become nonattached *(vairagya)* to worldly desires, and to realize that life's pleasures and pains *(kleshas)* are transitory. The qualities that need to be cultivated on this journey are equanimity, courage and the discipline *(abhyasa)* to practice meditation and other spiritually oriented activities in order to ultimately experience the Oneness of consciousness. The science of yoga provides several paths that culminate in the integration of body, mind and spirit.

The Four Main Paths of Yoga

At this point it is important to discuss the four main paths of yoga. Although my spiritual teacher, Swami Rama, taught us the four paths, he emphasized that the path of raja yoga was the most complete and organized of all the systems of yoga, and that all other yogic paths could be found within the eight limbs of raja yoga. Through the Sivananda organization, where I had studied and taught for ten years, I learned Swami Sivananda's philosophy. According to Swami Sivananda, there is a transition and continuum between the different paths of yoga that can lead the aspirant to the highest states of consciousness, and so he has combined the four major paths of yoga into the Yoga of Synthesis.

The four paths complement each other very well and together lead to the development of physical and mental discipline, concentration and meditation. They include the following: *karma yoga* (the path of serving others), *bhakti yoga* (the path of devotion), *jnana yoga* (the path of knowledge) and *raja yoga* (the path of meditation), as well as Tantric yoga and kundalini yoga, which are related to raja yoga. Mantra yoga is considered part of raja yoga, especially in the second rung of the niyamas (self-study). The ultimate goals of these paths are the attainment of physical and emotional health and well-being, joy, inner peace, freedom, increased awareness and expanded consciousness. Each path involves mental focus on a single thought, feeling or sound. This encourages the student to concentrate on one thing at a time, thus helping to set the stage for meditation.

According to one's temperament, a person can also focus on one path of yoga over the others. Karma yoga is more suitable for persons with active temperaments, who like to work hard and enjoy serving others. Bhakti yoga is best suited for emotional and devotional people, especially those who like to chant, pray and repeat sacred mantras. Jnana yoga is beneficial for philosophical people who like to inquire deeply about life and the reality of existence. Raja yoga is best for people who are systematic and organized in their approach to life, especially those who like a well-rounded approach to spirituality that involves body postures for meditation, mental discipline and spiritual techniques. This path is particularly good for doctors, healers and psychologists.

When I was staying at the Himalayan Institute in the early days of my training, we were introduced to and given the opportunity to experience all four paths. For example, we had classes in the evening on philosophy as an aspect of jnana yoga, would sing kirtan at night as part of a bhakti practice and do a great amount of work to maintain the ashram and serve guests as a dimension of karma yoga. As part of karma yoga, one of my most important jobs was to care for patients at our holistic medical clinic practicing homeopathy, advising on good nutrition and using yoga therapies. Also, as part of a well-rounded spiritual practice, Swamiji insisted that we do hatha yoga and breathing exercises daily, which were essential for the raja yoga part of our training. Following is a more detailed discussion of the different paths of yoga.

PATHS OF SPIRITUAL PRACTICE	
Karma Yoga	Path of Action and Selfless Service
Bhakti Yoga	Path of Devotion and Love
Jnana Yoga	Path of Knowledge
Raja Yoga	Path of Meditation
Kundalini Yoga	Path of the Primal Force
Mantra Yoga	Path of Sound
Trantric Yoga	Path of Expanded Consciousness

KARMA YOGA

The Law of Cause and Effect

Karma yoga is the path of action and selfless service. According to the teachings of Swami Rama, karma yoga is the most fundamental form of yoga, as one cannot progress on the spiritual path without it. The word *karma* refers to the law of cause and effect: for every action there is a reaction and a consequence. The major principles of karma yoga are: 1) to perform actions and fulfill one's duties, commitments and responsibilities skillfully, without dissipating energy in the process; 2) to not be overly attached to one's emotions, thoughts, actions and deeds; 3) to perform actions selflessly and lovingly and to give the fruits and results of one's actions to benefit all sentient beings; and 4) ultimately to give all the fruits of one's actions to the divine or to God.

As long as people carry out any actions in the world, the law of karma will come into effect. Since every breath one takes, every food item one consumes, every step one takes and every word one utters will have an effect on the world, it is of utmost importance that one's actions don't lead to chaos, disequilibrium or disharmony. Even one's emotions and thoughts, if projected outwardly, will generate actions. This is why it is essential to try to be ethical, humane and positive and to make effort to help others. Karma yoga emphasizes that everyone should strive to have as little negative impact on others, on the planet or on themselves. In addition, one should accept full responsibility and attempt to resolve any problems that may result from one's activities, speech and thoughts.

The Ego

The karma yogi realizes that generally the aim of even the most mundane of actions is the attainment of pleasure in the external world. The ego always has alternative motives lurking behind the scene. One needs to gradually step out of the ego to remove negative thoughts and actions.

Duties to Oneself

There are two types of duties, those to oneself and those to others. It is of vital importance to personally take care of oneself to remain healthy and productive. For example, it is mandatory to go to the bathroom, eat nutritional foods, drink enough liquids, keep the body clean and have adequate shelter. If one does not care for himself or herself, that burden will unnecessarily fall to members of the family, neighbors, friends or society. Since life involves constant relationship with others, caring for oneself is the first step in fulfilling one's duties in the world.

Selfless Service

Karma yoga is the path of selfless service to help remove the suffering of one's fellow human beings. In addition, every action needs to be carefully orchestrated so as to not create pain or suffering for oneself or another. Taking care of one's children, the elderly and the sick are fundamental actions on the path of karma yoga. Some examples of people who innately practice the path of action and selfless service are those who work in the healing, teaching, social services and environmental preservation professions as well as parents and other caretakers. Without any ulterior motives of the ego, such individuals devote their time and energy to help others. On a more mundane level, even washing dishes, doing the laundry, cooking food with care and attention and doing one's job with full intentionality are all forms of karma yoga.

More specific examples of karma yoga that involve fulfilling one's duty with selflessness in the world come from two stories from the great spiritual books. These describe situations where individuals needed to fulfill their responsibilities and destinies with great skill and discipline, even when there was great resistance.

In the Bhagavad Gita, Arjuna argues with his teacher Krishna that he doesn't want to go to battle against his cousins and teachers. Krishna prevails upon Arjuna that he must follow his lifelong chosen path of action as a warrior and fulfill his responsibilities in the world. Krishna instructs him not only to fight in the coming Great War, but to do it with discipline and courage. By doing so, even though he would be creating actions, he would not be generating karma for himself because he would be fulfilling his duty with skill and honor.

Similarly, in the Old Testament God told Moses to pass on the Ten Commandments to the Hebrew tribes as part of fulfilling his life's duties. Because initially he had lost his temper and distinctly disobeyed God and cooperated only after having experienced many trials and tribulations, Moses was not able to enter the Holy Land. Even though Moses eventually fulfilled his life destiny with determination and devotion, he was unable to experience the full joy and wonder of seeing the results of the distribution of the Commandments to his people. However, he was still able to experience the joy of having served others and having fulfilled his responsibility.

The Fruits

The karma yogi recognizes that the fruits of action are temporary and stem from the illusory part of the imagination of maya. Nonattachment to the fruits of one's actions leads to freedom from suffering. When actions are no longer based on selfish desires, one is free to experience the spiritual light of universal love and devotion.

Karma yoga also teaches that to be attached to the fruits of actions will lead to either wanting more to maintain happiness or to being fearful of losing what one has. Both of these perpetuate bondage to the never-ending cycle of desires and attachment. If there are positive fruits, one should not be attached to them but instead give them away to others and ultimately to Brahman. By doing this, one can become free of the law of karma.

The Four Noble Truths

The Four Noble Truths of Buddhism are similar to the path of karma yoga. According to the Buddha:

1. There is suffering, and all people suffer.
2. The cause of all suffering is attachment to the ideas and objects of the world and the desire to cling to those things.
3. By letting go of desires and attachments, one can be released from this suffering; and
4. The eight-fold path of how to actually let go of desires and attachments will ultimately lead to enlightenment and freedom, the state that is free of suffering.

Zen Buddhism

In Zen Buddhism, a Japanese spiritual tradition that also uses the practice of meditation along with the idea of living life skillfully, in the moment and with full intentionality is also similar to karma yoga. Individuals who devote their entire mind and body to develop a particular art or skill as a spiritual discipline are following the path of action.

Zen also teaches that one should live life with deep gratitude and be present and alert in every second of life. Susuki Roshi, the first Zen Buddhist priest to come to the West, wrote a wonderful book on this subject, *Zen Mind Beginner's Mind,* which details this endeavor. When a person is able to do this, he or she will have the energy, knowledge and learned discipline to serve others. Being purposeful, direct and honest with oneself and others is fundamental to serving humanity.

The Greater Whole

Within Vedantic philosophy, karma yoga propounds the importance of making effort to transcend all thoughts and actions that veil the truth of existence. These include:

1. *mala,* which is characterized by selfishness and impurities of the heart that make one egotistical and self-absorbed,
2. *vikshepa,* which is restlessness and tossing of the mind, and the constant flux of the mind in its innumerable and nonceasing thought waves, and
3. *avarana,* the ignorance that results when one becomes attached to one's ego and doesn't understand that he or she is part of a larger whole.

By being self-disciplined, performing the simple tasks of the day with full attention, and by giving the fruits of one's actions to others, a person generates few re-actions. At the same time, one recognizes that each action skillfully performed contributes to the overall harmony of the universe. When one performs one's duties without ego or attachment to the fruits of their actions, but instead offers those fruits to all sentient beings and to the divine, this leads to liberation from the suffering that results from attachments, unfulfilled desires and unnecessary cravings. Then the restless mind can calm down and move towards a constant state of peace and joy, and the veil of ignorance that covers one's true nature can dissolve to reveal the pure love of one's essential nature.

In Vedanta it is taught that the more one experiences true human and divine love, the more one becomes bonded to one's essential nature and feels more completely connected to Brahman. When a person understands they are part of a larger whole, they are ready to attain the true knowledge of the Self. Having accomplished this, one becomes free of suffering, even though continuing to act in the world. The practice in karma yoga of giving the fruits of one's actions to others as a form of selfless service and love naturally leads to bhakti yoga.

BHAKTI YOGA

Bhakti yoga is the path of devotion and love, especially divine love. The Sanskrit word *bhakti* means "devotion." A person who follows this path is dedicated to serving a divinity or a higher being. In bhakti yoga one surrenders one's mental and physical resources to attain the ultimate reality and channels all emotions towards feelings of reverence, love and selfless action. In the practice of meditation on this path one often uses divine images, a personal vision of God or forms of intense prayer as the object of concentration.

Devoting oneself to helping others is a form of bhakti. If one sees the divine in others and recognizes that everyone is part of the greater humanity, then loving others is the same as loving oneself. Other spiritual paths and religious sects echo the same ideas: the great concept of love and compassion in Buddhism; the idea of loving your neighbor as yourself in Christianity; and, the Zen Buddhist idea of gratitude for life itself, for every moment, every breath, every opportunity, and the experience of the fullness of the moment, whether pleasant or unpleasant. Similar ideas are found in the monastic traditions of the Christian religion, the Jewish path of Hassidic mysticism and the Sufi sect in the Islamic religion. Japanese archery training and tea ceremonies, Sufi rug weaving, Chinese martial arts training and Sufi dervish and Hasidic ecstatic dancing are more examples of devotional practices that lead one to unity with a higher being. The yoga practice of kirtan, devotional chanting, is a bhakti yoga practice. This is discussed in more detail in Part III in the section: "Chanting Forms of Meditation."

In Vedantic thought, once someone tastes the love of Brahman, they will want to remain permanently within this love. Self-surrender to the will of universal consciousness is by definition pure love and bliss. In such a state love becomes the motive behind all actions. The more one rests in this love, the more they want to think, talk about and sing to this love. People often choose a representative deity, such as Ishwara in the yogic tradition or God in the Abrahamic religions, with whom they desire to commune. When the aspirant is constantly communicating with a beloved god figure, they will ultimately merge and become one with this god figure.

An individual practitioner of bhakti yoga is called *bhakta,* and they often try to associate themselves with other devotees through satsang, a community of like-minded spiritual seekers. There are many distractions on the path of life and being able to share and support ideas and life's vicissitudes with others is often very helpful.

When Swamiji spoke about emotions he was not referring to sentimentality or emotionality. He emphasized that negative emotions like anger and envy should be minimalized, while positive emotions such as joy and love were to be strengthened. In his lectures he would often say to grease your actions with love. He repeatedly spoke about how to use emotions as a means to love and serve, and as an aid in the quest for enlightenment. Emotions can be sublimated into devotion. He also taught that it was imperative to work towards understanding one's deepest emotions and to transform them to serve and love others. This could best be accomplished through meditation and/or depth psychotherapy.

The Four Fountains or Primary Urges

Swamiji explained that one's actions were based on thoughts, thoughts were based on emotions, emotions were based on desires and desires were based on the four primary urges: the needs for food, sleep, sex and self-preservation. And with this in mind, he taught that the way to use emotions in an enlightened way was to channel them and to practice the eight limbs of raja yoga, where ethical standards and growth-promoting activities could be established, along with ways to maintain a healthy body, mind and spirit. Such intuitive and commonsense practices like eating quality and nourishing foods, sleeping when tired, devoting oneself to one's intimate partner and having a stable and clean home environment are all helpful to manage the four basic urges.

Seven Streams of Emotion

Swamiji also described the seven main streams of emotions that stem from the four basic urges and taught how to transform these streams. Desires *(kama)* bind us but can be transformed into a burning desire for truth, which is love in bhakti yoga. Attachment *(moha)* is changed by learning how to be attached only to love. Ego *(ahamkara)* protects the individual in worldly life and helps one develop a strong sense of self as a means to enlightenment. Anger *(krodha)* needs to be transformed as it represents suppressed and unfulfilled desires. When that emotional energy is released, it frees one to move forward on the path of love and devotion. Feelings of jealousy *(matsarya)* create unnecessary separation and inner tension through excessive competition and must be understood and released. Pride *(mada)* is having something and lording this over another person, which causes ill will. Greed *(lobha)* represents wanting more and more. In order to experience true and unselfish love one must overcome these emotional obstacles

To best accomplish transformation of the seven streams of emotion, the bhakti yogi uses *japa* (repetition of mantra), selfless prayer (not asking for things of the world but instead how to best serve and love), gentleness, kindness, tolerance, generosity, ahimsa (nonviolence of thought speech and action), healthy lifestyle, meditation on the heart chakra and selfless service. To practice bhakti yoga, one should avoid being boastful, conceited and rude. One does not have to live in a monastery but should live in the world with appreciation and devotion to others.7

JNANA YOGA

Jnana is a Sanskrit word that is translated as "knowledge" or "intellect." Thus, jnana yoga is the path of knowledge. The goal of this path is knowledge of the underlying truths of existence. Meditation by students on the path of the intellect often begins by contemplation of philosophical writings such as the Hindu Vedas and Upanishads, the Koran, the ancient Chinese treatise called the Tao Te Ching, the Jewish Talmud or the Christian Bible. When following this path, one uses the intellect to attain wisdom and to understand the mysteries of life. Questions such as "Who am I?" and "What is the meaning of life?" are pondered with great intensity. The ultimate goal of this path is Self-realization, where knowledge of one's internal states leads to a deeper understanding of the mysteries of the universe and all its manifestations. One can then let go of all preconceived notions of life so the higher functions of the mind can receive true knowledge and understanding.

Jnana yoga is the yogic path of inquiry and knowledge. It requires great strength of will to follow this path. Through one's intellect, the aspirant attempts to constantly inquire about one's true nature, beyond the ego, and to transcend the limitations of one's thoughts and emotions. The ultimate goal is to transcend false identification with one's body and mind, which are transitory and ephemeral and ultimately pass away. Through the practice of jnana yoga one can reconnect with the true reality by realizing that the individual soul (Atman) is the same as all souls and that this represents, in reality, the oneness of all life. When this happens, the aspirant achieves union with Brahman.

The Seven Bhumikas

In the Sivananda tradition, students are taught about jnana yoga with a focus on the seven *bhumikas*, the seven stages of knowledge of the true nature of the Self. The book *Yoga Vasistha* is comprised of a dialogue between the ancient Guru Vasistha and his disciple Rama on the seven bhumikas and jnana yoga. According to the Sivananda tradition, jnana yoga represents the culmination of the yogas. It is a very difficult path, but it is said to be the most direct path to Brahman and liberation. Whereas the yogas of karma, bhakti and raja train the mind to be pure and sattvic, jnana yoga is the final stage of spiritual knowledge and the evolution of the soul. The seven bhumikas represent the stages the soul goes through and provides a measuring stick to evaluate spiritual progression.

The first bhumika is *subheccha*, which means longing for truth. Subheccha has four aspects: *Viveka* is discrimination between what is real and permanent versus what is unreal and impermanent, with respect to objects, emotions and knowledge of the Self. *Vairagya* means nonattachment or dispassion. One realizes that desire for what he or she doesn't possess and the fear of losing what one has leads to frustration, unhappiness and suffering. *Shatsampat* encompasses the six main truths of jnana yoga: control of the mind and senses, eradication of subtle desires *(vasanas)*, devotion to the spiritual path, the capacity to endure hard work and hardships, faith in the teacher and preparation to experience universal consciousness. *Mumutkshutva* means to have a burning desire for liberation.

The second through the seventh bhumikas are as follows. *Vicharana* involves always using self-inquiry and listening carefully to and reflecting on the words and advice from one's teachers. *Tanumanasa* involves abandoning names and forms of the physical and mental worlds and focusing only on Brahman. *Sattvapati* is the attainment of the qualities of peacefulness and all things sattvic in nature. In this state of consciousness supernatural powers and siddhis become available to the aspirant. *Asamshakti* means transcendence of all creation. *Padarthbhavani* means that one only recognizes Brahman as real and sees Brahman everywhere. And finally, *turiya*, the state of liberation in which the individual is one with Brahman.8

RAJA YOGA

Because raja yoga is such an important and all encompassing path for the spiritual aspirant, it will be separately and more thoroughly covered in Part III: Raja Yoga, The Royal Path to Meditation.

PART III:

Raja Yoga, The Royal Path to Meditation

PATANJALI'S YOGA SUTRAS

Samkhya is the philosophy underlying the science of yoga, which was codified at least 2000 years ago by the ancient Indian philosopher, Patanjali Maharishi in the *Yoga Sutras. Ashtanga* yoga is included in this system of yoga. This short treatise explains yoga and meditation theory and introduces many spiritual disciplines and practices. The Yoga Sutras also describes the powers and experiences that result from attaining the highest states of consciousness. It is said that Ishwara is the originator of this great system and that Patanjali received this knowledge from a divine source. The more common nomenclature for ashtanga yoga in the West is raja yoga, or the royal path, and so I will use this terminology throughout this book. Yoga darshana is the underlying philosophical system of yoga, a way of seeing and making raja yoga comprehensible and available to the public.

Patanjali's Yoga Sutras is divided into four parts *(padas).* Each pada has a distinct philosophical and psychological orientation. Following is a brief description of the four padas.

The first pada is *Samadhi Pada.* It deals with the eighth limb of raja yoga, samadhi (superconsciousness). Those who are immersed in the philosophy of raja yoga consider this to be a very important chapter. Samadhi pada is for those students who have learned to still the mind. It describes the means to lead the practitioner to the higher practices and states of yoga. Samadhi pada begins with the statement, "Now Yoga is explained." *Now* reflects the readiness of the aspirant. Yoga is the union of the individual self with the universal Self. The goal is to live consciously in union with the

Infinite Self. The practice of meditation is the way to remain in samadhi.

Sadhana Pada discusses spiritual practices (sadhana) as a means to prepare the mind for the higher practices that lead to samadhi. In this part, chitta is described as the workings of the mind, both conscious and unconscious, and is sometimes called mind stuff. Chitta represents not only what the mind is made of, but also the mind taking shape. According to the Yoga Sutras, there are five categories of vrittis: right knowledge, wrong knowledge, imagination, sleep and memory. Each of these categories is colored by and affected by the three gunas. When a thought is rajasic, it is restless and painful. When a thought is tamasic, it is confused and deluded. The quality of sattva is pure and non-painful. When a person is under the influence of rajasic vrittis they are so busy physically and mentally they do not even notice they are suffering. *Ekagrata* represents the one-pointed mind and is the state of mind where tamasic and rajasic vrittis are restrained, while the sattvic vrittis remain active. Thus, when the sattvic vrittis predominate, the tamasic and rajasic vrittis are controlled. An important sattvic thought is: *I am not the mind.* Another sattvic vritti is: *I do not want to be a slave to my thoughts. I want to have positive thoughts and incorporate love and forgiveness in my life.* The most important aspects of sattvic vrittis are discrimination and dispassion.

Nirodha is the mental process that restrains all the vrittis. When the thought waves/vrittis are restrained, one reaches the first stages of samadhi and beholds the ultimate reality with a still, clear and one-pointed mind. This experience is like looking at a very clear mirror but realizing this is only a reflection of the truth. This process represents the state when chitta/mind is absolutely still and one-pointed. This reflection is an indication that mind still remains, but at this point in the practice the meditator is able to clearly distinguish the difference between mind/matter and consciousness. When one becomes completely absorbed in pure consciousness, ultimate reality is attained. At this stage there is no mind, just consciousness aware of itself without reference to mind/matter.

Vibhuti Pada deals with powers called divine glories, which are the beneficial and collateral physical, emotional and psychological manifestations of samadhi. However, it is advised to be careful not to use these powers for one's ego. In the higher state of samadhi where all vrittis are restrained, the spiritual aspirant rests in their true nature, Self-realization.

Kaivalya Pada deals with spiritual liberation. As long as the vrittis are not restrained, the perceiver will identify with every vritti of the mind because it is very easy to become attached to these vrittis. With spiritual liberation, all thought waves are transcended. Now the question arises, how to restrain the vrittis.

Chitta Vritti Nirodha is an important aphorism in the Yoga Sutras. It can be translated as "controlling (nirodha) the stuff of the mind (chitta) and the thought waves (vrittis) within the stuff of mind." All the practices of yoga are the means to do this. By doing these practices, the rajasic/tamasic vrittis are weakened to allow only the pure sattvic vrittis to remain. Abhyasa (sadhana or spiritual practice) means to do regular practice over a long time and with detachment as the means to success in yoga/samadhi. This is similar to the ideas in the sixth chapter of the Bhagavad Gita when Krishna talks to Arjuna about spiritual practice. The second is constant and regular daily practice to help the aspirant to always be on guard to replace tamasic and rajasic vrittis with sattvic ones. And the third is to be inspired in one's daily life to continue spiritual practices.

This process should be effortless, nonmechanical, devotional and done with enthusiasm. Satsang with fellow devotees is essential. It is best to create or join a spiritual community such as a yoga group, ashram or kirtan community. Vairagya (non-attachment) is also a very important part of the process of control of the mind and progression on the raja yoga spiritual path. Here vairagya means nonattachment to the suffering that is due to the five *kleshas* or poisons. These are: ignorance *(avidya)* ego *(asmita)*, likes *(raga)*, dislikes *(dvsha)* and fear of death *(abhinivesha)*.

Living in the world with all its mundane needs and impressions can make human beings lose touch with the true Self that is present within each person. Vairagya is a mental attitude and involves the use of practices to purify the mind and make it possible to be in the world but not of the world. One should always keep awareness of the divine behind all thoughts and actions.

RAJA YOGA

Raja yoga is a very systematic path that leads to meditation because it has practices that span the three realms of existence: the physical, mental and spiritual and helps us gain mastery of these dimensions. Following this path, one embarks on an internal journey to the innermost levels of consciousness.

When we were living at the Himalayan Institute, Swamiji would guide us in meditation and teach us various spiritual practices where we would learn how to focus on the seven major chakras. He also instructed us how to use mantras to deepen our meditation practice according to the Himalayan tradition. These teachings represented the essence of raja yoga, the path of meditation as well as related philosophical ideas regarding Samkhya, the Yoga Sutras, Vedanta and Tantra. As a physician, raja yoga became an extremely important medical paradigm to understand various health related practices and how diseases manifest on the multiple dimensions of our existence.

Raja yoga is a path of meditation in the Indian tradition that accepts the underlying intellectual principles of Samkhya philosophy. Patanjali has summarized the technique of meditation in the eight rungs of ashtanga yoga (raja yoga) in *Sadhana,* the second pada of the Yoga Sutras. The raja yoga path of meditation is an exact science that has been developed over thousands of years. This systematic path serves as a guide on the internal journey from the external body to the deepest levels of consciousness and shows the way to lead a healthy life at all levels: physical, emotional, mental and spiritual. The benefits said to be gained from the practice of raja yoga can be verified by anyone who accepts the prescribed methods as a hypothesis and then tests them by his or her own experience. The practices of raja yoga and meditation are systematic disciplines that do not require unquestioning faith but instead encourage healthy decision-making and discrimination.

Eight Steps of Raja Yoga	
Yamas	Regulations
Niyamas	Observances
Asanas	Hatha yoga and meditation postures
Pranayama	Control of prana and breath
Pratyahara	Sense withdrawal
Dharana	Concentration
Dhyana	Meditation
Samadhi	Absorption, enlightenment

There are eight steps or rungs in the ladder of raja yoga. In the practice of raja yoga, the student learns to systematically prepare for meditation by first encouraging wise and healthy habits. In addition, one practices physical and breathing exercises to help focus the mind and learn to direct the desires, emotions, thoughts and subtle impressions that lie dormant in the unconscious. These practices steady the mind, make it one-pointed, lead to increased awareness and to an expanded state of consciousness.

The first two rungs on the path of raja yoga, the *yamas* and the *niyamas,* represent the highest moral and ethical values of human beings. These principles help to create sattvic vrittis by leading the mind from ego obsession and selfishness. They are essential prerequisites before undertaking the more advanced practices of yoga. While seemingly simple in nature, each has great depth and complexity. The yamas and niyamas set the stage for growth and internal observation by encouraging discipline, self-study, honesty, continence of speech and action, and contentment. Discipline need not connote rigidity or stoicism but can provide a channel for creative energy. Learning to be content in any situation eliminates the torment and obsessiveness that often lead to emotional or physical ailments. An attitude of receptivity and self-study enable the student of yoga to understand which habits and conditions inhibit wellness. Having gained such awareness, he or she learns to avoid certain psychological conflicts, reinforcing instead those patterns or ideas that lead to psychosomatic balance. The five yamas, along with the five niyamas, are the foundation of raja yoga. Without strong roots, a tree can easily fall over, as will a house collapse that does not have a sturdy foundation.

Yamas (Restraints)

The yamas help guide the student to establish regulations in relationships with others. These regulations all lead to modifications of behavior to replace negative habits with ethical values. When these restraints are practiced, one remains free of guilt and remorse and experiences a greater sense of self-confidence, fulfillment and peace of mind. Regulation of attitudes helps to conserve and direct one's energy to higher spiritual practices. These restraints help to control rajasic and tamasic thoughts, speech and actions. The five yamas are presented below.

Yamas: Restraints	
Ahimsa	Nonviolence of thought, action and speech
Satyam	Truthfulness to oneself and others
Asteya	Nonstealing
Brahmacharya	Control of sexual and sensual desires
Aparigraha	Nonpossessiveness and nonattachment

Ahimsa

Ahimsa is the Sanskrit word for nonviolence. The first and most fundamental regulation is nonviolence in thought, action and speech. In the practice of nonharming, one purposefully avoids hurting another person physically or emotionally and also avoids self-condemnation. This is similar to the Hippocratic Oath in which physicians make the pledge to "First, do no harm." Even if it is not possible to help another person in one's community, it is important to not cause more pain or suffering in another's life.

There are two aspects to this most important yama. The negation of violence and cruelty is of utmost importance not only for humans but for all sentient beings. Selfish love, where one tries to manipulate or control another person they care about, is not ahimsa. On the positive side, ahimsa is the cultivation of selfless love for all, the essence of bhakti yoga.

When practicing ahimsa, one should always try to understand and release negative and even violent thoughts about themself, as these destructive thoughts could be projected outwards to another person and possibly lead to harmful actions. One can injure another person with a word, glance, gesture or blink of an eye. It is well known that a kind word can lift another's spirits and a hostile or sarcastic comment can be quite harmful. A single word or sentence can be as destructive as any action. For example, if a parent degrades a child, this can lead to permanent issues of self-esteem and self-confidence. If a national leader states he will attack another country, this will send the stock market reeling and perhaps encourage a first strike by the country feeling threatened. Words are indeed powerful. This is why gentle speech is always encouraged.

The bodhisattva principle that permeates Buddhist philosophy is a form of ahimsa. This refers to the idea that enlightened ones return to earth to reincarnate in order to help others. According to this philosophy there can be no real enlightenment unless all sentient beings are free from the bondage of identification with their physical and mental bodies and thus can experience the bliss of pure consciousness. Since everyone is part of a larger whole, true freedom is possible only if pure consciousness is experienced and realized by all. Loving all humanity and serving individuals as divine, no matter their race, caste, gender, social status or religion, is essential on the path of yoga and represents the selfless love that is part of ahimsa.

Satyam

Satyam means to be truthful and honest with others. It also means to be honest with oneself, which often involves careful and thoughtful self-inquiry. Journaling, psychotherapy and meditation can all be helpful in this process. Satyam not only means to not tell lies, but also to not deliberately omit feelings or actions that another person would want to or needs to know. Omission can be as problematic as outright lying.

To palter is another form of not being truthful. The word *palter* means "to use words and highly literal statements to create an incomplete version of the truth and convey a false impression." People who do this may feel more ethical as it falls somewhere between the truth and a total lie. But the problem is the person on the receiving end doesn't feel the same way. They may feel just as deceived as if you had told a blatant and bold-faced lie.

Even though I consider myself to be an honest person, about ten years ago I omitted something important about my life to one of my children, who expressed deep disappointment with me. It caused needless distance between us, but over the years, after I apologized and explained the reasons for my mistake, our relationship recovered, and we are as close as ever. I learned a valuable lesson.

It requires strength and courage to practice satyam, which allows for the development of trust between people. The truth must be expressed in a careful and kind way so others can hear and understand the message. Being gentle with the truth is essential, as ahimsa must always accompany honest communication. One can hurt another if truth doesn't include ahimsa and wisdom.

While I try to practice nonviolence in thought speech and action and to be truthful and clear in my communication with others, I do mess up at times. I have had moments of anger, jealousy, suspiciousness and envy in my life. I do, however, constantly try to understand, release and redirect these feelings into forgiveness, peace, compassion and wisdom. I am committed to try to continue this transformation for the rest of my days.

Ultimately satyam is about seeking the true and absolute reality, Brahman/God.

Asteya

The third yama is asteya, which means to not steal. Both lying and stealing inevitably lead to more deception to cover up the original lie or theft. A great amount of time and energy is wasted in these attempts to cover up misappropriations. In addition, the conscience will often be affected, which can lead to preoccupation and troublesome thoughts. Asteya also means to not be covetous or cultivate feelings of jealousy. It involves not stealing from others or acting on negative desires, and also not hoarding or having more than what is needed. The act of stealing is not congruous with the practice of ahimsa or satyam.

Brahmacharya

Control of sensual and sexual desires is the fourth yama. Brahmacharya actually means always walking with Brahman, which can be achieved by moderating and carefully directing sensual and sexual energy. Preoccupation with satisfying sexual urges can be distracting when one is on a spiritual path. Being moderate with such desires, not manipulating another for sexual control and directing one's affection to a mutually loved one, all represent control of the sensual desires. The practice of brahmacharya helps to transform the spiritual force ojas to be used in deeper meditative practices. In monastic traditions this can mean celibacy. Householders practice relative brahmacharya by being faithful in love relationships. Seeing the divine in one's loved one is a form of walking with Brahman.

Aparigraha

The fifth regulation is aparigraha, which means nonpossessiveness. A great amount of time is wasted in accumulating possessions that are useless or unnecessary in daily life. Attachment to material wealth leads to discontentment because one either worries about what they don't have or fears they will lose what they already do have. Aparigraha also means to not be greedy and to not take bribes or gifts of persuasion.

Niyamas (Observances)

Niyamas: Observances	
Saucha	Cleanliness of body and mind
Santosha	Contentment and equilibrium
Tapas	Practices for a healthy body and mind
Svadhyaya	Study of philosophy and inspiring readings
Ishvara Pranidhana	Surrender and devotion to a higher consciousness

The niyamas are observances of body and mind that enable the development of self-awareness and self-control to prepare for more advanced practices. The niyamas are sattvic ways of conduct to help one to live a spiritual life. The five niyamas include the following principles:

Saucha

Cleanliness and purity of body and mind make up the first observance. *Saucha* means "purity, inside and out." There are two ways to practice saucha. One is external, which includes cleanliness of clothes, body and environment such as taking regular showers, dressing modestly and using kriyas for inner cleansing. It also includes doing puja, a ritual that involves purification of mind and heart. In the yoga tradition, wearing yellow represents study and white represents purity.

To be clean physically is an easy task to accomplish, but purity of the mind involves being discriminating and mindful at all times. Mental purity means to cultivate sattvic ideas and thoughts by purifying the thought processes. One way to purify the mind is the Buddhist form of meditation called Mindfulness. This involves maintaining continual awareness of the origins of negative, impure or harmful thoughts and using breathing techniques to allow these thoughts to dissipate.

Santosha

Santosha means "contentment." Contentment is a state of mind that encourages tranquility and equilibrium in all circumstances. Learning to be content in life regardless of wealth or personal status is the goal of this observance. The practice of aparigraha helps to cultivate contentment by eliminating the desire to accumulate more possessions than is necessary for healthy and comfortable living. Santosha involves the cultivation of happiness and humility as well as restraint from complaining. It requires the desire to help other people and to aspire for the contentment of all souls. As part of being content, santosha involves dedicating oneself to serving others, as in the practice of karma yoga.

A good sense of humor is very important in the path of raja yoga. If everyone could learn to laugh at themselves and the surrounding world, they would no longer consider what is impermanent as reality or take life too seriously. The great masters have been described as people who would laugh, tease, joke and sing and who were light-hearted in general. I often talk with my friends, students and colleagues about the healthy and spiritual aspects of a sense of humor. I believe it is a great cosmic joke that people take their small selves so seriously, while physical existence is so ephemeral. The reality, from the yogic and Vedantic perspective, is that all of life is unreal and only Brahman is real. By developing a sense of humor about this, people practice yoga, meaning union, so everyone can become one, in a sense, with the great cosmic joke!

Tapas

Tapas means "austerity." Tapas is sadhana or spiritual practice performed with will power and self-control. Raja yoga practices are tapas, as are the devotional practices of bhakti as well as jnana yoga, which involves devoting great amounts of time to study spiritual teachings.

Tapas also means "fire," fire being the result of the friction created by sadhana. This results in the burning of the ego, which in turn leads to the fire of inner purification that is so essential for yoga. In this context, sometimes pleasantness and easy success can create a sense of numbness on the spiritual path. This is why it is often very important to have the opportunity to overcome challenges. Mistakes and failures can act to instigate the student to try harder, become more resourceful and face life with determination and gratitude.

Svadhyaya

Reading books of philosophy and religion and studying the writings of inspirational spiritual leaders are examples of this observance. Such study leads to understanding of the nature of truth.

Ishwara Pranidhana

Devotion to the higher Self and ultimate reality is the fifth niyama. This involves devoting one's whole being to the pursuit of knowledge, truth and wisdom. Ishwara pranidhana represents a desire to experience the higher Self that connects all sentient beings. It involves a conscious and active form of surrender of the ego along with openness to guidance from spiritual teachers.

Asana

In this discussion I will focus on the sitting postures used in meditation. The hatha yoga postures as well as bandhas, mudras and kriyas will be discussed in Part V: The Practice of Holistic Medicine. According to Patanjali, the main criteria for a meditation sitting posture are it should be steady, comfortable and still. There are several sitting postures that are conducive to steady and comfortable sitting for the practice of meditation. All positions should allow for the natural curves of the spine with the head in alignment with the chest and torso. The hands are placed on the lap, thighs or knees with the palms placed either face down or upwards. In the yogic system, the fingers are situated so that the thumb and index finger of both hands lightly touch each other to form a circle, as will be described in the section on mudras under hatha yoga. The eyes are gently closed.

If you are more comfortable sitting on a chair, it is best to sit away from the back of the chair so that the spine can be properly aligned. The feet should be placed comfortably on the floor. If you need to sit against the back of the chair for added support, use a straight back chair with a small pillow placed against the small of the back.

There are five main postures that involve sitting on the floor. Because people raised in the Western world are often unaccustomed to sitting in this manner, it is recommended that a folded blanket or firm cushion be placed under the hips and buttocks. The height of the cushion should be adjusted according to individual need. A daily practice of hatha yoga can help prepare the body to sit comfortably and for longer periods of time in meditation.

Sukhasana (the easy pose) is the simplest of the cross-legged postures. It causes the least amount of strain on the hips, knees, ankles and feet. Beginners, people with stiffness in their back or lower extremities and the elderly often find this position comfortable. Here the right foot is placed below the left knee and the left foot is positioned below the right knee. Each knee can then rest on the opposite foot.

Swastikasana (the auspicious pose) is also a cross-legged sitting posture but is a bit more complicated. Here the left leg is bent at the knee and the left foot is placed against the right thigh. The right foot is placed on top of the left calf with the outer edge of the foot and toes tucked in between the thigh and calf muscles. Only the right big toe should be visible here. The toes of the left foot are pulled up between the right thigh and calf, with only the left big toe being visible. The ankle bones and heels are not lined up in this meditation posture.

Siddhasana (the accomplished pose) is a more advanced sitting posture and can be stressful on the lower limbs, especially for beginning students. It is particularly helpful when practicing locks (bandhas), breath retention (kumbhaka) or when attempting to more vigorously activate the latent energy (kundalini) at the first chakra. Here the root lock is applied by contracting and holding tight the anal muscles and the muscles of the perineum. The left heel is placed between the genitals and the anal area. The right heel is placed against the pubic bone above the genitals. The ankle joints are placed so they are in a line one on top of the other. The toes are positioned in the same manner as in the above-mentioned auspicious pose.

Ardha padmasana (the half lotus) is sometimes used in meditation and can be used as a preparation for practicing the full lotus. One foot is placed on the opposite thigh with the heel resting firmly against the abdominal wall. The other leg is bent and tucked comfortably under the top leg.

Padmasana (the lotus pose) is a more strenuous cross-legged sitting pose for meditation. Only people with very flexible ankles and knees can use this position in meditation. The legs are stretched to a great extent and long meditation may become difficult. Because of the stress on the lower extremities, this posture is seldom recommended for meditation. The right foot is placed on the left thigh and the left foot is placed on the right thigh. The heels are placed against the lower abdominal wall.

In the Zen Buddhist tradition (Zazen practice), *seiza* is the meditation posture most often used, although it is less commonly practiced in the yoga tradition. In this position, the practitioner sits on their knees and heels with a straight back. Hands are folded in the lap with the thumbs touching and with the right hand placed inside the left. This hand position is called Dhyana mudra. There is a wooden bench that a person can sit on to help keep the back straight in this meditation posture. This Zazen bench also helps take pressure off the knees.

Common problems that occur while doing the sitting meditation postures are aching or discomfort of the back, hips, knees or ankles. Paresthesias (pins and needles sensations) of the feet are also a fairly common occurrence. If any of these problems occur, it is often best to gently move and switch positions, rather than suffer discomfort or pain.

Sitting Postures for Meditation

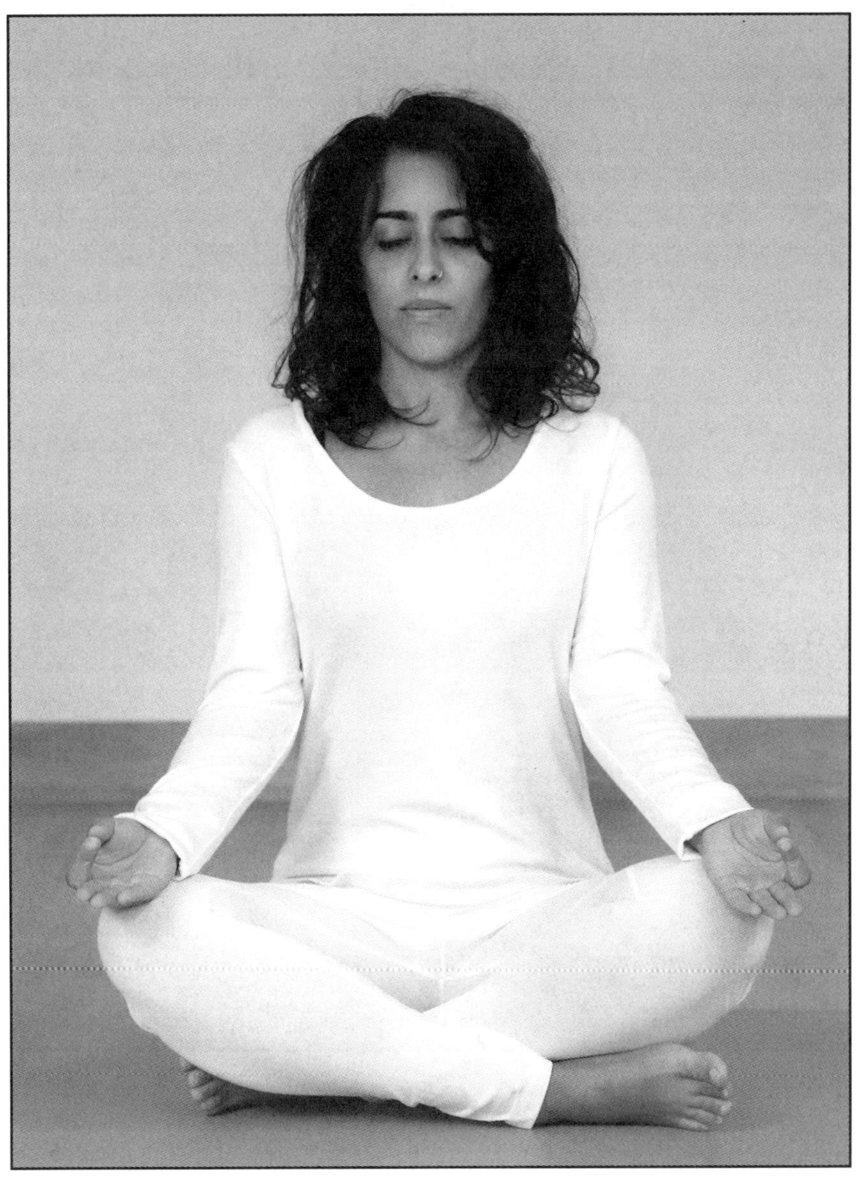

Sukhasana, the easy sitting posture

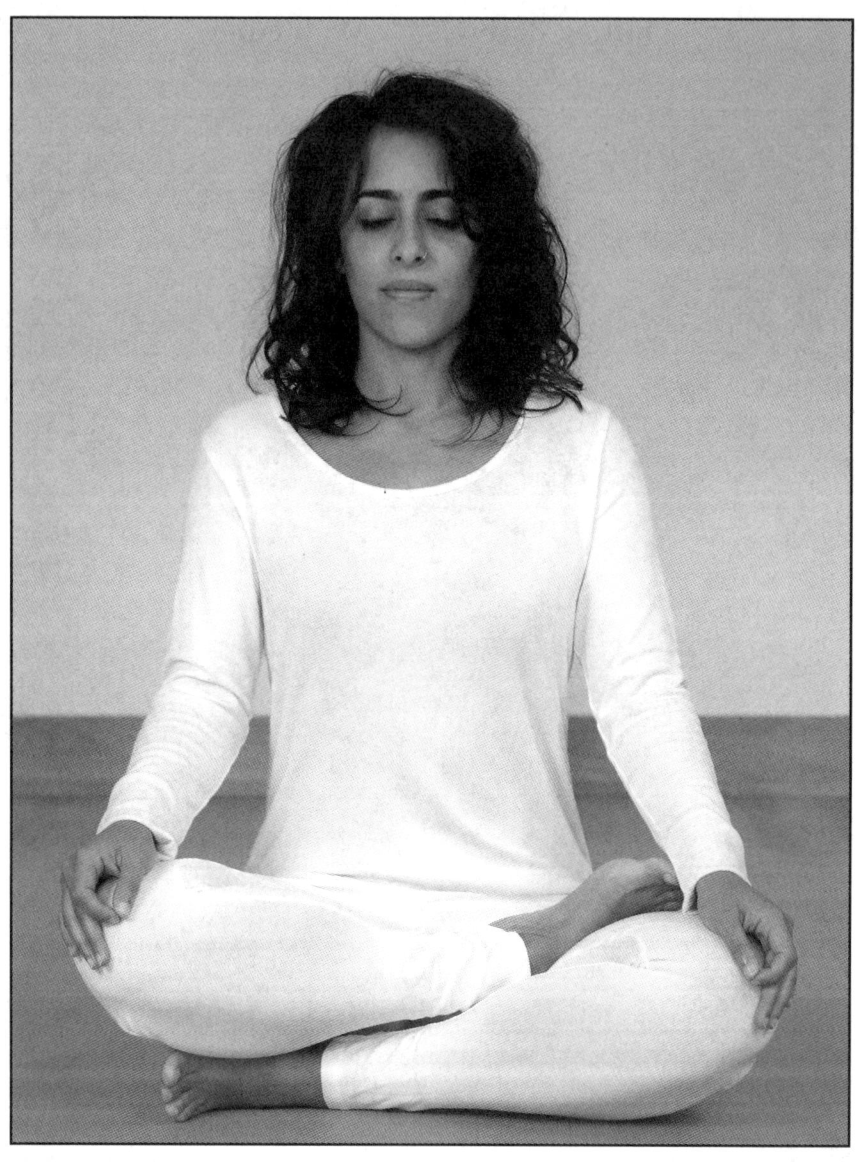

Ardha padmasana, the half lotus

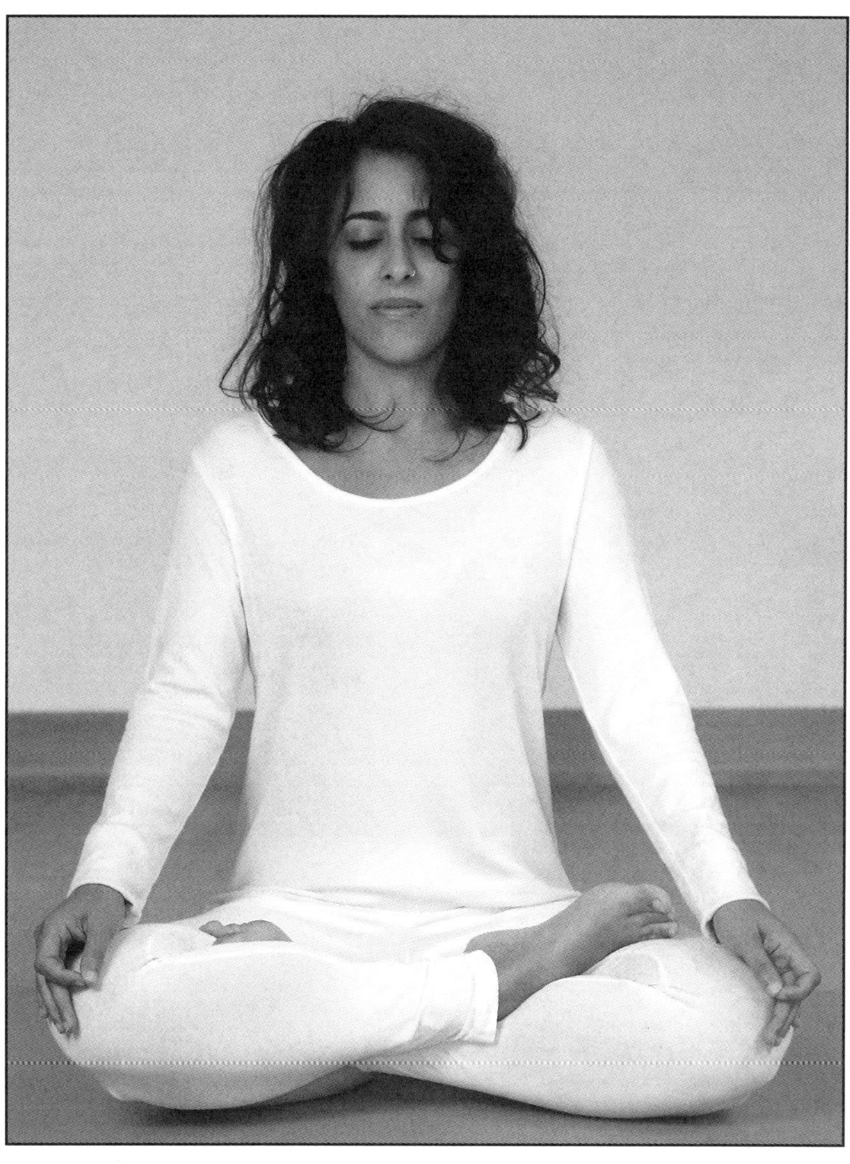

Padmasana, the full lotus

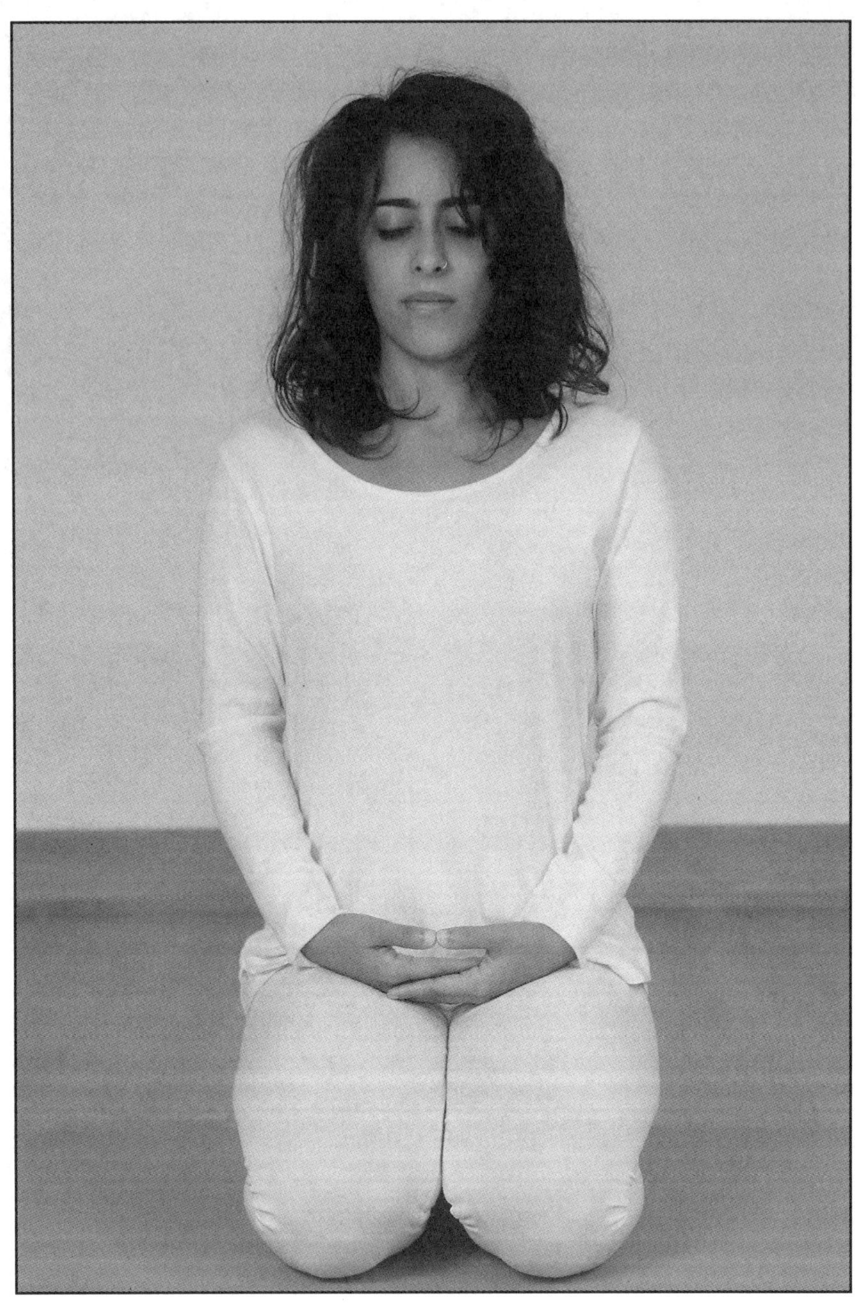

The Zen meditation pose

Pranayama

Pranayama is the fourth step in raja yoga. In Sanskrit, pranayama is a composite word consisting of *prana,* which means "energy" and either *yama,* meaning "control," or *ayama,* which means "expansion." Therefore, *pranayama* means "a practice in which the flow of energy is expanded and brought under control." To break it down even further, *prana* is composed of "pra," which means first unit and "na," meaning energy. Therefore, *prana* refers to the first and the subtlest form of energy that animates the body and mind as well as the entire universe. All inanimate objects, life forms, and all human sensations, thoughts, feelings, ideas, desires and knowledge are possible because of prana.

While prana underlies and sustains all aspects of human functioning, the main vehicle that allows for its control within the body and exchange with the outside world is the breath. This is the reason that breathing techniques are most closely associated with pranayama. Although eating also represents a vehicle for exchange of prana with the outside world, it occurs only a few times daily, while breathing occurs many times every minute.

From a spiritual perspective, the veils that obscure pure consciousness and the impurities of rajasic and tamasic tendencies can be destroyed by pranayama, allowing the light of sattva to shine. When prana is consciously directed or restrained, the mind becomes steady. Though prana is by nature rajasic, it can also be tamasic. Pranayama involves doing controlled breathing exercises where the physical nerves are not overly or under stimulated. Through the practice of pranayama the nadis become strong enough to contain the energies that arise during meditation. A more detailed description of pranayama can be found in Part V: The Practice of Holistic Medicine.

Pratyahara

Classically pratyahara refers to the withdrawal of senses from the external world as well as control and mastery of the senses. The five senses (hearing, touch, vision, taste and smell) are tools of the mind. Sense withdrawal from external desires and objects is an essential preliminary to deeper concentration and meditative techniques. It involves control of body, breath, senses and mind.

Prati means "mastery or control" and *ahara* means "food." Here food refers not only to physical food but also to the food of impressions that nourish the mind and senses of the individual. In this context, the practice of pratyahara includes ways to withdraw from the environment's constant stimulation of the senses, such as avoiding too much TV, radio and internet.

Selfless service for others helps to withdraw the mind and senses from distracting activities. Another aspect of pratyahara involves moving one's mind towards positive impressions that encourage concentration and meditation, such as by going to spiritually oriented events and having more quiet time during the day. One can create positive impressions for the senses by burning pleasant smelling incense, having a special meditation room in one's home or by chanting with others. In general, pratyahara is also practiced by encouraging one's creative side, such as doing art or listening to uplifting music. By practicing pratyahara, one can concentrate the mind and direct thoughts and emotions to higher spiritual truths.

Pratyahara represents the crossroads between the inner and outer aspects of raja yoga. Some yogis who focus on raja yoga believe that with the practice of pratyahara the external limbs of raja yoga end and the inner essence of the deeper practices of meditation begins. In this context, the sixth to eighth limbs of raja yoga—concentration, meditation and samadhi—form a continuum. *Concentration* means "to focus the mind on a single object," while meditation is a state that results from sustained, prolonged and uninterrupted concentration on a single object; samadhi is absorption with the object.

Dharana

Dharana means "concentration" and includes practices where the distracted thoughts of the mind are gathered together and directed inwards towards an object of concentration through continual voluntary attention. In the practice of concentration, the mind is focused on a single object. This object can either be internal, like the breath or a mantra, or external such as a candle or yantra. Generally, one attempts to allow no other thoughts to arise. Neutral and nonjudgmental observation of the content and experiences of the mind should accompany the process of meditation. It is important to avoid being attached to the contents of the mind during meditation, because the desire to attain something or to have certain types of experiences distracts the mind from its focus and will interfere with continued concentration. This can lead to disturbance of the calmness and contentment that normally characterize a steady mind.

Dhyana

What is Meditation?

Systematic approaches to meditation in the Eastern traditions began in India. The Sanskrit word for meditation is *dhyana.* The practices later spread through Tibet to China and the word became "chan." The word was further transformed in Japan to "zen."9 Throughout the last one hundred years, spiritual teachers from Asia came to the West to share their knowledge of meditation techniques with those students who were eager and prepared.

Meditation is sustained and uninterrupted concentration that leads to a highly focused mind. Concentration precedes meditation to make the mind steady. When prolonged concentration leads to the continuous flow of the mind towards one object, this becomes meditation.

Meditation has three key components: the person who is meditating, the technique of meditation and the object of concentration during meditation. As focus on the object of concentration becomes steady and automatic, awareness of the technique diminishes until finally one ceases to be conscious of it at all. Next, awareness of the meditator's individual self dissipates as the mind identifies completely with the object of concentration. Ultimately, the object of concentration itself disappears as the mind becomes completely permeated with the object by constant association with it. After all three components have disappeared, one experiences a state of expanded consciousness.10

While the stated goal of meditation, to attain an enlightened state of consciousness, seems difficult to achieve, it is actually always close at hand. Meditation philosophy teaches us that human beings are special beings, full of light and constantly and intimately connected to the underlying forces of the universe. However, people individuate and separate as they grow, losing their sense of wholeness. The underlying philosophic premise of meditation is that the individual human is both a separate being with an individual consciousness and also an inseparable part of the greater universal consciousness. The body and mind are vehicles through which the universe reveals itself. All energy and matter that exist in the universe also exist in the individual. Thus, by analyzing and exploring the body and mind, one can understand the entire universe. In this context, the purpose of meditation is to explore the inner self (microcosm), thereby unfolding the basic reality of the universe (macrocosm).

Thus, everyone is already enlightened and complete, but awareness of this is obscured by the endless train of thoughts, desires and emotions. In this sense, the transformation brought about by meditation is a process of peeling away the layers of illusion to awaken to one's true Self. Even striving for enlightenment is itself an illusion.

Misconceptions about Meditation

In meditation there is sustained focus on an object and unbroken mental flow towards the true Self, away from the distractions of the senses. Although concentration techniques are used extensively to prepare for deeper meditation by making the mind steady and one-pointed, concentration is not meditation. Contemplation also is not meditation. The statement, *I will contemplate on that idea,* declares an intention to reflect on a concept with some intensity. But without the systematic regulation of the breath, the focus of the mind and the constant, nonjudgmental awareness of consciousness, it is not meditation. In meditation the mind is centered and focused for an extended period of time on a single point of concentration and is not distracted by random thoughts, emotions or desires. Such a one-pointed mind then pierces through the conscious and the unconscious beyond all thoughts to expand to a higher state of awareness.

Meditation does not create a high such as one might experience when taking a hallucinogenic drug. Those who explored Eastern forms of meditation in the 1960s and '70s often experimented with drugs but quickly found out there was no similarity between drug-altered states of consciousness and expanded consciousness associated with the meditative experience. In actuality, mind-altering drugs inhibit a person's ability to concentrate, making deep meditation more difficult.

The goal of meditation is not to achieve altered states, to see colors or to have unusual auditory or visual experiences. While extrasensory experiences may occur, nonattachment to these events is encouraged. It is best to simply observe these inner phenomena and to let the images go, gently returning to the focus of concentration.

While the ultimate goal of meditation is not to experience altered states of consciousness, there are some experiences that result from meditation that are life transforming. Barriers between the senses are blurred and people sometimes describe being able to "see" sounds and fragrances or to "hear" colors. Extrasensory perception, including clairvoyance and telepathy, can also be an outcome of intense concentration practices. Advanced teachers of meditation always warn their students to view these phenomena with simple curiosity, neutrality and dispassion and never to use these abilities to impress, manipulate or harm another person.

Meditation does not require withdrawal from the world but rather from dependence on objects and people as sources of gratification. One comes to recognize that all human beings are part of the same underlying universal consciousness and they all share similar feelings, experiences and qualities. Other people are seen as fellow travelers on similar life paths.

Meditation is not a religion, although religion and belief in a higher force can inspire a person to pursue the path of meditation. Meditation can also enhance one's understanding of religion. All the great religious traditions practice some form of meditation, though this may not be commonly known or frequently taught.

Similarly, meditation is not prayer, but certain prayers can be used as a focus of concentration. Prayers are tools to change one's attitudes or to inspire higher spiritual ideals. Meditation philosophy teaches that true prayer should not be an appeal to receive something or to become happier. Sincere prayer focuses on self-surrender and offering oneself to others, to a higher principle or to God. Prayer helps a person to be less self-centered and can lead to increased humility and feelings of forgiveness. All these attributes and experiences of prayer can enhance the meditative process.11

Benefits of Meditation

As the power of concentration develops through the practice of meditation, one's physical and mental abilities may also increase. It is important not to use these abilities for selfish purposes because this would interfere with the development of compassion and humility. Self-indulgence and the need for self-gratification limit most persons to the narrow confines of the individual mind and inhibit the experience of expanded states of awareness.

Self-acceptance and learning to be less judgmental become possible through a regular practice of meditation. Sitting quietly in meditation, one becomes aware of breathing irregularities, unpleasant emotions, physical pain or a myriad of fears, such as fear of death, disease, poverty or injustice. Through meditation one learns to cultivate an accepting attitude towards each of these negative feelings and experiences. As meditation progresses, one learns to let go of the pain and sorrows of past losses and betrayals. With the development of a tolerant attitude towards one's fears and unease, one realizes that all humans have similar anxieties and apprehension. Seen in this light, compassion is an intense and sincere feeling that rises spontaneously in the heart to help relieve the pain of others. In this way one learns to direct loving kindness even to people who are disliked or who have been hurtful.

While practicing meditation one learns to slow the rapid movement of thoughts through the conscious mind. In this way meditation can train the scattered and disorganized mind to become more focused and creative. Thus, the mind becomes more like the concentrated and powerful light coming from a laser beam and less like the scattered light of an ordinary light bulb.

With a regular practice of meditation each moment is experienced more fully with heightened awareness and greater clarity. For example, when viewing a beautiful sunset, ordinarily the mind may be distracted by thoughts of work, feelings of hunger or worries of being late for some future obligation. As a result, one's attention does not stay completely focused on the scene of the setting sun, and so the total experience of the scents in the air, the sound of birds singing and the palette of colors in the sky is diminished. Alternatively, a proficient practitioner of meditation can use the skill of concentration to turn off mental interference and concentrate totally on the whole sensory experience.

By practicing meditation, one learns to stay in the present, to let go of troublesome memories and to release anxiety about the future. Meditation helps to experience the fullness of the moment and realize its full potentiality. In the philosophy of Zen Buddhism, this is called beginner's mind. Each moment becomes a new and life-enhancing experience and each experience of sitting to meditate becomes fresh and alive.12 Meditation is not about acquiring new experiences or getting to any different place, but rather, it involves acceptance of what one already has and being where one already is. In other words, it involves learning to be here now.

Meditation helps to explore the four levels of consciousness: waking, dreaming, deep sleep and sleepless sleep (turiya). Turiya is a fully conscious state similar to deep sleep except one remains totally awake and aware. Every human has the potential to access this peaceful state of consciousness, but most individuals are too distracted and preoccupied by their thoughts and desires. Turbulence of the mind is based upon the types of desires one has, especially when one wants more than what is necessary for healthy and comfortable living. Through the practice of meditation, one can become truly content when free from desires. Likewise, one realizes the true source of happiness does not reside in attained objects and goals but in a state of mind that is independent of these objects.

Meditation is helpful both during life as well as in the process of preparing for death, the state of consciousness between death and the next birth and in preparation for future incarnations. Those who believe in reincarnation maintain that positive thoughts and memories at the time of death will influence their rebirth so they can continue with the process of spiritual growth. Also, meditation practices that focus on the chakras allow the dying person to experience the phenomenon of the dissolution of the five elements (space, air, fire, water, earth) that occurs during the dying process. This can lead to a state of emptiness, openness and a conscious rebirth, which is considered by yogis to be an extremely advanced state of consciousness.

Meditation and the Mind

Meditation has positive effects on each of the components of the mind. For example, meditation helps to develop the higher qualities of buddhi such as intuition, wisdom and the ability to reason carefully. In this way, meditation facilitates clearer decision-making by buddhi and enhances the ability to disregard distracting impulses that normally flow through manas. Thus, decisions are made quickly and effortlessly.

In addition, meditation has important effects on ahamkara by helping the practitioner develop a strong inner center, confidence and a healthy sense of oneself. At the same time, during meditation one learns not to be restricted by or overly identified with the sense of self that separates each individual from other persons and from the world. In effect, meditation teaches the practitioner to expand the sense of individual self to experience a more unified universal consciousness.

Meditation has the effect of slowing sensory impressions and information from the external world that can inundate and overwhelm manas. It is not advisable to try to force the thoughts to stop. Thoughts (vrittis) should be allowed to gently rise in the mind and then to pass out effortlessly. Ordinarily, a thought wave arises in the mind, lasts for a few moments and is quickly replaced by another thought. During meditation, a succession of identical thought waves is consciously raised in the mind with such rapidity that no new thought wave can take its place. Perfect continuity of concentration is the ultimate result, where all thoughts become fused into one. As the process of letting go and refocusing become easier, meditation deepens naturally. With persistent practice, the mind gradually becomes identified with the object of concentration. This allows the individual to experience deeper and more refined states of consciousness.

In meditation, thought waves are quieted, allowing the mind to rest and become more focused so that the memories and unconscious impressions from chitta can rise to the surface of the conscious mind where one can observe their nature and content. After some time, one will be able to observe the activities of the mind without being distracted or affected by any thoughts or emotions that arise.

Forms of Meditation

Sitting Meditation

This is the most widely practiced form of meditation. Besides the yogic system of sitting meditation, there are other Eastern meditation systems that use the seated position during meditation. Tibetan Buddhists have several different techniques of meditation including some brief practices to quickly center the mind and others that are more complex. One interesting technique involves instructing students to listen quietly both to the sounds around them and to the space between the sounds in order to become aware of the void. The void implies having an empty mind, free of distracting thoughts and desires. Only when the mind is empty, can a person be completely filled with higher forms of knowledge. In Zazen, the sitting form of meditation in Zen Buddhism, one counts the breath as a focus of concentration. To focus on the breath is a way to create "space" in which one can learn more about the mind. In Jewish sitting meditation one often concentrates on the four Hebrew letters *Yod-Heh-Vov-Heh* that mean "God." Other Judaic meditation practices include concentrating on the *Shema* prayer, on *Shalom,* a mantra-like word, or on the sefirot of the tree of life, a concept with similarities to the chakra system.

The sitting meditation practices presented in this book represent an integrated approach based on the great Indian philosophies of Tantra, Samkhya and Vedanta. These philosophies also provide the theoretical and practical foundation of chakras, mantras and yantras, the objects of concentration used in this form of meditation.

Tantra is a philosophy that emphasizes personal experimentation and specific meditative practices. Tantric meditation focuses on the subtle energy centers (chakras) and the nadis through which energy is channeled to the highest centers of consciousness. It describes how pure consciousness has manifested into individual beings.

Samkhya is accepted by those on the raja yoga path as an important philosophical system. Raja yoga represents a powerful and systematic path for uniting individual with universal consciousness by incorporating specific physical exercises (hatha yoga postures), breathing techniques (pranayama) and concentration and meditation practices.

Vedanta incorporates sitting forms of meditation with philosophy and describes the theoretical foundation of the mind and how it is affected by meditation as well as the mind's relationship to expanded states of consciousness.

Moving Forms of Meditation (including tai chi)

These include tai chi as well as Sufi dancing, which uses turning and spinning movements to create an ecstatic state of consciousness. My first encounter with tai chi was in the early '70s in San Francisco's Golden Gate Park. I remember being moved by its slow, rhythmic, dance-like motion and was captivated by its beauty. I knew instantly that I had to study this art form. Much to my delight, I soon discovered that hidden within tai chi were both a powerful martial art form and the practice of meditation through movement. When I returned to Ann Arbor, my study of tai chi (Yang style) was initiated with a local, colorful and soft-spoken Volvo mechanic, Bob Thorson, and his teacher, Phil Ho. The opportunity to learn this ancient practice was very exciting to me.

I had been studying tai chi for several years before I moved to the Himalayan Institute. Because I had heard that Swami Rama had great expertise in martial arts, I was hopeful that he would teach me his form. When I asked him about it, he said I would be very busy studying yogic meditation, pranayama and homeopathy as well as teaching classes and raising a family. But he said that perhaps later on he could work with me on the more advanced form of his martial arts. While this never happened, I continued to practice the form I had learned in Ann Arbor during medical school. He always encouraged me to continue my practice and smiled when he saw me doing tai chi on the Himalayan Institute grounds.

In the late '90s, back in Ann Arbor, I decided to expand my study and learn other forms of Chinese martial arts. I had heard that Richard Miller was very skilled in martial art forms and, coincidentally, I happened to see him practicing with his group in a park in my neighborhood. I was very impressed, and soon my daughter Ari and I began to study tai chi with him in the Chen style, which is the original and oldest form of tai chi. I have also studied *bagua zhang*, another Chinese internal martial art, which is fast, crisp, very strengthening and powerful.

My good friend and lawyer, Marty Kriegel, and I have had many discussions about the interface between tai chi, qi gong and yoga. Several years ago, Marty asked me if I'd like to learn a short form of Yang tai chi that he had learned in Hong Kong. In the summer of 2009, I studied and practiced this short form with Marty. It is the form the Chinese government had developed so that the Chinese people would have an exercise option that was shorter and less complex than the longer traditional Yang form.

The philosophy of tai chi is to avoid using violence in response to a violent opposing force. Injury is a natural consequence of meeting hard force with hard force. To avoid this, students are instructed not to resist an incoming force but instead to meet it with softness, follow its motion and remain in physical contact until the force of attack exhausts itself or can be safely redirected. Done correctly, the balancing of soft and hard forces brings about a balance of yin and yang principles in the combat aspect of tai chi. This is one of the primary goals of training. This principle is also a metaphor for the mind and how one can best deal with emotional and psychological resistance. Spiritual growth often involves gently transforming the many obstacles one faces on the path to liberation. In the famous Taoist classic text, the Tao Te Ching, it is stated that, "The soft and the pliable will defeat the hard and strong."13

There are many physical, mental and spiritual benefits of tai chi, but some people say the main intention is to still the mind through movement. During the practice of tai chi, one can attempt to create a state of emptiness that promotes a state of unattached centeredness. Body, breath and mind are fused into an integrated whole. One learns to use the breath to focus power, to heal oneself and to raise consciousness. This is why some view tai chi as meditation in movement.

Tai chi is very powerful, especially when the graceful and spiraling movements are sped up and used to fight. But this type of battle is a metaphor for the process used to master and conquer inner psychological and emotional battles. Tai chi teaches to adapt and change effortlessly, which helps the person deal with the natural flux of the universe and life's vicissitudes. It teaches to be hard or soft and active or receptive as things unfold. It also teaches to be egoless and devoid of expectation and at the same time to be fully aware of the moment and the current event as it unfolds, similar to the goal of meditation.

In addition, there are important physical benefits from twisting the spine and stimulating connections in the nervous system. Certain types of tai chi stretch and tone muscles, massage the internal organs, move spinal fluid along the spinal column and promote fluid exchange between cells. Practitioners also use the dance-like movements in tai chi for artistic and creative expression.

There have been many studies on the positive health effects of tai chi. One such meta-analysis, *"Health benefits of tai chi: What is the evidence?"* found excellent evidence that tai chi helped improve balance and prevent falls in the elderly, lessened the pain of osteoarthritis of the hands, hips and knees, improved mobility and balance in people with Parkinson's disease, decreased the shortness of breath due to emphysema (COPD) and improved cognitive function. There was also good evidence that tai chi was helpful with depression, cardiac and stroke rehabilitation and increased functional capacity after heart attack and dementia. There was also fair evidence that tai chi improved the quality of life for patients with cancer, fibromyalgia, hypertension and osteoporosis. Tai chi improves aerobic capacity, especially in sedentary people, increases strength conditioning and improves flexibility, thus improving the quality of life. Tai chi was also found to be correlated with better sleep, an overall sense of well-being and improved quality of life in hemodialysis patients.14

A recent report summarizing three studies that was published in *The Pain and Medicine News* found that tai chi was more effective than standard exercise for nonpharmacologic management of the pains of fibromyalgia. A longer duration of practice and training was more beneficial than a shorter duration. In this study comparing the two groups, people expressed a strong preference for the multidisciplinary approach of tai chi, which includes physical, mental, mindfulness, balance and social support.15

Standing and Walking Forms of Meditation

These practices include a tai chi posture, the horse stance, where one stands with legs apart and arms extended out with elbows and knees slightly bent. This can be used to focus the body, breath and mind. If one empties the mind and attends to gentle smooth breathing, it can become a meditation practice. I practice this, especially at the beginning of doing the entire tai chi form.

Another classic meditation is the yogic and Buddhist practice of walking slowly, taking each step with total awareness of the moment. Coordinating one's breath with taking steps is a very nice practice, especially as the sun is rising. One can also walk slowly in a garden labyrinth with breath awareness. In Hassidic mystical Jewish meditation practices, congregations often sway from side to side as they recite prayers. In Pentecostal Christian churches, the dancing and clapping during religious services also has a meditative effect.

Chanting Forms of Meditation (including kirtan)

Chanting and singing forms of meditation focus on sound. For instance, Christian meditation uses prayer along with music, such as Gregorian chanting, as a focus of concentration. Native Americans use drums, singing and dancing as a form of meditation.

Kirtan is yogic chanting; yoga means union and kirtan chanting enables a sense of unity. Born from one of the oldest sacred sound traditions of the world, kirtan or call-and-response chanting comes from India. Chaitanya Mahaprabu (1486-1533) began spreading congregational call-and-response chanting throughout India and started the sankirtana movement that continues worldwide today. He brought chanting to the streets, to the temples, to the common person and to communities. Kirtan involves *satsang*, a Sanskrit term meaning "community." Kirtan is part mantra and nada yoga (the yoga of vibratory frequency and sound) and part bhakti yoga (the yoga of devotion of the heart).

From a Tantric yoga perspective, as mantras are chanted, energy from the sound current creates a channel of healing energy, which travels through the spinal cord to stimulate the chakras, the energy centers of the body. In nada yoga, mantras are chanted or repeated mentally and practiced in a relaxed state of mind. Thus, through the practice of nada yoga, one can enhance efficient cellular communication, stimulate the immune system, improve physical health and calm the mind.

Kirtan uses a combination of sound, vibration, melody, harmony and Sanskrit mantras to lead one into meditation, an expanded state of consciousness and state of unity and inner connection with oneself and the community. Chanting can be moving and exhilarating, and at the same time, quieting and meditative. All sound comes from a divine source and, because kirtan is sung with devotion, its vibrations have a universal impact. Chanting is a form of spiritual self-expression and can help a person experience mental calmness and a sense of unity with all creation and consciousness. Its primal sounds help connect the physical body to the subtle qualities of the mind.

As I look back, my journey into the ancient world of yogic chanting actually began a bit awkwardly. As a young physician drawn towards Eastern thought and spiritual practices and alternative methods of healing, I felt embarrassed about chanting. Adding to my self-consciousness, was the then common sight of orange-robed and shaven-headed Hare Krishna devotees chanting loudly, dancing and clanging their cymbals on the streets and in airports. Did I want to be like them? At the same time, however, I enjoyed the Beatles' and particularly George Harrison's foray into Indian music. And I was fascinated by the wonderful tones and rhythms of the Indian drum, the tabla.

When I lived at the Himalayan Institute, we would chant late at night and sometimes Swami Rama would lead us in kirtan. While I didn't know it at the time, kirtan would become a major meditation practice for me many years later. Even though I enjoyed the kirtan with Swami Rama, I never really connected to it deeply and didn't feel comfortable singing in a group. Even in the following years the only times I sang, often Jewish melodies, was when I was putting my two youngest children, Ethan and Ari, to bed.

It wasn't until years later that I realized that what was missing in my spiritual practice was how to relate to the divine and to others and the world around me with greater love and compassion. Bhakti yoga, the path of the heart, was a path I had not really developed well in my early years of the study and practice of yoga and meditation. When I rediscovered kirtan, I found that singing and chanting divine names with people in a group created a state of joy and love that began to nurture and heal my heart. Also, my separation and subsequent divorce were a very difficult time for me. Kirtan helped me get in touch with the loss and to face the world with gratitude and love. I learned how to meditate on my heart and relate to the world of inner meditation in a new and powerful way.

In kirtan, names of Hindu deities are chanted. As a Jewish person who was taught that there is one God, I initially felt uncomfortable about chanting multiple names of the divine. What I came to understand is that the deities represent different aspects

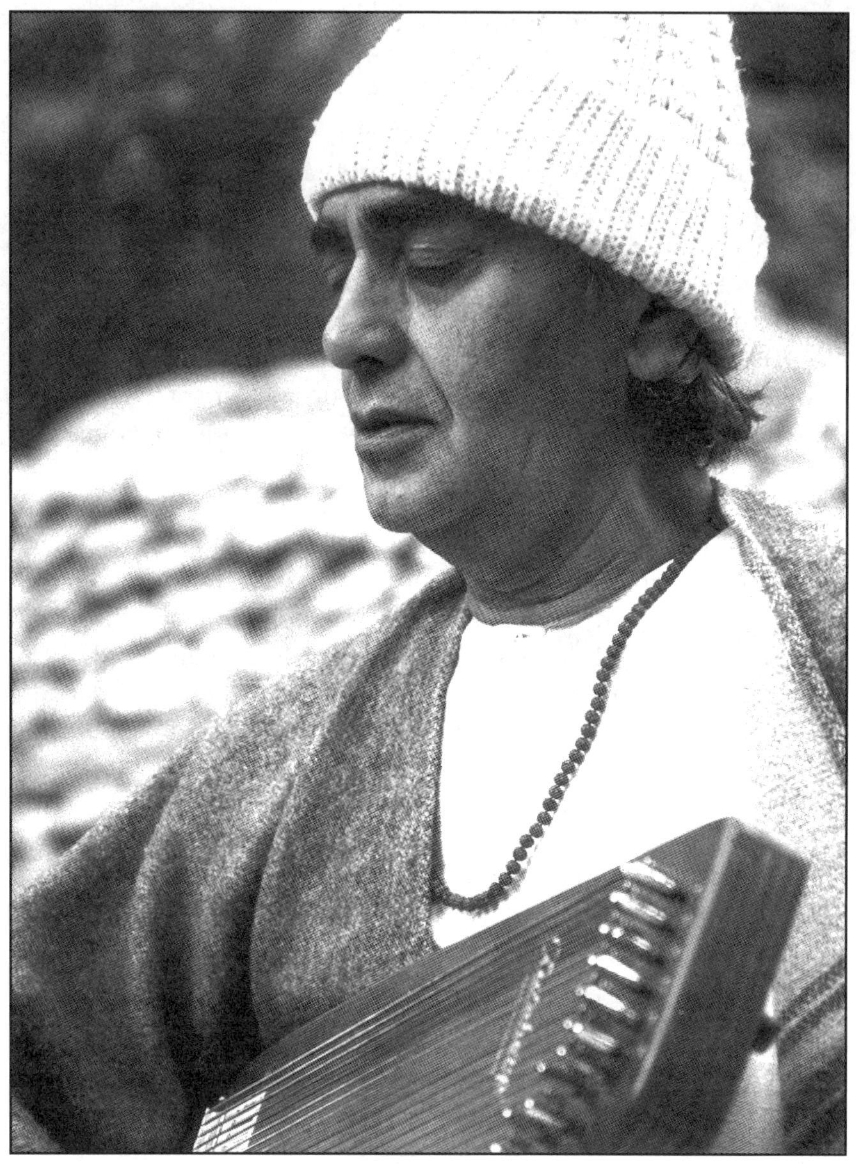

Swami Rama chanting

of divine consciousness that pervade our inner psyche and nature. The deities endow universal energies and forces with voices, faces and personalities that touch us personally. Deities also represent the various aspects of Brahman: existence, consciousness and bliss. In essence, deities are symbolic and poetic anthropomorphic representations of all sentient beings. They mirror the diverse attributes and functions of both the seen and unseen universe. They have different personalities, powers and weaknesses that reflect similar qualities in human beings. On a higher level, kirtan enables the unfoldment of deity energies as symbolic forces of universal consciousness.

In 2005, my friend Glenn Burdick and I decided to share our passion for meditation, mantra and chanting with the local community. This led to the creation of Ann Arbor Kirtan. Our vision was to create an opportunity for people who love chanting to come together in a setting that was not affiliated with any religious group. Ann Arbor Kirtan combines Indian and Western instruments and melodies, including guitar, dulcimer, cello, tambura, harmonium, flute, cymbals, tabla, khol drum and an assortment of other percussion instruments. Kirtan is a participatory and cross-cultural musical experience in which the participants are equally as important as the chant leaders and musicians.

When I first began to meditate, I felt quite at ease repeating Sanskrit mantras quietly during my practice and I soon began to have powerful and life-transforming inner experiences, hearing beautiful inner sounds during my meditation practice. Later on, teaching meditation and participating in kirtan became wonderful vehicles to share these mantric sounds with others. While I still dress in Western garb, now I enjoy chanting many of the same Hare Krishna chants I heard on the streets many years ago.

Goals of Meditation

There are several specific goals of meditation. The first is to liberate the mind from disturbing and distracting emotions, thoughts and desires. In other words, the mind is transformed from a state of unrest and disharmony to a state of calmness and equilibrium. Another important goal of meditation is to bring the unconscious mind into conscious awareness in order to gain greater control over thought processes and emotions. However, the ultimate goal is to attain expanded states of consciousness in which not only is there increased awareness of previously unconscious thoughts and feelings, but also awareness of more subtle and universal principles. In this state, one experiences great joy and inner peace.

Meditation and the Kundalini

The object of meditation in the Tantra and yoga traditions is to awaken, move and then unite the feminine individual kundalini (Shakti) with the masculine kundalini energy (Shiva) that permeates the larger cosmos. Shakti is located within the first chakra, while Shiva is within the seventh chakra. As the word yoga means "union," kundalini yoga involves using practices that include meditation and advanced breathing and pranayama exercises that instigate the movement of kundalini upwards through the chakras to unite with the pure consciousness of the crown chakra.

The word *kundalini* is derived from the Sanskrit word *kundala*, which means "coiled." It is also described as a "bowl of fire." Kundalini is the subtlest form of prana and is often called the primal energy of consciousness. The latent energy of kundalini is not only present in each human being but also in every particle, atom and molecule in the universe. Within each human, kundalini is associated with both active (kinetic) and latent (potential) energy. The active form of kundalini maintains the mental and physical functioning of the organism. There is also a vast amount of surplus energy not utilized by the mind or body and this is described as being stored as potential energy within the first chakra. In most individuals the kundalini lies dormant throughout their lifetimes and they are unaware of its existence. In meditation the kundalini can be visualized as a resting or sleeping serpent that is coiled up, whose inner heat and power are stored as potential energy. Through meditation and other yogic practices, the kundalini moves up the chakras in its journey to the higher centers of consciousness. 16, 17

Three Granthis

There are three knots, called *granthis,* where energy in the chakras tends to stagnate or get blocked. These represent obstacles in the path of kundalini in its inexorable movement upwards through the energy centers. These granthis are areas in the pranic body where illusion *(maya),* selfishness *(mala),* mental restlessness *(vikshepa),* attachment *(moha),* ignorance *(avidya)* and desire *(kama)* are particularly strong. These knots need to be unblocked and transcended to free kundalini on its ascension through the chakras. Asanas, kriyas, pranayama, meditation, nutrition, homeopathic remedies and herbal medicines can all be helpful to work through the granthis.

The first block is called *Brahma granthi* and is associated with the first chakra. It represents over attachment to the pleasures and pains of the physical world. Selfishness and the desire for excessive material possessions are seen when there is stagnation here. With respect to the gunas, the first granthi is dominated by tamas and its characteristic sloth, laziness, resistance and general emotional negativity.

The second granthi is called *Vishnu granthi* and is associated with the fourth chakra. Here there are blockages that lead a person to become overly emotional and excessively attached to ideas and people. The guna most closely connected to Vishnu granthi is rajas, which causes one to become assertive and ambitious at the expense of interpersonal relationships.

The third granthi is called *Rudra granthi* and is associated with the sixth chakra. Here the bondage that manifests in this knot is attachment to one's personal power and the concept of oneself as an individual being.

Three Bandhas

There are specific hatha yoga and breathing techniques that help stimulate kundalini from its latent state. The three physical locks (bandhas) force prana to move in opposite directions. This creates tension as well as internal heat, which arouses kundalini from her quiet slumber.

Jalandhara bandha (the chin lock) is practiced by swallowing first and then placing the chin onto the chest. This forces the normally upward moving prana to move downwards.

Mula bandha (the anal lock) involves contracting the perineum and anal muscles and holding them in this position. This forces the normally downward moving apana to move upwards.

Uddiyana bandha (the abdominal lock) is practiced by first exhaling and then holding the breath on exhalation. Drawing the abdominal muscles upwards towards the spine follows this retention of breath. As the forces of prana and apana merge, the abdominal lock is used to increase the compression of the energies and activate the energies of the third chakra that can be used in more advanced breathing exercises.

A more intense variation of uddiyana bandha is *agni sara*, which means "fanning the fire." Swami Rama repeatedly emphasized the importance of the practice of agni sara and said it should be done even if no other exercise was possible on any particular day. This exercise involves the lower abdomen and pelvis. To do the practice of agni sara, one stands with the feet about six inches apart while resting the weight of the body through the arms on the knees, keeping the back straight and relaxed. After exhaling, the lower abdominal muscles are contracted and pulled in and upwards. This is immediately followed by inhalation along with a gentle release of the abdominal muscles to allow the lower abdomen to return to its normal position. Pulling the abdomen in and upwards helps to expel stagnant air CO_2 from the lungs, and when the abdomen is allowed to move back out on inhalation, oxygen automatically refills the lungs. Work at your capacity and start with ten to fifteen repetitions, then gradually increase to 100 to 150 times to achieve the most benefits. Agni sara should not be done by women who are pregnant or menstruating.

Pranayama and Kundalini

Meditation is most easily practiced when prana is flowing through sushumna. This leads to a relaxed body and a calm and focused mind. There are several breathing techniques that facilitate the entry of prana into sushumna. For example, the practice of *nadi shodanam* (alternate nostril breathing) involves mentally shifting the breath from one nostril to the other with the goal of stimulating the ida and pingala nadis, so that the physical and mental functions associated with each become regulated and balanced. This breathing technique also helps to equalize the flow of breath and prana so that prana will begin to travel through sushumna. During the process of intense concentration and deep meditation energy is redirected from ida and pingala into sushumna because the pathway through the central nadi to the crown chakra is more direct and straightforward. When this occurs, the kundalini that is stored in the first chakra is activated to move upwards through sushumna.

Kumbhaka is a technique of holding the breath either at the end of exhalation or the end of inhalation. When breath holding is practiced at the same time as the three locks, this has the effect of further intensifying the compression. This is especially true when holding the breath at the end of exhalation. The union of the pranic forces created by applying the locks along with breath retention is analogous to a hollow tube that has a piston working at both ends. This prevents air from escaping and creates internal heat, which activates the kundalini to rise up into sushumna on its journey to the higher chakras.

Surya bheda kumbhaka is an advanced pranayama technique that can also help activate kundalini. This breathing technique involves inhaling through the right nostril and at the end of inhalation, applying the chin lock and holding the breath. Before the breath retention becomes uncomfortable, the abdominal and anal locks are also applied for a few seconds. Then the breath is exhaled slowly through the left nostril. Following complete exhalation, inhalation begins, and the process is repeated three times. This process should not be forced, the breath should not be uncomfortable and the number of repetitions can gradually be increased. This is a complex technique and should only be done under the guidance of a teacher and after having developed a regular meditation practice in which the mind is stable and content.

Signs of Kundalini Awakening

During meditation there are various physical and mental changes that may be associated with activation of kundalini. True signs are always accompanied by a sense of joy, integration and increased awareness. Some of these signs are automatic movements of the body into yoga postures and spontaneous occurrences of advanced breathing exercises with breath retention and the application of locks. Breathing may stop without any willful effort, neither being in inhalation nor in exhalation. Electrical currents may be felt traveling up the spine. Often the spontaneous recitation of mantras or other unusual sounds occurs. The eyes may roll upwards, or the tongue may curl back towards the throat. Sounds such as bells, drums or waterfalls may be heard, especially in the right ear. Beautiful and inspiring images may appear in the mind.

As the energy rises through the chakras, each center becomes activated, and the physical, mental and spiritual qualities of each chakra are experienced. For example, when the first chakra is activated, one feels more grounded and secure. An energized second chakra is associated with healthy sexual identity and expression, the third chakra with a strong sense of self and ego, the fourth with the ability to love and feel compassion, the fifth with the qualities of communication and creativity and the sixth with intuition and insight. When the seventh and highest chakra is pierced and energized, one experiences the highest state of consciousness associated with feelings of union, pure joy, freedom and inner peace. In deep meditation, the lotus petals associated with the different chakras are sometimes seen to be hanging downwards, and as the energy rises and activates a chakra, the petals turn upwards. There may be deep insight into profound or obscure philosophies or concepts or momentary feelings that the mind and body are dissolving into infinity. During and after these experiences there is no fear and a perpetual sense of awe, peace and feelings of unity remains.

On the other hand, there may be no obvious or extraordinary experiences at all when the kundalini energy becomes activated. Instead, some people experience sudden surges of mental or physical energy, increased enthusiasm, a burst of creativity, peak experiences or a wonderful sense of well-being. These subtler experiences are accompanied by a slow and gradual evolution of growing wisdom, courage and patience, and an enhanced ability to be intimate and have compassion for others. The actual experience of kundalini activity depends on one's personality and inner nature. The awakening of kundalini is determined by one's samskaras from previous lifetimes along with one's present karma, deeds and desires.

Shaktipat is the transfer of energy to the student by a teacher who is advanced in meditation and has learned to concentrate his or her mind and will. Shaktipat acts as a catalyst to rouse the kundalini from its dormant state. Only a teacher with a pure heart and pure intentions can impart the true experience of shaktipat, and only a sincere and prepared student can receive it.

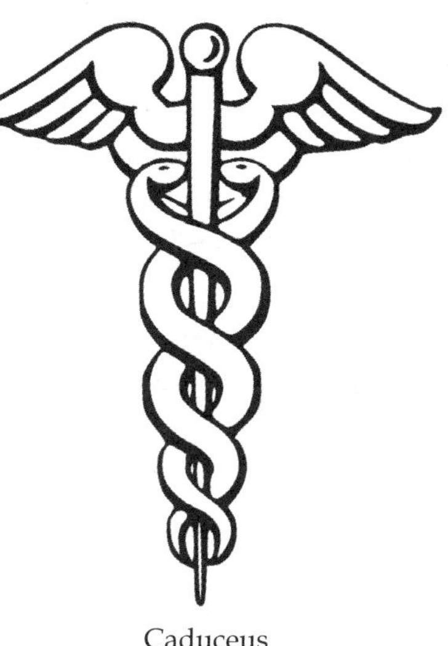

Caduceus

There is an interesting simi-larity between the concept of kundalini, the nadis, and the chakras and the symbol often used for the practice of medicine. This symbol is called the caduceus and has come from Greek mythology. It is pictured as two serpents wrapped and intertwined around a central staff, intersecting at several points as they travel upwards. At the top of the staff are two wings. This symbol looks almost identical to the image of the chakras and nadis described in this book. The staff represents sushumna within the spinal cord, the snakes represent ida and pingala as they crisscross upwards, the points of intersection represent the chakras, and the wings appear like the two lotus petals of the sixth chakra. The whole picture represents the path of the kundalini as it rises upwards towards the highest stage of consciousness. Since the caduceus represents the symbol for health and healing, its similarity to the traditional imagery associated with meditation reflects the ancient awareness that the ultimate form of health is the spiritual unfolding of consciousness.18

The Shekinah

While yoga describes the most latent form of energy within the subtle body as kundalini shakti, Jewish mysticism names this feminine force the *Shekinah,* or the Divine Presence. Like kundalini's journey upwards from the first chakra to the crown chakra through the middle nadi, the sushumna, the Shekinah rises up from the lower sefirot to the higher and spiritual sefirot by passing through the middle channel called *rachamin* (compassion).

In yoga, energy and consciousness also rise through two of the main nadis, pingala (left, active male principle) and ida (left, passive female principle). The other two pathways in the kabbalistic system are called *chesed* (right, quality of mercy) and *din* (left, quality of judgment). Metaphorically, chesed represents thoughts and decision-making that is discriminating and life affirming, while din (judgment energy) represents actions and thoughts that are neutral objective forces. When these forces are balanced, then rachamin (compassion) manifests, which is described as consciousness traveling upwards through the sefirot within the central channel.

With life's many decisions, a healthy balance between objective and subjective, as represented by chesed and din, leads to positive growth and outcomes. For example, the simple act of stealing to survive in war or famine versus stealing because one covets another person's possessions can both be judged (din) simply as being a crime subject to the same punishment. But when mercy (chesed) is added to the equation, one would understand the unique differences and not punish the former, or at least be much more lenient. In this case, compassion is shown (rachamin). From this example it is apparent that psychological concerns and decision-making are inherent in the different concept of the energy channels in Jewish thought.19

The Chinese Taoist Idea of Chi

There is a close association between tai chi and the microcosmic orbit meditation practice, as they both are part of the Taoist spiritual system. Both the physical movements of tai chi and the concentration practices of the microcosmic orbit move energy and clear energy blockages from the circulation of chi in the subtle body. Specifically, the chi is moved through the two major channels, the governing spinal channel, which goes up the back part of the body and the conception channel, which travels down the front part of the body with special focus on the major dantian. As people become more deeply engaged with Taoist practices, they will do both tai chi and meditation on the microcosmic orbit as part of their spiritual practice. This is analogous to the way in which many hatha yoga practitioners do a yoga-based meditation to move energy through the chakras. Breathing practices are also part of all these complementary systems.

In yoga, the kundalini moves through the chakras upwards in a vertical way. Although there is some movement helically through the ida and pingala nadis as the energy winds through and around the individual chakras, the idea is to consciously move the energy through the central sushumna in its ascent towards higher chakras and more evolved states of awareness. On the other hand, the energy practice in the microcosmic system is more circular in its movement through the dantian towards the higher states of consciousness. This is in line with the Chinese spiritually oriented physical practices like tai chi and qi gong, which encourage rounded, circular and spiral movements.

In order to prepare for the microcosmic orbit of meditation through the dantian, the individual must get ready for increased energy needs as these meditation practices put a considerable strain on the nervous system of the physical body as well as on the subtler energy body. These practices include tai chi, qi gong and Taoist yoga techniques. Like the pranayama techniques in yoga, Chinese breathing practices are a necessity in this energy journey. Deep and full abdominal breathing is very important. As in yoga, where the third chakra represents the main energy storehouse, in the microcosmic orbit the center of the abdomen is considered the power center. In the microcosmic orbit configuration, this dantian is called *shen guan.* When using tai chi or its cousin bagua for fighting, the power comes from this energy center. During microcosmic meditation practices, the shen guan dantian stores energy as well as creates heat and energy, which helps propel the energy through the circular microcosmic orbit. This orbit is called the "golden stove."

The practices of meditating on the microcosmic orbit involve the conscious movement of chi towards higher dantian in the individual's journey to more expanded consciousness and enlightenment, which is called "following the essence of the Tao" in Chinese philosophy. This, as mentioned earlier, is a bit different from yogic kundalini movement. The essence of chi is called *jing,* which is similar to the idea of kundalini in yoga. Jing is encouraged through meditation and other spiritual practices to flow upwards along the major meridians (nadis in yoga) through the dantian (chakras in yoga). The major upward flowing meridian is called the governor vessel. The movement of subtle energy up through the governor vessel through the spinal column is coordinated with the breath through the act of inhalation and begins in the lowest dantian, *hue yin,* and is further energized in the *ming men,* located in the back.

Through exhalation, the energy is moved back down to the base of the spine, this time through the middle organs of the body and frontal dantian. The downward directed great meridian that directs this flow of jing, called the conception vessel, now completes one cycle of the microcosmic orbit meditation. The continual practice of raising and lowering jing through the nine dantian purifies the jing and transforms this subtle chi into spiritual essence. Some practitioners of the microcosmic orbit, instead of visualizing the dantian and the movement of jing in the spine and inner organs, visualize the movement up the back, experiencing the governor vessel on the surface of the skin. The downward movement through the conception vessel is then visualized moving down the front of the body, also on the surface of the body. This makes sense as the chi energy in the microcosmic orbit is the same energy that is stimulated in Chinese acupuncture, which uses needles that are placed on the surface of the body, creating a response even in the deepest organs and within the nervous system.

Three centers that tend to create inhibition or stagnation in this flow are called the three gates, like the three granthis described in the yoga tradition, which are the first, fourth and six chakras. The three gates are *Wei-lu* (tailbone gate), the *Jai Ji* at the heart center in the back of the spine and *Yu Jen* located in the back of the head. Purification practices and continual meditation through the microcosmic orbit will act to keep these dantian open. As in yoga practices that require guidance from a teacher to help with movement of kundalini through the chakras, the microcosmic orbit meditation should likewise be practiced only under the guidance of very competent practitioners.20

Meditation in Action: Application to Daily Living

Meditation is not simply sitting quietly for twenty to sixty minutes once a day but is also a process of learning to be poised, strong and focused amidst the dramas and vicissitudes of life. In order to have real practical value, meditation should provide direction and inspiration to one's daily life as well as help cultivate a sense of calmness, peace and joy throughout the waking hours. By learning to apply the principles of meditation to daily activity, one can transform the entire day into a meditative experience.

In sitting meditation, one learns to focus the mind, while in meditation in action one applies the ability to concentrate to the various activities and responsibilities of life. Meditation in action involves being constantly mindful and fully present in the moment, whether the actions or circumstances are enjoyable or unpleasant. Because meditation in action involves always returning to the moment, one learns to appreciate the fullness of the now. This can be accomplished by momentarily reflecting on life's most simple activities such as: pausing to think about the wonders of language before reading the newspaper; appreciating how fortunate it is that there is money in the bank before writing a check; smiling about having a car to drive when stuck in a traffic jam; giving thanks for the gift of food before eating; or stopping for a moment to appreciate life and health when sending love to a sick friend.

Meditation as applied to daily living teaches to let go of negative habits and addictions. During meditation the restless mind is calmed. This allows one to see clearly without the distortions of fear and worry. By practicing this attitude during everyday life, one learns how to navigate through difficult times with a sense of clarity and purpose. This improves the ability to quickly assess a situation by seeing the whole picture more clearly and leads to making appropriate and intelligent decisions.

Through meditation in action one learns to see value in all situations and finds meaning in both positive and negative life experiences. For example, one comes to realize that even illness, loss or pain can create opportunities for growth. Life becomes a learning process and one takes responsibility for one's actions in all situations and accepts the consequences. One learns how to use and enjoy the objects of the world, but at the same time does not get attached to them. By practicing meditation in action, one comes to realize that happiness is independent of a big house, a new car or other material possessions. One remains deeply immersed in life, yet remains free from the desire to accumulate more than necessary for healthy living. In this way, one can enjoy the complexities of daily life but avoid getting bound by its many entanglements.

Meditation in action involves enjoying the world with a sense of lightness and humor. As the impermanence and changeability of life become obvious, one recognizes how pointless it is to take oneself too seriously. Because meditation leads to a more concentrated mind, one learns to think more clearly and to act and react in the world with greater skill and more precision. The ability to communicate becomes more honest and direct, often resulting in improved and more trusting interpersonal relationships. As one commits to the meditative path, one practices loving kindness and compassion and becomes devoted and truthful with family and community.

Meditation in action can also involve self-study and introspection, such as reading books and poetry written by inspiring people and keeping a diary or journal. One can also visualize the coming day upon awakening in the morning, or practice retrospection before going to sleep, recollecting the events of the day.

Another way to practice meditation in action is to stay focused on the mantra or breath. This can be done any time of the day and can be especially useful in stressful situations or during periods of anxiety. Breath awareness or mental repetition of a mantra can also be practiced while walking, exercising, driving a car or eating. This helps keep the mind centered, so one can fully enjoy the present, make good decisions and remain calm in the face of life's many challenges.

Samadhi — Absorption

Turiya (samadhi, sleepless sleep) is similar to deep sleep, except one remains totally awake and aware. Samadhi is a state in which one is absorbed with the object of concentration (mantra, yantra or chakra) through intense and prolonged effort. In this state one exists beyond the bondage of time, space and causation. As the focus of concentration deepens, associated sounds and visual images fade. A conscious and calm state ensues, devoid of extraneous thought. As the state of samadhi deepens, all experiences of duality and separation are lost, sense of self dissolves and one experiences union with the underlying forces of the universe. Every human has the potential to access this highly peaceful state of consciousness, but most individuals are too distracted and preoccupied by their thoughts, desires and dreams.

There are several other states of consciousness that one cycles through each day throughout the expansion of a lifetime and after death: waking, hypnogogic (state of awareness between waking and dreaming), dreaming, deep sleep, moment of death, states between death and rebirth (bardo) and moment of rebirth, to name a few. Meditation helps to explore these states of consciousness and can provide the necessary techniques to consciously experience sleepless sleep. As the sincere student of meditation progresses, he or she becomes more aware of the innermost levels of consciousness and realizes that the subtlest domains are truly the very basis of life itself. Only through the consistent practice of meditation over a long period of time can one reach this level of consciousness. In the meditative process, as consciousness is directed more and more inwards, the narrow confining ego is cast off, and one pierces through the final sheath to merge with the Self, which is nonchanging and eternal. Besides samadhi, this state has many names such as: enlightenment, illumination, atonement, God, Christ consciousness, Self-realization, nirvana or the Tao.

While it is impossible to adequately verbalize such an experiential state, it has been described as a state of ultimate wisdom and knowledge, waves of tranquility, boundless and transporting joy and overwhelming feelings of bliss. This enlightened state of consciousness leads to a deeper understanding of spiritual truths, and one experiences complete knowledge, absolute peace, indescribable joy and ultimate bliss and love. A person who has reached the state of samadhi has continual access to these experiences and at the same time continues to live simply in the world to help others.

There is a discussion of the two types of samadhi in the first pada of the Yoga Sutras, aphorism 17. The first superconscious state is called *samprajnata,* which means "with seed." In this state of consciousness, there is very deep meditation, absorption and the experience of bliss, but duality still exists. There is awareness of oneself meditating as well as being aware of the object of meditation (mantra, breath or chakra). A true sage in this stage would be able to understand and experience the subtleties of each chakra and could be able to direct energy through the centers to the higher chakras. The Yoga Sutras goes on to describe the other type of samadhi, *asamprajnata,* which means "seedless." Here all awareness of the self as meditator and all objects of meditation are transcended. There is no duality in this state as the person in meditation has totally merged with Brahman.21

PART IV:

How to Meditate

QUALITIES NECESSARY TO PRACTICE MEDITATION

To sit quietly and concentrate on an object may seem to be a simple thing to do, however, a dedicated practice of meditation can actually be difficult and demanding. Therefore, it is necessary to cultivate several important qualities, not only to prepare for the practice of meditation, but also to sustain an ongoing practice and to ensure consistent progress on the spiritual path.

When embarking on the path of meditation, one needs to practice simplicity of thought, deed and action. Because human beings tend to be distracted by the pleasures, attachments and habits associated with life, it takes a great amount of effort and discipline to foster healthy habits and avoid entanglement in unwholesome lifestyles. The accumulation of more luxuries and external comforts than necessary to satisfy one's basic needs is distracting and interferes with attaining a concentrated mind. On the physical level, eating simple foods low in saturated fat, salt and sugar allows for better health and greater clarity of thought. Getting enough exercise and sleep as well as directing one's sexual energy appropriately free the mind to go inwards. The practice of simplicity on the mental and emotional levels means to avoid useless gossip and dwelling on irrelevant or disturbing thoughts, all of which dissipate one's energy. Balance and moderation are essential to create an inner environment conducive to meditation.

It is also important that body, breath and mind settle down and remain silent and alert. The quality of tranquility ensues when one gives up the futile effort to control everything and instead greets each moment with openness and calmness, remaining centered and unaffected by changing circumstances. Tranquility is the ability to remain calm in the busy, modern world. One can also gradually strengthen this quality through a consistent practice of meditation.

One also needs an inherent curiosity and desire to learn more about oneself, one's relationships with other human beings and with the universe. The questions "Who am I?" and "Where have I come from?" are of paramount importance. In addition, one needs to have an intense desire to investigate the underlying mysteries of life and to know the inner essence of things.

Next, one needs to be open to seeing things from a larger perspective. Being open also means to allow oneself to be vulnerable, to admit to having weaknesses and to acknowledge one's insecurities. Because meditation involves self-observation, one may experience uncomfortable moments of anger, greed, jealousy, fear or sadness. It takes courage to free one's heart and mind from these emotions and to maintain a spiritual and meditative practice and lifestyle.

Patience is vital on the path of meditation. There are moments when a person feels like nothing is happening in spite of regular and intense meditative practice. Progress is often slow and so it is quite common to become discouraged. The desire for sensory or sexual pleasures, laziness, boredom, restlessness and feelings of doubt all can disrupt the process of meditation. These thoughts and feelings are to be expected. One needs to learn to be patient and confident that with consistent practice these hindrances will be overcome in time.

Persistence is important to maintain an ongoing meditation practice as there are innumerable obstacles and doubts on the path to enlightenment. For example, one may question the process: *Why am I sitting here watching my thoughts, being aware of my breath and mentally repeating a sound?* With a regular practice of meditation there is always progress, but the transformation process occurs unconsciously and continuously. The journey on the path of enlightenment is ongoing and one must be persistent, sincere and diligent. It is often said that breakthroughs to higher perception levels occur when one is finally able to let go of the need for results.

The cultivation of mindfulness helps to deepen the meditation practice. Mindfulness means to have clear awareness of what is happening at all times. It is the ability to see things as they really are and to listen carefully to what is being said. Mindfulness means to be fully present and to practice conscious living at all times with respect to body, senses, mind and emotions. If a person consistently drifts or is distracted during meditation and does not practice mindfulness, meditation will be less effective and will seem more difficult. Each time the mind wanders in meditation, one must gently bring it back to the object of concentration.

The quality of joy that arises during meditation and provides inspiration for continued practice is unlike the temporary pleasurable feelings that come from having a desire satisfied. The feelings of true joy that come from meditation result from the integration of body, heart, mind and consciousness with universal consciousness. This unlimited joy is described as bliss or rapture. Joy that is cultivated by a meditative practice also involves living life with a lightness of heart and gentleness of action, speech and spirit. By learning not to take life and its innumerable experiences too seriously, one can enjoy each moment more fully.

Qualities Necessary to Practice Meditation
Simplicity
Discipline
Tranquility
Curiosity
Openness
Courage
Patience
Persistence
Mindfulness
Joy

CREATING THE ENVIRONMENT FOR MEDITATION

Try to find a place for meditation that you can use regularly. It should be dry, quiet and slightly cool and free from distractions. Try to face the north or east. It is important to meditate at the same time each day. Early morning or late at night are particularly quiet times and thus are auspicious for meditation, but if this is not possible, any time is fine.

It is best not to meditate if you are tired or drowsy because sleep is not the goal of meditation. Avoid eating before meditation because meals can also lead to sleepiness. Consider doing yoga postures before meditating to stretch the muscles and strengthen the spine. The practice of alternate nostril breathing, the complete breath, ujjayi or bhramari (bee breath) before meditation can also help enhance concentration.

As a beginner, you may want to gradually increase the time spent in meditation. Ten to fifteen minutes is a reasonable amount of time to begin with, gradually building up to twenty to sixty minutes. As you gain more experience, you may spend as much time as you want in meditation. Be realistic about how much time you have to spend in meditation, especially if you have small children to take care of or you are particularly busy at work or school. It is not necessary to change your general habits or activity patterns to adopt a meditative lifestyle. Create an internal state of mind where you look forward to your practice each day. If you miss a day, don't be discouraged. Simply resume your practice the next day.

The technique of meditation is actually quite simple and systematic. When practicing meditation, sit on a chair or on the floor with an erect spine and with hands placed comfortably on the lap, thighs or knees. Find a comfortable sitting posture that suits you. If you choose to sit in a chair, sit so that your feet touch the ground. If you sit on the floor, have a folded blanket under your hips so that your head, trunk and hips are lined up. Carefully place your feet in a position so they don't fall asleep. You may want to wrap yourself in a blanket or shawl to stay comfortably warm.

Gently close your eyes. Using the mind, systematically relax each body part, beginning at the head and ending at the feet. Then regulate the breath by using the abdomen and diaphragm to move air in and out of the lungs. During inhalation the upper part of the abdomen moves out and away from the body in coordination with the contraction of the diaphragm, and on exhalation that part of the abdomen moves inwards towards the body, along with the relaxation of the diaphragm. Next, adjust the rhythm of your breath to become efficient, slow, smooth, deep and without pauses. The next step is to withdraw the senses from the outside world and direct all attention inwards, while mentally affirming: *I have a body but I am not the body; I am a breathing being, but I am not the breath; I have senses to experience the external world but I am not the senses; I am a thinking being but I am not the mind; my essential nature is peace, happiness and bliss.* Follow this by focusing on a chosen or given object of concentration.

OBJECTS OF CONCENTRATION

Meditation involves focusing the mind on a single thought or object. There are some objects of concentration that not only center and calm the mind but also are intrinsically connected to higher states of consciousness, and therefore have inherent power to lead the practitioner of meditation to experience those states. The objects typically used for meditation are images (chakras or yantras), sound (mantras), light, breath or prayer. Chakras, mantras and yantras are of particular importance to my practice of meditation.

Chakras as Objects of Concentration

Meditation on the chakras is of fundamental importance in the Tantric and raja yoga systems of meditation. Swami Rama taught a form of meditation that uses the chakras to move spiritual energy to higher centers of consciousness. When a person focuses attention on a specific chakra, they learn to integrate the physical, emotional, psychological and spiritual energies of that center. As this energy rises upwards through the major chakras during meditation, pranayama and various other spiritual and yogic practices, one gains increasingly greater mastery of the qualities of each center.

Swami Rama imparted energy to me through the process called shaktipat through initiation and instructed me to use specific chakra-focusing techniques by using various concentrative techniques, visualizations and mantras. Sometimes we would meditate together, and I have also experienced initiation during deep sleep and dreams. I learned several ways to meditate using the chakras as centers of focus. The full process begins by focusing attention on the sixth chakra, moving to the seventh, then down the spine to the first and then traveling back up through the second, third, fourth, fifth, sixth, seventh and finally back down to the sixth chakra where one remains for the rest of the meditation. One can remain momentarily at each center or focus attention on each chakra for a longer period of time. One can also remain focused on a specific chakra if there is need to work on that center's physical, psychological and spiritual qualities to counter illness or emotional difficulties, or if one feels they have excess or deficient energy at that center.

During meditation on the chakras, I always use the breath to take the mind from one center to the next, inhaling as I move up to the next higher chakra and exhaling as I descend to a lower chakra. When stopping at an individual chakra, I also use the breath to steady my concentration. When I focus my attention on a specific chakra, I can use one or more of the following objects that are characteristic of that chakra: an element, one of the senses, a bija mantra, a mantra associated with the various lotus petals, a prayer of two or more mantras recited together, a spiritual quality or a yogic deity that has the qualities I want to enhance or purify. During meditation, the object of meditation that I choose to focus on depends on my mood, health concerns or the amount of time I have to meditate.

When I lived at the Himalayan Institute ashram in Glenview, Illinois, I was asked to meditate at midnight every day. I was also instructed to meditate in the morning after my hatha yoga practice and after doing various pranayama practices. During the breathing exercises, I was instructed to use breath retention on exhalation and

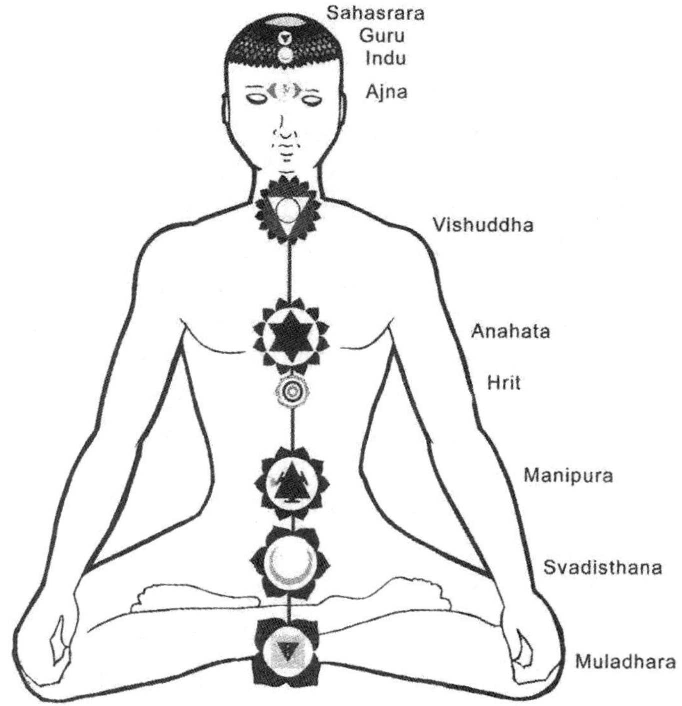

Seven Major and Three Minor Chakras

to practice the three major bandhas (locks) to activate the latent kundalini energy that lies dormant in the first chakra of every human being. When this energy is awakened and directed upwards through the central sushumna nadi, one experiences spiritual insight and expansion of consciousness. At first, I consciously practiced these techniques as instructed, but eventually the locks and breathing techniques occurred on their own as the kundalini energy became activated. These experiences continue to this day and I feel my maturity and familiarity with the process has made these inner experiences even richer and more fulfilling.

Mantras as Objects of Concentration

The word *mantra* is a Sanskrit word composed of the root *man* meaning "mind" and *tra* meaning "instrument to liberate one from bondage." Thus, the word *mantra* means "an instrument of the mind that can liberate one from bondage."

Mantra underlies all manifestation from the unformed to the formed and from the unity of consciousness to individual consciousness. The sound that resonated from the initial vibration of manifestation occurred before other energies such as light and gravity manifested. The subtle hum of the Big Bang is akin to the idea of mantric vibration. The great religious texts also recognize this reality. In the Old Testament, God said, *"Let there be light."* In the Gospel of John in the New Testament, it is similarly stated, *"In the beginning was the word."* And the Hindu text, *Shatapatha Brahmana* states that, *"In the beginning was God through the power of speech."*

Yoga teaches that the entire universe is continuously vibrating, extending from the deep tones of the Milky Way to the medium tones of cellular activity, and from the inaudible frequencies of brain waves to the ultrafast frequencies of light. Yoga philosophy believes that the human body represents the crystallization of sound and light. For example, yogis say the mantra *So Ham* (pronounced like hum) is the collective sound that emanates from all the cells of the body. Thus, repetition of this mantra in coordination with the breath can energize the entire human organism.

The mantra itself may be a single word or phrase. Ancient practitioners have described hearing subtle sound vibrations or mantras while in deep meditation. These were condensed forms or seeds of vibratory experiences. Being a latent force or seed, it has a very powerful effect and can be nurtured to grow into the entire experience. These mantras have been passed on to us through a long line of teachers who have acted as transmitters to distribute them to receptive students.

Mantra and the Power of Vibratory Frequency

Mantras are likened to fire in that they can burn and purify. This is why the chanting of prayers and mantras, whether they are from the Hindu, yogic, Buddhist, Christian (especially Gregorian), Jewish, Sikh, Jain, Muslim or native traditions, can relax and clear the mind and make it receptive to inner creativity, love and compassion. Mantras that are chanted or meditated upon with intention energize the physical and the subtle body. Similarly, the chants, prayers and meditation that people have done in sacred spaces, such as cathedrals, temples or pyramids for many years have filled those spaces with so much energy that the experience of just being there or meditating there has become very meaningful and powerful.

There is immense power in sound, which includes speech, the sounds of nature and music. For example, the sounds of poetry, national anthems and words expressing love or anger all have deep effects on the mind and body. Emotions are often associated with sounds: people sing when feeling joy, shout when angry, cry when sad, groan in pain and scream in fear. The sounds of their words and voice carry emotional force. Yogis maintain that mantras have even greater power than other types of sounds. While words can evoke great feelings on a physical and emotional level, mantra evokes its power on the subtler bodies of the inner koshas—the pranic, mental, unconscious and blissful sheaths.

Mantra and Meditation

When the conscious mind has been cleared, the mind can concentrate on a single object such as a mantra. The coordination of the sound of the mantra with the breath flow helps the body, breath and mind function as an integrated whole. The power of mantra derives not only from its meaning, but also from the vibrational effects created through its repetition. The repetition or recitation of mantras is actually an experience of moving energy, as mantras are not tangible objects. Mantras thus represent energy forces rather than simply being words imbued with particular meanings. Just as a plucked string on a violin or guitar can cause other strings in the instrument to vibrate in unity, so can the vibratory frequency of mantra cause other forces within the human to vibrate in harmony.

Through consistent practice, the mental repetition of a mantra can help to concentrate the mind and to replace distracting conscious thoughts and disturbing memories from the unconscious. Mantras can also redirect emotional energy. Through their vibratory and frequency effects, mantras can break up negative energy patterns stored in the mind, emotions, breath and body and replace them with healthier patterns. As the meditator advances, his or her concentration becomes absorbed with the sound. Because the mantra's vibration is a subtle manifestation of the deepest levels of inner existence, prolonged repetition of a mantra gradually pulls individual consciousness towards universal consciousness. In this way, mantras connect us with spiritual wisdom and the energy of consciousness hidden in the vast cosmos.

According to both Ayurveda and Chinese medicine, the palate, much like the foot, hand and ear, has many reflex points on the meridians throughout the body that connect to other parts of the body. When the rich vibrating sounds of mantras are combined with the stimulation of these reflex points in the palate during mantra recitation, it subtly stimulates the pituitary gland and the hypothalamus that are situated above and very close to the palate. The pituitary is the master gland in the body that regulates the release of many hormones and modulates psychological and physiologic functions.

Mantras as sacred sounds need to be energized through intense practice, pranayama, heart-centered devotion to a deity, mental concentration, ritual or puja. Once energized, the mantra resonates by itself and can even reveal itself internally through its own power. Mantras can also activate and raise the kundalini up through the vortices of the energy-transforming centers (chakras) by clearing blockages and causing the lotus petals of the chakras to vibrate at the higher and more subtle frequencies of the higher centers. The teacher who passes a mantra to a student should understand the deeper aspects and the inner essence of the sound and vibratory frequency of the mantra and how they can be used to expand consciousness. When there is great trust between teacher and student, a realized teacher through shaktipat can help activate the kundalini in the prepared student. This can be done through mantras as well as through touch, a glance, a thought and/or in dreams. It is the student's responsibility to be ready for the increased energy levels that accompany kundalini awakening.

How to Use Mantras in Meditation

Swami Rama taught us four ways to use mantras in meditation. The first way is to repeat the sound out loud. For example, when using *OM,* beginning students of meditation may want to verbally repeat *OM* on three consecutive deep exhalations to become familiar with its tone, rhythm and vibration. The second way is to whisper the mantra under the breath. The third way is to mentally repeat the sound in coordination with the breath. For example, one can repeat *OM* with each inhalation and exhalation, with one whole round of breath or with several breaths in sequence. If the practitioner is able to experience the mantra resonating deep within, the fourth way is to simply listen for the sound and vibrations of the mantra.

When one continually repeats a mantra over a long period of time, it will begin to rise up into conscious awareness on its own, sometimes seeming to call to the person who is meditating. After living with the mantra for several years, the student will come to appreciate its latent power of transformation. Meditation on a mantra ultimately leads to awareness of the underlying unity of all things.

OM: The Mother of All Mantras

There are several types of mantras, including seed or *bija* mantras, mantras associated with the chakras, mantras that correspond to the yogic deities and longer mantras that have many syllables that are chanted together. The mantra *OM* in particular is considered to be the manifestation of the universal vibration in its most subtle and sublime form. *OM* is the primordial sound of timeless consciousness, which has been vibrating within people since the beginningless past. *OM* was the sound that resonated from the vibration of the initial separation of universal consciousness into the manifest universe. Therefore, *OM* is considered to be the mother or the source that contains within itself all sounds and vibrations. The vibrations of *OM* can be heard in deep meditation, reverberating through the mind and the surrounding universe. A sound that approximates *OM* is heard when a seashell is put to the ear or when one speaks with lips closed. Through concentration on the mantra *OM,* the reverse process of manifestation takes place — the gathering of the scattered energy and drawing it back towards the ultimate source.

The mantra *OM* is most closely associated with the sixth chakra and is also used in meditation while moving concentration upwards through the chakras. *OM* is chanted at the beginning of most Hindu prayers and rituals. Many other religious and spiritual traditions incorporate a similar sound in prayer or meditations. For example, in both Christianity and Judaism, prayers end with the word *Amen,* similar to the sound of *OM.* In Islam, prayers often end in *Ameen,* while in Jewish meditation, *Shalom* (peace), is often used as a mantra. *Shalom* can be coordinated with the flow of breath, with the *sha* and *lom* repeated silently during inhalation and exhalation, respectively. The *l* sound quickly becomes silent with the long and gentle exhalation focused on the *OM* sound.

OM is the signifier of the ultimate truth that all is One. All that can be comprehended by humans is *OM.* By living in harmony with nature and one's fellow human beings, by eating whole and nutritious foods, by coordinating the breath with the rhythms of one's physiology and environment and by promoting quiet and peaceful thoughts one experiences *OM.* Feeling love for others as reflections of ourselves, having compassion for all sentient beings, practicing loving kindness, promoting feelings of nurturance, forgiveness and generosity of spirit are all part of *OM.* All that there is, namely Brahman, the absolute reality and pure consciousness without an object is *OM.*

OM can also be written as *AUM.* The letter *A* (*A* sounds like "a" in the word about) represents the act of manifestation of the universe (yogic idea of Brahma), the waking state and the gross body. The *A* sound permeates all the other sounds of *OM* and represents all the gross objects of the phenomenal world such as all the celestial bodies, the earth, plants and all sentient beings.

The letter *U* (the *U* sounds like the double "oo" in root) represents the preservation of all manifestation (yogic idea of Vishnu), the dreaming state and the subtle or energy body. In this second state, consciousness is turned towards the inner world. The *U* represents the formless or shapelessness of mind, air, fire and water.

The letter *M* (*M* sounds like "mmm") represents the transformative power of life (yogic idea of Shiva), deep sleep and the causal or mental body. In this third state there are no dreams nor any desire for or attachments to objects of the world. In deep sleep all such experiences recede and merge into the state of undifferentiated consciousness where one is filled with the experience of bliss.

The silence that follows enunciation of *AUM* represents the fourth state of sleepless sleep or *turiya*, which means "the fourth." In the fourth state consciousness is absolute. It is associated with the sound of *OM* and represents the Vedantic idea of Brahman, that which cannot be experienced through the senses or thought. This state is indescribable and cannot be comprehended by the mind. Turiya represents pure consciousness, the real Self and the cessation of all phenomena. Turiya is like the dreamless sleep of the third state, but here the practitioner is fully aware and awake, not only to the mental world, but also to the greater cosmos. Swami Rama demonstrated the turiya state of consciousness when he was doing experiments at the Menninger Foundation in 1969-70. 22

An advanced method of meditation on the sound *AUM* is to break it into its component sounds. One can begin by concentrating on the first chakra and visualizing the latent energy of kundalini becoming activated and starting to move up the central nadi. While mentally repeating the sound *A,* one can bring the now activated energy up to the third chakra with inhalation. Keeping the concentration there for many breath cycles, the practitioner continues to focus on the *A* sound. Then with a subsequent inhalation, one can move the energy up to the fourth chakra, coordinating the sound of *U* with the breath and maintaining awareness on the "*U*" sound. Then after several breaths, on inhalation one moves the focus along with the "*M*" sound up to the seventh chakra. Then one can simply rest in meditation, bringing the OM sound back together and either repeating OM with the breath or simply listening for the sound in stillness and in openness.

The Katha Upanishad states: "*The goal, which all the Vedas declare, which all austerities aim at and which humans desire when they live a life of conscience, I will tell you briefly, it is AUM.*"

The Chandogya Upanishad states: "*The chanting, that is, the syllable OM, is the best of all essences, the highest, deserving the highest place, the eighth.*"

The Mandukya Upanishad says, "*All this, whatever is visible, whatever is cognizable, whatever can come within the purview of sense-perception, inference or verbal testimony, whatever can be comprehended under the single term, creation — all this is OM.*"

In addition the Bhagavad Gita states, "*Uttering the monosyllable AUM, the eternal world of Brahman, one who departs leaving the body (at death), he attains the supreme goal and he reaches God.*" Also in the Bhagavad Gita, Lord Krishna says to Arjuna, "*I am the father of this universe, the mother, the support and the grandsire. I am the object of knowledge, the purifier and the syllable OM.*" And: "*OM, tat and sat have been declared as the triple appellation of Brahman, who is truth, consciousness and bliss.*"

When one chants *OM*, one creates within a harmonious vibration in the body mind system that is in resonance with the cosmic vibration. When this takes place, instead of thinking independently as jiva, an individual soul, one starts to think universally as Ishvara.

Bija or Seed Mantras

Teachers frequently use bija mantras to initiate students into the practice of meditation. To assist with the selection of the mantra the teacher examines the student's personality and life circumstances. The teacher selects the mantra just as a physician prescribes a medication, except in this case the diagnosis and prescription are made on the spiritual level. The personal mantra can then be used not only to help focus concentration but also to help the student with specific difficulties they be experiencing.

Before describing the individual seed mantras, a brief discussion of the sounds of the Sanskrit letters is necessary:

- The *k* sound creates energy or prana and helps manifest ideas and desires.
- The *l* sound has a magnetic and holding energy.
- The *r* sound is associated with light, heat, friction, fire and transformation and helps prepare the practitioner for the spiritual path and dharma. It also represents shakti energy and drives the kundalini force.
- The *ee* sound represents insight, vision and imagination.
- The *h* or *ha* sound represents air and prana and is associated with exhalation and letting go.
- The *sa* sound is associated with inhalation and the power of holding on and the development of power.

The following mantras are the most common and most powerful bija mantras for use during meditation.

Aim (pronounced *I'm*) is the syllable for "teacher." It is often called the feminine aspect of the mantra *OM*. The mantra *Aim* helps the practitioner gain knowledge of the unknown and is associated with learning, art and self-expression. It is the seed mantra for Saraswati, the goddess of knowledge, speech, art, learning and communication. By repeating *Aim*, a person can gain higher truths. *Aim* can enhance the vocal cords, the singing voice and help correct problems within the throat. As it is connected most closely with the fifth chakra, one can meditate on this center using the mantra *Aim* to improve communication and creative receptivity to one's higher Self.

Hrim (rhymes with *cream*) is the syllable for energy, light, activity, empowerment and motivation. *Hrim* represents the spiritual heart mantra and repetition helps dissolve illusions of perceived reality. It is sometimes a component of longer Vedic and Tibetan Buddhist chants. *Hrim* is often chanted or mentally repeated during concentration on the fourth chakra. It is a feminine energy associated with Shakti and with the inner flame of devotion to the spiritual heart. It also is said to represent the soul's abode and the *Hrit* chakra, located just below the fourth chakra. Repetition of *Hrim* creates a fiery type of energy, helping to direct circulation of blood, breath, lymph and cerebral spinal fluid. This mantra can be used to help strengthen the heart, for general vitality and immune functioning.

Klim is the syllable for desire. It has a magnetic type of energy where it consolidates, holds and draws things in and because of this, it is said to attract objects of one's desires. It is especially useful for people wanting to attract the divine, spiritual teachers or companions on the road to truth and liberation. *Klim* is a mantra for devotion and love and is a soft and more feminine energy. It is most associated with the second, third and fourth chakras. The yogic deities of Krishna and Sundari are associated with *Klim.* This mantra helps balance the watery (kaphic) parts of our body, especially the digestive fluids, skin, reproductive tract, urinary organs and blood. It also calms the heart and the nervous system.

Krim is the syllable for union. It is a stimulating and focusing mantra, creating a type of energy that is associated with the powers of work and action. *Krim* combines the qualities of air and fire, which create active forces and dynamic energy patterns and is especially useful to activate the circulatory, nervous and digestive systems. It is associated with the feminine kundalini energy, which when activated moves upwards through the sushumna nadi to merge in union with the male Shiva energy located in the crown chakra. The yogic deity Kali is most closely connected with *Krim.* Kali is the feminine aspect of Shiva, the great destroyer and transformer.

Shrim is the syllable for delight. It is the mantra for spiritual abundance, health, inner peace, material wealth, friendship and love of family. It is connected to the goddess Lakshmi who is associated with abundance. She is the wife of Vishnu, who represents the preservation and stability of the universe. Repetition of the mantra *Shrim,* brings the guru's grace and devotion. Calmness of the mind and happiness result and this mantra is particularly good for female reproductive issues. It is good to meditate on the heart chakra when repeating *Shrim* because of its connection to faith and the emotional expression of love and devotion. It often precedes or follows the mantra *Hrim* when several bija mantras are chanted together. For example, *OM Hrim Shrim Klim Aim Swaha.*

Trim is the syllable for fire. This mantra is often used to increase inner energy and direct activity. It helps overcome obstacles in life whether they are physical, emotional or spiritual and gives courage to face difficulties. This mantra can be used when focusing on the third chakra as a means to transform kundalini as it ascends up the chakras.

Strim is the syllable for peace and stability. It helps the individual to stand on their own two feet and protects and guides the student through stresses and traumas. It is considered a feminine mantra and helps with creative endeavors.

Hlim is a mantra for protection and helps to stabilize in the face of negative or harsh influences. This mantra is helpful when practicing yoga postures and pranayama as it helps stabilize and slow down movements.

Gum is a masculine mantra associated with Ganesha, also known as Ganapathi. This mantra bestows the energy of benevolence and brings success to beginning endeavors. The mantra *OM Gum Ganapatayei Namaha* means "salutations to the removal of obstacles."

Glaum is another seed mantra of Ganapathi and is related to Ganesh as the energy of will power. This mantra helps remove emotional obstacles between the throat and base of the spine and can be meditated upon when focusing on the first chakra.

Dum is the seed mantra for Durga and is for protection. It activates the feminine energy and helps a person be less fearful. *OM Dum Durgayei Namaha* means "*OM* and salutations to Durga," who is beautiful and protective to seekers of truth, but terrible in appearance to those who injure devotees of truth, which generally refers to one's ego, that part of oneself that interferes with the path of spirituality. This aspect of Durga is depicted by her many fierce weapons. This is an excellent mantra for meditation on the third chakra.

Hoom energizes other mantras and can be used to activate the mantras associated with the chakras. For example, to activate the physical, emotional, mental and spiritual qualities of the third chakra, a person could repeat *OM Ram Hoom.* I will discuss the chakra-based mantras below.

Mantras Associated with the Chakras

Other bija mantras are the syllables that correspond to each of the five lower chakras. Beginning at the first chakra and moving upwards, the sounds are *Lam, Vam, Ram, Yam,* and *Ham* (each of these sounds rhymes with the word rum or numb). While meditating on the visual image (yantra) of each chakra and repeating the associated seed mantra, the student activates the physical, psychological and spiritual energies of that chakra.

So Ham is the universal breath mantra that corresponds to the quiet sound of breathing. *So* is mentally repeated on inhalation and *Ham* on exhalation. *Ham Sa* is the mantra in reverse, with *Ham* repeated on exhalation and *Sa* on inhalation.

There are a few other mantras that activate the chakras and/ or their elements directly. These include two important Sanskrit mantras, the Gayatri mantra and *OM Namah Shivaya,* both of which can activate all the chakras. A well-known Tibetan mantra, *OM Mani Padme Hum,* awakens the fourth chakra. In the Jewish tradition, using the names for God (*Adonai* and *Elohim*) while visualizing the tree of life has a very powerful effect. *Amen, Shalom* and the *Shema* prayer can also be used with visualizations. *Yod Hey Vav Hey* are the Hebrew letters for God. In Jewish mysticism, this holy name of God can only be written but never spoken. When the Hebrew letters are placed one on top of the other, it looks like a human form. Thus this image links humans and the divine.23

Specific letters in the Sanskrit and Hebrew alphabet are themselves important mantras and yantras. The letters associated with these great languages are not merely building blocks for constructing spoken and written words. They also represent the sounds, vibrations and forms that ancient practitioners heard and saw in deep meditation. Thus, the internal repetition and

Chakras and Bija Mantras with Sanskrit Letters/Symbols

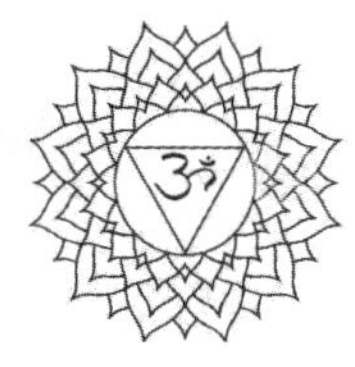 Sahasrara
OM

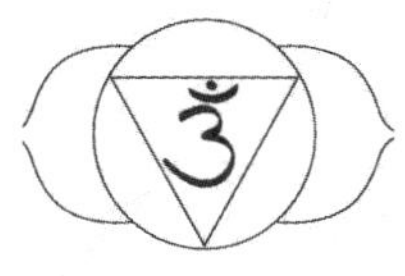 Ajna
OM

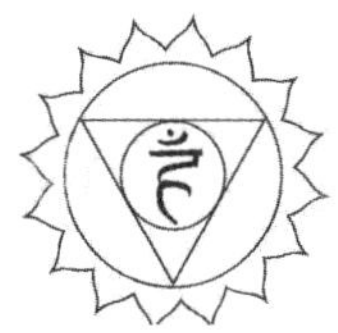 Vishuddha
HAM

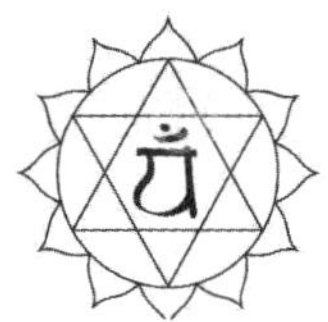 Anahata
YAM

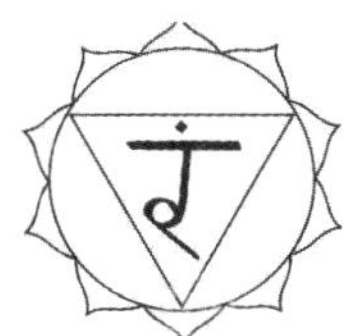 Manipura
RAM

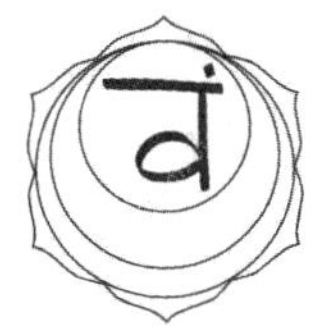 Svadhisthana
VAM

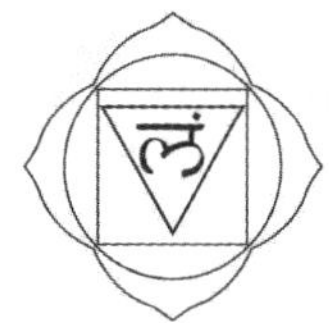 Muladhara
LAM

visualization of letters as yantras in meditation can lead the mind back to the ultimate source.

Deities as Mantras

In English the word *deities* refers to gods and goddesses, but in Sanskrit, deity comes from the word *devatas* which means "divine principle." The deities reflect the divine consciousness that pervades the inner psyche of all humans and all of nature. Deities reflect the chakra energies: earth, water, fire, air, ether/space, mind and consciousness. Deities also represent the various aspects of Brahman: existence, consciousness and bliss (satchidananda).

Deities represent the divine within each individual. They are symbolic representations of the powers inherent in life and the qualities and characteristics of consciousness. Deities are cosmic, symbolic, poetic anthropomorphisms, representing human beings as God and God as a human being. Deities are like actors in the great cosmic play of life with the cast of characters reflecting the karmas of one's individual soul that has incarnated in one's present human form. Like the characters in the great mythologies, deities reflect the rhythms of life and represent symbols and archetypes in one's unconscious and conscious quests for higher knowledge. Kirtan often uses the names of deities as mantras.

Specific Deities

The trinity of deities that govern creation, preservation and dissolution have both masculine and feminine qualities and are: Brahma (male) and Saraswati (female), Vishnu (male) and Lakshmi (female) and Shiva (male) and Devi/Kali (female).

Devi denotes the divine mother who has many forms: Shakti, Saraswati, Lakshmi, Kali, Durga, Parvati, Sita, Sundari, and Bhairavi. Shakti is the feminine divine energy that leads to the unfoldment of consciousness. Shakti energy resides in the root chakra and represents the kundalini force. Shakti guides the individual through the evolution of the soul.

Saraswati is the feminine version of Brahma and represents the creative power of the universe as well as wisdom, intelligence, memory, speech, communication, poetry, knowledge of mantra, music, art, dance, literature and learning. *Aim* is the bija mantra of Saraswati and is meditated upon on the fifth chakra.

Lakshmi grants health, wealth, beauty, fertility, happiness, abundance, grace and fulfillment of worldly desires. Lakshmi's incarnations are Sita, the wife of Ram and Radha, Krishna's consort. *Shrim* is the bija mantra of Lakshmi.

Kali guides one through the dissolution of worldly attachments and towards the higher self. Kali helps clear emotional and physical barriers and obstructions, especially when meditation focuses on the first chakra. Kali energy helps to transform grief, fear, jealousy and resentment into the positive qualities of compassion and caring. As the kundalini begins to awaken, Kali helps move this energy in a coordinated way through the higher chakras.

Durga is beautiful to behold but is also frightening because of her many arms and weapons. She attacks and slays intruding forces such as the ego on the spiritual path, and protects against harm. Durga is invoked during meditation and kirtan for strength. Durga energy enhances leadership qualities. Durga helps in the drive for purposeful activity and the development of personal power for physical, emotional and spiritual transformation. *OM Dum Durgayei Namaha* is chanted for protection with a focus on the third chakra.

Radha represents pure love and absolute commitment in relationships. Radha was Krishna's consort and her complete devotion to him epitomizes the path of bhakti yoga. Radha helps to overcome jealousy, possessiveness in relationships and fear of separation as well as provides support during the experience of loss.

Sita was Rama's consort and also represents complete devotion to the loved one. Fidelity is an important characteristic of the Sita energy. One invokes Sita to develop compassion, empathy, commitment in partnership, patience and the ability to love.

Shiva represents pure awareness and the forces of transformation through destruction. Rudra is the fierce form of

Shiva and rules fire, heat, fevers, infections and contagious diseases. Nataraja is the dancing form of Shiva who represents the creative forces inherent in transformation. One invokes help from Shiva to begin and sustain a meditation practice and a yogic lifestyle. His mantra is *OM* or *Haum*.

Vishnu represents peace and preservation of the universe. Vishnu is invoked through chants to Rama, Krishna or Narayana to help one love and serve and for help on the path to enlightenment. *OM Namo Narayanaya* is a chant for peace.

Krishna, an incarnation of Vishnu, represents God as man. Krishna is the magnetic energy of divine love. Krishna's teachings to Arjuna are embodied in the Bhagavad Gita. On the path of bhakti yoga one invokes Krishna for the love that is necessary to expand one's consciousness. Krishna also represents the path of action, karma yoga, as he encourages Arjuna to follow the path of a warrior as he had committed himself to, even though this would entail many hardships. Two mantras that are commonly used in kirtan to invoke Krishna's energy are *Hare Krishna* and *Om Namo Bhagavate Vasudevaya*.

Rama is an incarnation of Vishnu who represents the ideal king who leads an ethical life. Chanting to Rama protects us from negativity in the external world and in our hearts. Rama is like the sun's energy, epitomizing warmth and nurturance rather than burning and destruction. Rama helps to empower and preserve an ethical life. *Shri Ram Jaya Ram* is an important kirtan that invokes Rama energies.

Hanuman is the monkey-faced god who is an incarnation of Vishnu and also is the son of Vayu, the god of wind. Hanuman is the ideal yogi and embodies the qualities of loyalty and devotion. Hanuman signifies the higher force behind prana, and singing to Hanuman promotes healing and longevity. Meditation on the fifth chakra using *Ham*, the seed mantra for Hanuman, helps to open up the voice. One invokes Hanuman for courage, for the ability to serve others in a nonegotistical way and for devotion to the spiritual path.

Ganesha is the elephant-headed deity, who rules over time and dispenses the fruits of karma. Ganesha removes all obstacles on the path and grants health, wisdom, skill and success. He is to be invoked before initiation of tasks. Ganesha is the first son of Shiva and Paravati and, being very close to his mother, carries the grace of the goddess. Meditation on the first chakra using *Glaum*, the seed mantra for Ganesha, stabilizes and directs the kundalini shakti energy. *OM Gum Ganapatayae Namah* invokes the power and consciousness of Ganesh.

Yantra

The term yantra derives from the Sanskrit root word Yam and means "a device or instrument that sustains or supports the energy inherent in a particular element, object or concept." Yantra is an abstract geometric design that functions to support and enhance mental focus and increase inner awareness. Yantras represent visual images of consciousness, encompassing the underlying organization of the physical universe and the underlying order of the conscious and unconscious mind. It is a graphic representation of the energies of the universe as they manifest into visual form.

Each chakra has a yantra, a geometric form that is associated with specific colors. Inside the yantra for each chakra is a Sanskrit letter that corresponds to the associated bija mantra. The lotus petal is another simple pictorial representation and varying numbers of petals surround each of the chakra yantras, adding up to the fifty letters in the Sanskrit language.

In a sense, a yantra is a mathematical symbol of consciousness in geometric form. The shapes of these building blocks are mostly simple geometric forms, including points, lines, triangles, squares, rectangles, pentagons, circles and spirals. These simple shapes are seen even in the smallest physical particles such as molecules, atoms, electrons and other subatomic structures.

The different shapes in yantras have specific meanings. The circle in a yantra represents the cyclic and rhythmic contraction and expansion of universal energy. The square represents the four directions of nature, which bind the universe in space. And the lotus represents the outward movement of consciousness, the power that unfolds the universe.

Of all the different shapes in yantras, the points or bindis are perhaps the most important. Points represent the center, the nucleus of potential energy from which kinetic energy radiates outwards towards manifestation. A point is the symbolic representation of the all-embracing reservoir of consciousness. It is the seed of the universe, where male and female energies are united. It is the center of the Shri Yantra. 24

Shri Yantra

Transmutation of the vibratory resonance of *OM* into form generates the Shri Yantra. The Shri Yantra is the most perfect representation of how the human being reflects the underlying forces of the universe. Its complex mathematical and geometric structure represents a map of the union of the opposing but complementary forces in the cosmos, including male and female, expansion and contraction and positive and negative energy.

There are three major branches in Tantra. The kaula school uses more external practices such as pujas, rituals and occasionally sexual practices. The mishra school uses a mixture of rituals and inner meditative practices. And the samaya school is an almost entirely inner process, which uses meditative practices similar to the meditation I learned and have described in this book. Meditation on the Shri Yantra is considered to be the most advanced practice in the samaya path of Tantra. This meditation is very complex and is associated with mantra recitation while visualizing the shapes and patterns of the yantra. Meditation on the Shri Yantra leads the student to experience and energize the nine chakras (the seven major chakras and the two minor chakras located between the sixth and seventh chakras). Only a highly skilled teacher is qualified to guide the student in this meditative practice.

Vedic Astrology

A few years ago, I decided to study Jyotish, also called Vedic astrology, an ancient system of knowledge that is connected with other bodies of Vedic knowledge such as Ayurveda and yoga

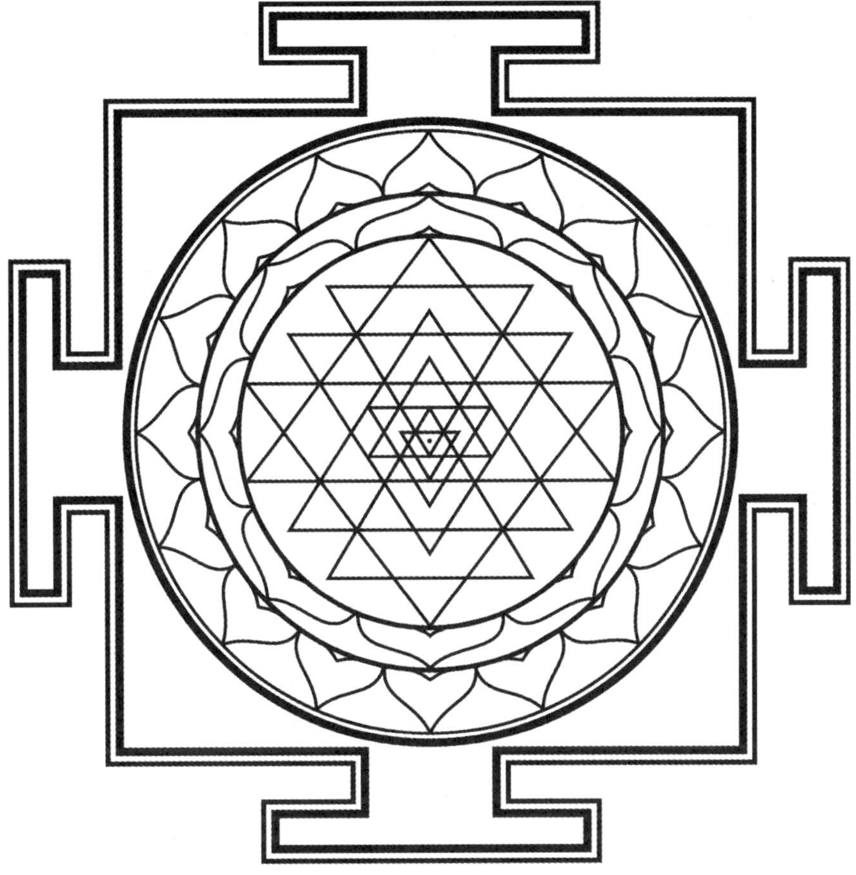

Shri Yantra

philosophy. While I am a novice in this science, it has helped me understand some of the patterns in my life and karmic connections on my healing and spiritual journey.

The Vedic astrological chart is said to represent the karmic DNA of the incarnating soul. Vedic astrology mirrors the fact that all aspects of the universe exist in patterns, whether it be the solar systems or the organization of genes in DNA. From this perspective, karma from previous lifetimes forms patterns and these are depicted in the Vedic astrological birth chart. My understanding of Vedic astrology is that the planetary alignments at the time of one's birth represent a pictorial and symbolic pattern of one's past karmic tendencies as well as offer a blueprint for moving forward in life. There are four types of karma:

Sanchita karma reflects the sum total of all previous actions in individual incarnations and past lives.

Prarabdha karma is the portion of sanchita karma that results in one's present birth and is reflected in the planetary positions at the time of birth.

Kriyamana karma results from one's present actions and affects one's current lifetime. This type of karma is akin to the idea of free will, where one's everyday choices affect how one's life will unfold.

Agami karma results from the totality of one's thoughts, speech and actions in this life that will affect future incarnations.

Vedic astrologers say that mantras can affect the four types of karma. For example, mantra repetition with conscious intention can help remove some latent tendencies present within an individual so that the planetary cycles will have less effect on the individual, thus allowing one to change through the exercise of free will one's present and future karmic experiences. Besides mantra, spiritual practices can also help alter certain karmic tendencies. These include karma yoga, through which one selflessly serves others; bhakti yoga, through which one devotes oneself to higher divine principles; and meditation, through which one tries to raise one's awareness and consciousness.

Recently Ruma and I were discussing with heaviness in our hearts about being present with my sister during her passing. We both felt strongly that we could feel her pranic life force slowly leaving her physical body as her breathing slowed. We were so grateful to be with her, holding her hand, sending her love and saying both the great Jewish prayer of belief in the oneness of God, the *Shema*, and the Hindu prayer for easy transition from life to death, the *Mahamrityunjaya Mantra*, which we hoped would help her spirit release easefully from her body.

It seemed inconceivable to us that this vibrant life energy could simply be lost forever. Remembering that modern physics states that energy is neither created nor destroyed and can only be transformed, we both felt that the vital energy force that was once my sister Donna, had been transformed and was in the process of connecting and reconnecting with those who loved and cared for her during her physical life here on this planet.

Ruma once shared her view that she sees astrological charts like a yantra of our lives, a pictorial and geometric representation of our past, present and future karmas. As one looks at the many intersecting lines and planetary aspects, the constellations, yogas and dashas in a chart, patterns that are unique to the person become apparent.

Swamiji, who we were told had studied Jyotish, did not encourage his students to pursue this science. I'm not entirely sure I understand why, though I suspect it had something to do with him wanting us to focus on areas of knowledge that were compatible with Western medical practice. He also stated at one point that through the practices of yoga and meditation, one could transform one's karma and the astrological chart. One of my ashram friends from the Himalayan Institute, Linda Johnsen, did immerse herself in the study of Jyotish and has written *A Thousand Suns* among other books.

MEDITATION TECHNIQUES

There are many meditation techniques. For example, a meditation practice in Tibetan Buddhism and in some yogic traditions concentrates on the dissolution of the five subtle elements. It is a visualization practice in which the meditator focuses on merging and dissolving one element into another, beginning at the first chakra and its associated element, earth. As one ascends to the sixth chakra, ether is dissolved into mind and at the seventh and highest chakra the mind is dissolved into pure consciousness. The purpose of this meditation technique is twofold: to consciously practice identification with the subtler forces and pure consciousness as well as to prepare one for the dying process when the soul (jiva) leaves the human body as it dissolves upwards through the chakras and their associated elements. It is said that the more one practices the dissolution of the elements through meditation, the more conscious will be the experience of leaving the body and the conscious mind, which allows the soul to move on.

The form of meditation presented here is based on the philosophies of Tantra, Samkhya, and Vedanta and closely follows the eight steps of raja yoga. It is a system that has been practiced for thousands of years in the Himalayan Mountains. To begin with one prepares mentally for the practice of meditation by following the lifelong systems of yamas (regulations) and niyamas (observances). Next, a daily practice of hatha yoga asanas can help strengthen the back and make the body more limber. After establishing a sitting posture suitable for meditation, one begins to mentally relax the body. The next step is to practice some simple breathing exercises to begin to focus the mind. More advanced pranayama techniques, which include nadi shodanam, bhramari, and ujjayi, can be used to clear the nadis and sushumna. Sense withdrawal (pratyahara) follows as one lets go of thoughts, feelings and desires and moves inwards to the deeper aspects of mind. Then one begins to concentrate (dharana) on a specific object. The objects of concentration used in this form of raja yoga-based meditation are chakras, mantras, yantras, light, color and breath. Concentration on these objects leads to more sustained and intense meditation (dhyana) and ultimately to the highest level of consciousness, samadhi.

The goal of this meditative practice is to move the latent kundalini energy from the first chakra where it is stored, upwards through the chakras to the higher centers. This is basically done through mental effort and sometimes with the help of more advanced physical practices such as locks and breath retention. An experienced teacher can also help activate kundalini in a student through shaktipat, the transfer of highly focused energy.

One need not be concerned with results after each time one meditates. Because of the sustained mental concentration, the process itself automatically stimulates the kundalini to ascend upwards. It is not necessary to dwell on the attributes of an individual chakra to try to change a particular concern or attitude that might be associated with that center. To specifically activate or stimulate a chakra, there are certain other concentration techniques that can be practiced under the guidance of a knowledgeable teacher.

With this form of meditation, one simply should visualize the chakra along with awareness of the breath and the mantra. At the same time, observe whatever feeling, thought, or sensation may arise and then gently let it go. This meditative technique leads to the slow and steady transformation of physical, psychological and emotional problems as well as to the refinement of spiritual qualities, and ultimately to the highest states of consciousness.

As one progresses in the practice of meditation, there will be a growing sense of competence, an inner calmness and feelings of a stable inner center. Constant mental activity slows, the mind becomes quieter and emotions become steadier. Decision-making becomes easier and one becomes more intuitive and creative. One develops a greater capacity for compassion for others and an increased ability to let go of hurt, resentment and anxiety. There is a strengthening of the ego and at the same time a sense that one is not defined or restricted by the ego as one begins to realize everyone is intimately interconnected with the entire universe. As one progresses with consistent practice, the inner sounds and vibration of one's mantra flow effortlessly into the mind, resulting in the experience of greater peace and joy.

The following meditations are appropriate for both beginning and more experienced students. Until one feels comfortable with meditation and has established a steady and consistent practice, one should progress slowly through the seven phases. One may decide to stop at any phase or may want to work with a more complex practice. This will help one to remember the progression of the meditation. Spend two to four weeks on each phase before progressing to the next. The complete meditation is presented in Meditation VII. As outlined, it is important to become familiar with the geometric form of the chakras before adding color to them. I have recorded these meditations on two CDs when I wrote my previous book, *How to Meditate Using Mantras, Chakras and Breath.*

Seven Sequential Meditation Practices

Note: Each time a person sits for meditation they should follow the same preparation steps as given below. These include:

1. Body posture and awareness
2. Progressive relaxation
3. Abdominal and diaphragmatic breathing
4. Breath awareness
5. Sense withdrawal

Body Posture and Awareness

Sit comfortably on a straight-backed chair or on the floor with a firm cushion under you so that your hips are elevated a few inches off the floor. The purpose of the cushion is to encourage the natural curves of the spine, particularly at the lumbar region. You may find that a cushion is not necessary. Be sure your back is straight, with your head, chest and pelvis all in alignment. Your hands are placed comfortably in your lap, or on your thighs or knees with your palms faced either down or upwards. Touch the tips of your index fingers with the tips of your thumbs, forming a small circle with each hand. Gently close your eyes. Give yourself permission to let go of thoughts of your daily activities and concerns. Be aware of your body and the space your body occupies.

Progressive Relaxation

Begin to relax your body. Send warm relaxing energy to each body part. Let all the muscles soften. Begin at the top of your head and move down to your face and relax your eyes, eyelids, jaws, mouth, lips, teeth, tongue, throat and neck. Let the muscles of your shoulders soften and send warm energy down your arms to your fingers. Move down and relax your chest muscles, heart and lungs. Then relax the abdominal muscles and the organs inside. Relax your entire back and spine. Then send this relaxing energy to your pelvic area, buttocks and down your legs to your toes.

Abdominal and Diaphragmatic Breathing

Be aware of your breathing. Be sure to breathe quietly through your nose. Breathe deeply, slowly, smoothly and evenly without strain. Eliminate any pauses or hesitations while breathing and especially avoid the tendency to pause during the transition between inhalation and exhalation or between exhalation and inhalation. Visualize for a moment a perfectly round circle and imagine that you are inhaling with half the circle and exhaling with the other half. As you inhale, allow the lower part of the chest and upper part of the abdomen to move out away from the body. Then, as you exhale, allow your abdomen and lower chest to move inwards towards the body. Continue this diaphragmatic breathing for about one minute.

Breath Awareness

Bring your attention to the flow of the breath through your nose. With your mind, follow your breath from the bridge between the two nostrils to the point between the two eyebrows as you inhale. Then follow your breath back down again as you exhale. Notice the coolness as the breath flows up the nose on inhalation and the warmth as the breath flows down on exhalation. Continue this breath awareness for a few extra moments. Then follow your breath up to the area between your two eyebrows, in the center of your forehead and slightly above the level of your eyebrows and keep your concentration there.

Sense Withdrawal

Remind yourself that you have a body to use and enjoy the world, that you are a breathing being and your breath connects you to the world, that you have senses to experience the world and that you have a conscious and unconscious mind to understand the world. But remember that you are also more than all this; you are both an individual yet part of a larger whole, like a wave that has its own form but is also part of the greater ocean. You are a wave of beauty and bliss merging with the waves of universal consciousness.

After having completed these five steps, the practitioner can proceed to the visualizations. For each successive meditation practice, I have described a progressively more complex visualization. The reader can move on to each succeeding meditation technique when they have practiced the preceding one for some time and feel comfortable with it.

Closing

After the meditation is completed, one can proceed to the closing as follows: As you slowly come out of the meditation, be aware of your breath flowing through your nostrils for a few moments. Feel the coolness of the breath rising up the nose and the warmth of the breath as it flows back down. Now feel the movement of your abdomen as it moves away from your body as you inhale and back towards your body as you exhale. Finally, be aware of your body and the space that your body occupies. Tell yourself that you will take the same feelings of calm awareness, peace and joy that you experienced during this meditation back into your everyday life. Slowly bring your hands up to your face, cover your eyes with the center of the palms and then gently open your eyes. Gently bring your hands down to your lap while continuing to look at the center of the palms. Slowly look up and enjoy the moment.

Meditation I: Awareness of the Sixth Chakra

Sit quietly with straight posture and practice progressive relaxation, abdominal breathing, breath awareness and sense withdrawal.

Keep your concentration at the point between your two eyebrows and be aware of the inflow and outflow of your breath for a few more minutes. Watch your thoughts, worries, memories and feelings float by with nonjudgmental awareness. Each time your mind is distracted, gently bring your concentration back to this area.

Meditation II: Awareness of and Visualizing the Sixth Chakra (Third Eye)

Sit quietly with straight posture and practice progressive relaxation, abdominal breathing, breath awareness and sense withdrawal.

With your focus of concentration continuing at the center of your forehead between your eyebrows at the sixth chakra, visualize a circle with one lotus petal on each side of the rim of circle. This is what is referred to as the third eye, the center of insight, intuition and wisdom. This eye sees inwards, watching your thoughts, worries, memories and feelings float by. It is accompanied by non-judgmental awareness. Gently bring your concentration back to the image of the third eye each time your mind is distracted. Allow your attention to remain at the center of the sixth chakra and visualize the third eye for the rest of the meditation and for as long as you wish.

Meditation III: Awareness of and Visualizing the Sixth Chakra with Mantra

Sit quietly with straight posture and practice progressive relaxation, abdominal breathing, breath awareness and sense withdrawal.

With your focus on the sixth chakra, visualized as a circle with one lotus petal on each side of the rim of the circle, begin to mentally repeat the sound of your mantra. You can use one of three different mantras: the mantra *OM*, the mantra *So Ham* or a personal mantra if your meditation teacher has given you one. At this point you may want to coordinate the mantra with the breath. You can repeat your mantra with each separate inhalation and exhalation, with one round of breathing (one inhalation and exhalation) or with several rounds. If you seem to hear the mantra resonating deep within, you may also simply listen to the inner sound and vibration of the mantra. Allow your attention to remain at this center, listening to the mantra for the rest of the meditation and for as long as you wish.

Meditation IV: Awareness of the Seventh Chakra (Crown Chakra)

Sit quietly with straight posture and practice progressive relaxation, abdominal breathing, breath awareness and sense withdrawal.

Be aware of the third eye, visualized as a circle with one lotus petal on each side, and mentally repeat or listen for the mantra *OM, So Ham* or your personal mantra. As you inhale, follow your breath, mind and mantra upwards and bring your concentration to the seventh chakra at the top part of your brain (cerebral cortex). Here, visualize a lotus flower with a thousand petals emanating light upwards above your head. Imagine your individual self-identity and the entire field of universal consciousness blending into one indissoluble whole. Keep your focus here for one to five minutes. Then let your concentration gently move back to the sixth chakra (third eye). Allow your attention to remain at this center, listening to the mantra, for the rest of the meditation and for as long as you wish.

Meditation V: Awareness of the First Chakra and Kundalini

Sit quietly with straight posture and practice progressive relaxation, abdominal breathing, breath awareness and sense withdrawal.

Be aware of the third eye, visualized as a circle with one lotus petal on each side, and mentally repeat or listen for the mantra *OM, So Ham* or your personal mantra. Then be aware of the seventh chakra. As you exhale, follow your breath, mind and mantra down the center of the spine to the first chakra at the base of the spine near the tailbone. Now concentrate on the image of an inverted, downward directed triangle situated inside a circle. In the center of the triangle, where the latent kundalini is stored, visualize an awakening serpent that is coiled around itself three and one-half times with its head facing upwards. As you concentrate on this chakra, experience the feelings of being grounded, the sense of physical and emotional stability and the inner security associated with this center. While listening to the mantra, feel the energy slowly moving upwards through the spine to the top of your head as you inhale and follow the energy back down the spine to the first chakra as you exhale. You may continue this awareness of energy movement for as long as you wish.

Meditation VI: Awareness of All the Chakras

Sit quietly with straight posture and practice progressive relaxation, abdominal breathing, breath awareness and sense withdrawal.

Be aware of the third eye, visualized as a circle with one lotus petal on each side of the rim of the circle, and mentally repeat or listen for the mantra *OM, So Ham* or your personal mantra. Then be aware of the seventh chakra. Next allow your awareness to come down to the first chakra, visualized as an inverted, downward directed triangle situated inside a circle. In the center of the triangle, where the latent kundalini is stored, visualize an awakening serpent that is coiled around itself three and one-half times with its head facing upwards. As you inhale, follow your breath, mind and mantra up to the second chakra located within the spinal cord. This center is directly opposite and slightly above the genital region. Visualize a crescent moon within a circle. Feel the balance of masculine and feminine qualities within and the inner strength to appropriately direct sensual and sexual energies. Continue to concentrate on this chakra from one to five minutes.

Then as you inhale, follow your breath, mind and mantra up to the third chakra located across from the navel within the spinal cord. Visualize an upward facing triangle inside a circle. Feel the heat and power here as the rising energy is amplified and concentrated at this important energy transformation center. Experience your individuality and the strength of your ego. Continue this concentration from one to five minutes.

Then as you inhale, follow your breath, mind and mantra up to the fourth chakra located across from the heart within the spine. Visualize two intersecting triangles (Star of David) situated inside a circle. In the center of the triangles, visualize yourself sitting in a meditative posture in a dark cave gazing at a flame from a candle that does not flicker. This light is described as being the reflection of the soul. Feel the calmness, sense of love and compassion associated with this center. Remain at this center from one to five minutes.

Then as you inhale, follow your breath, mind and mantra up to the fifth chakra across from the throat within the spine. Visualize a full moon on a dark blue sky inside a circle. At this center experience feelings of being nurtured by the higher consciousness that lies within. Feel your openness to accept creative impulses from an inner, unlimited source. Continue this focus from one to five minutes. If you tend to be a creative, artistic or musically talented person, you may want to spend extra time at this chakra.

Then as you inhale, follow your breath, mind and mantra up to the sixth chakra. Visualize the third eye being across from the center of the eyebrows in the deeper part of the middle brain. Experience the inner vision, insight and intuitive knowledge associated with this center. Allow the focus to remain here from one to five minutes.

Then as you inhale, follow your breath, mind and mantra up to the crown chakra located deep within the cortex of the brain. Again, visualize light from a thousand lotus petals shining brightly. Imagine your individual self-identity and the entire field of universal consciousness blending into one indissoluble whole. Continue this visualization from one to five minutes.

Then as you exhale, follow your breath, mind and mantra back to the third eye. Allow your attention to remain at this center, listening to the mantra, for the rest of the meditation and for as long as you wish. You may also maintain your concentration on the heart or throat center. The chakra you remain at for the rest of the meditation depends on instructions from your teacher and upon your own personality, emotional needs or spiritual strengths or weaknesses.

Meditation VII: Awareness of All Chakra Colors: the Complete Meditation

Sit quietly with straight posture and practice progressive relaxation, abdominal breathing, breath awareness and sense withdrawal.

With your focus of concentration continuing at the center of your forehead between the eyebrows (sixth chakra), visualize a third eye, seen as a white circle with one pale blue lotus petal on each side on the rim of the circle. Inside the circle is a small white inverted triangle. This is the center of insight, intuition and wisdom. This eye sees inwards, watching your thoughts, worries, memories and feelings float by. It is accompanied by non-judgmental awareness. Each time your mind is distracted, gently bring your concentration back to the image of the third eye.

Then begin to mentally repeat the sound of your mantra. You can use one of three different mantras: the mantra *OM*, the mantra *So Ham* or a personal mantra. You may want to coordinate your mantra with your breathing. You can repeat your mantra with each separate inhalation and exhalation, with one cycle of breathing that includes one inhalation and exhalation, or with several cycles. If you seem to hear the mantra resonating deep within, you may also simply listen to the inner sound and vibration of the mantra.

As you inhale, follow your breath, mind, and mantra upwards and bring your concentration to the top part of your brain, the cerebral cortex. Visualize a lotus flower with a thousand petals emanating either white light or the colors of the rainbow, four inches above your head. Imagine your individual self-identity and the entire field of universal consciousness blending into one indissoluble whole. Keep your focus here from one to five minutes.

As you exhale, follow the breath, mind and mantra down the center of the spine to the first chakra, located at the base of the spine near the tailbone. Visualize a red inverted, downward directed equilateral triangle surrounded by a yellow square, both shapes resting inside a circle. Resting on the rim of the circle are four crimson red lotus petals. In the center of the triangle, where the latent kundalini is stored, visualize an awakening serpent that is coiled around itself three and one-half times with its head facing upwards. In the center of the triangle, concentrate on the great amount of latent energy (kundalini) located here. Experience the feelings of being grounded, the sense of physical and emotional stability and the inner security associated with this center. Feel the energy slowly moving upwards through the spine from one to five minutes.

As you inhale, follow your breath, mind and mantra up to the second chakra located within the spinal cord. This center is directly opposite and slightly above the genital region. Visualize a silver-white crescent moon within a white circle. Resting on the rim of the circle are six crimson red lotus petals. Feel the balance of masculine and feminine qualities within and the inner strength to appropriately direct sensual and sexual energies. Continue to concentrate on this chakra from one to five minutes.

As you inhale, follow your breath, mind and mantra up to the third chakra located across from the navel within the spinal cord. Visualize a crimson red, upward facing triangle inside a white circle. Resting on the circle are ten dark blue lotus petals. Feel the great heat and power here, as the rising energy is amplified and concentrated at this important center of energy transformation. Experience your individuality and the strength of your own ego. Continue this concentration from one to five minutes.

As you inhale, follow your breath, mind and mantra up to the fourth chakra located across from the heart within the spine. Visualize two intersecting triangles (Star of David) that are a blue-green color inside a white circle. Resting on the rim of the circle are twelve dark crimson lotus petals. In the center of the triangles, visualize yourself sitting in a meditative posture in a dark cave gazing at a flame from a candle that does not flicker. This light is described as being the reflection of the soul. Feel the calmness, sense of love and compassion associated with this center. Remain at this center from one to five minutes.

As you inhale, follow your breath, mind and mantra up to the fifth chakra across from the throat within the spine. Visualize a white full moon against the background of a deep blue sky resting within a white triangle. A circle surrounds this and resting on the rim of the circle are sixteen purple lotus petals. As you concentrate on this center experience feelings of being nurtured by the higher consciousness that lies within. Feel your openness to accept creative impulses from an inner, unlimited source. Continue this focus from one to five minutes. If you tend to be a creative, artistic or musically talented person, you may want to spend extra time at this center of consciousness.

As you inhale, follow your breath, mind and mantra up to the sixth chakra, which is visualized as a white circle with one pale blue lotus petal on each side. Inside the circle is a small, white triangle that is pointed downwards. Inside the triangle is the symbol for *OM*. Visualize the third eye being across from the center of the eyebrows in the deeper part of the middle brain. Experience the inner vision, insight and intuitive knowledge associated with this center. Allow the focus to remain here from one to five minutes.

As you inhale, follow your breath, mind and mantra to the crown chakra, located deep within the cortex of the brain. Again, visualize white light or the colors of the rainbow emanating from a thousand lotus petals shining brightly upwards. Imagine your individual self-identity and the entire field of universal consciousness blending into one indissoluble whole. Continue this visualization from one to five minutes.

As you exhale, follow your breath, mind and mantra back to the third eye. Allow your attention to remain at this center, listening to your mantra, for the rest of the meditation and for as long as you wish. You may also maintain your concentration on the heart or throat center. The chakra where you remain for the rest of the meditation depends on instructions from your teacher and upon your individual personality traits, emotional needs and spiritual strengths or weaknesses.

Advanced Meditation Techniques

As you advance in your practice, attempt to spend longer periods in meditation. There are also several techniques that can be incorporated into your practice that can deepen your meditation. These more advanced techniques are directed at intensification of the previously described meditations. Some of these techniques help to activate the kundalini directly. This is particularly true when you apply the locks and practice breath retention. These latter physical techniques should be undertaken with caution because they tend to amplify and exaggerate physical, emotional and spiritual concerns that you may be experiencing at the time. Before you decide to make your practice more complex, it would be wise to seek advice from your meditation teacher. It is best to work closely with a meditation teacher who is skilled in these practices and who can discuss the wisdom of your doing these more advanced meditation techniques. If you have a strong inclination or intuition to attempt a new technique, try it slowly and methodically. Experiences in your own meditation can sometimes lead you to the next level and practice of meditation. This may occur if you spontaneously hear an inner sound or mantra, visualize a specific image or yantra or automatically begin to practice certain advanced breathing techniques or hatha yoga asanas.

Following are five examples of more advanced meditation techniques. You should have carefully and gradually completed all phases of the above-mentioned meditation practices before you consider undertaking these more advanced techniques.

1. Repeat the bija mantra as you concentrate on each chakra. As you ascend through each chakra, mentally repeat the following mantras: *Lam* at the first chakra, *Vam* at the second chakra, *Ram* at the third chakra, *Yam* at the fourth chakra, *Ham* at the fifth chakra, and *OM* at the sixth chakra.

2. After moving through all the chakras described in the complete meditation and having concentrated on the sixth chakra for some time, slowly let all inner visualizations disappear. Simply be present. Experience the mantra and the sounds of silence within. Continue this for as long as you wish.

3. After moving through all the chakras described in the complete meditation, bring your final concentration point to the guru chakra, located within the brain between the sixth and seventh chakras. This lesser known chakra is an extremely subtle center associated with experiences of fine vibrations, sublime mental images and feelings of bliss.

4. After practicing the complete meditation, visualize the entire universe and all of its creation dissolving into light. Breathe in this light and imagine the light dissolving into you. Visualize yourself dissolving from above and below simultaneously, with only the clear light of the flame in the center of the heart chakra remaining. This is the reflection of the soul that is constant and never changing.

5. After practicing the complete meditation, visualize a tiny transparent pearl of pure crystal at the sixth chakra. When the vision of this is totally clear, imagine yourself looking deeply through this pearl of pure, colorless light, with the transparency extending to infinity. Move this image to the crown chakra. Hold on to this perception of clear light and emptiness with single-pointed concentration. Realize that this infinite empty space has no category of the mind into which it can be placed. This is the experience of the void and the state of nothingness. It is in this state of total emptiness where you are most sensitive, open and receptive and where you can then be filled with the higher knowledge of universal consciousness.

PERSONAL EXPERIENCES WITH MEDITATION

When I was a student at the University of Michigan Medical School, about two years before my first meeting with Swami Rama, I noticed an advertisement on the Student Union message board. It stated there would be a demonstration of spiritual transmission by an Indian yogi later that day. Since I was already immersed in meditation practice, I decided to go to the event. As we were waiting for the program to begin, an Indian man walked in, followed by what appeared to be several of his students. He instructed us to lie down and relax.

After about ten minutes, I began to feel my mind leaving my body and traveling through a dark space at a very rapid speed. I could hear angelic voices and I could see light at the end of what seemed like a spiral tunnel. I felt a great sense of peace, joy and wonderment at where I was headed. Then all of a sudden, the lights went on in the room and the experience ended. The Indian yogi just smiled and left.

An older woman had stayed on and she and I discussed our experiences, which were somewhat similar. We felt that we had been in the same tunnel. This was my first out of body experience, and it both startled and excited me. It provided me a glimpse into an altered state of consciousness and motivated me to learn more.

Meditating with Swami Rama

When I was living at the ashram, Swamiji always seemed to know when I was meditating. He had told me to meditate at midnight. I remember once he told me that he knew I hadn't meditated one night. I told him that he was correct, and he smiled. That was the last time I didn't meditate at midnight while I was at the ashram.

One night I began to have an out of body experience and my body started to move spontaneously into advanced yoga postures that normally would have been very difficult or impossible for me to achieve. I also began to do advanced pranayama techniques with long periods of breath retention. Inner vibrations and energetic movements traveled up my spine and I felt great bliss and joy. I heard beautiful sounds that seemed like they were coming from another dimension. I began to speak in another language that I thought was Sanskrit. I also began to repeat certain mantras that I experienced as a form of initiation and I received a spiritual name. These experiences recurred nightly for several weeks and became more intense. I experienced great euphoria during that time. Ideas rushed into my head, and my studies of yogic, Tantric and Vedantic literature deepened. After many nights like this, I rushed to tell Swamiji and to share my experiences with him. But he wouldn't speak to me. Not even one word. He wouldn't even look at me or acknowledge my presence.

After weeks of ignoring me, I finally grabbed his meditation shawl and said, "Swamiji, why won't you talk to me?" He spun around like a top, looked directly into my eyes, looking quite annoyed. Then a sweet smile appeared on his face and he said,

"Sonny, don't you know that I know what is happening? Just do your practice and let meditation be your guide." Then he calmly walked away. We never spoke about this again. But I knew that he knew where my meditation was leading me and that he had something to do with these wondrous experiences.

I was learning that the spiritual teacher could transmit subtle energy to his students to help them on their journey towards expanded consciousness and deeper self-awareness. This transmission is called shaktipat and can be transferred from the teacher to the student through various intentional means, including meditation, thought, touch, gaze, mantra repetition, selected herbs or simply through an act of grace. Yogis can transcend the boundaries of time and space when the student is receptive and prepared and can transmit knowledge and experience to them.

In my case, Swamiji seemed to use several of the above methods to impart energy to me. Sleep and dreams also were vehicles of consciousness through which I experienced initiation. I learned that this subtle, latent spiritualized energy, which is transformed and directed, is called kundalini. This stored energy lies dormant within the pranic body of every human being. Spiritual insight and expansion of consciousness occurs when this energy is awakened and directed upwards through the body. This kundalini force resides in its potential form near the base of the spine in the first chakra, the lowest of the subtle body's energy centers. Once activated, it is said that the student's capacity to learn expands and spiritual experiences occur.

OM: **A Personal Experience**

At a large yoga conference that the Himalayan Institute had organized, Swami Rama guided a meditation using the mantra *OM*. After the meditation ended, I continued to hear the *OM* sound for many hours, deep within myself. The mantra kept reverberating and got louder as time went on. I felt great ecstasy and total immersion in something much larger than my individual self. Gradually, as the internal *OM* sound faded in intensity, it left me in a calm and joyful state of mind.

It was then that I more fully understood the great power of mantra and sound vibration and this has been a guide for me ever since. The experience of *OM* has continued to the present time, so that sometimes, the universal and beautiful *OM* sound spontaneously arises and permeates my consciousness. This is especially true during deeper and longer meditation sessions. The experience is always exhilarating.

Teaching Meditation

I have continued to practice and teach meditation in the style that Swamiji taught me. I have taught classes on various aspects of meditation, including pranayama and meditation, the use of mantra in meditation, bhakti yoga and kirtan, the interface between homeopathy and yogic philosophy, meditation and healing consciousness, meditation and energy medicine and meditation and tai chi. I have taught very large groups, workshops and seminars and I have also taught very small groups and individual sessions. I have some students who meditate with me in my medical practice. I have also taught raja yoga in workshops in my hometown of Ann Arbor. Since I often accompany Ruma to her scientific conferences on biochemistry research, I have sometimes been invited to teach tai chi in the mornings to her busy colleagues. I especially enjoyed teaching in Spain, on a boat journey through Russia and in Uruguay. Each of these settings offered the students and me different kinds of experiences. Also, I often lead a meditation practice after my lectures, and this affords an opportunity to learn and grow from the practice.

Teaching something that is intimate and yet practical like meditation has helped me to deepen my practice so that the experiences during meditation have become my guide. Knowledge of the traps, pitfalls and wonderment that can be experienced during meditation have helped me to guide others, to understand the obstacles they are experiencing on the path and to help them incorporate emotionally and psychologically the experiences characteristic of alternate or expanded consciousness.

I always mention that what I'm teaching has been handed down to me from Swami Rama and that it is a Himalayan Mountain tradition. It was through teaching meditation and pranayama that I met Ruma. In a sense, Swami Rama had a hand in helping me pick up my life and to find hope and love again after my divorce. Now, besides my own biological nuclear family, I am also part of a large and supportive Indian family that is spread across three continents.

From 2008-2018, I taught meditation and healing at the Sivananda Ashram in the Bahamas, Grass Valley, CA, Woodbourne N.Y. and in Kerala, India. I found resonance with Swami Sivananda's teachings because the emphasis on the eight-fold path of raja yoga in the Sivananda organization was similar to Swami Rama's teachings.

An Ongoing Life of Meditation and Medicine

The meditative techniques and medical approaches like homeopathy that Swami Rama imparted to me form the basis of my meditation and healing approaches today. This meditative tradition is based on the Eastern philosophies of Vedanta, Samkhya and Tantra and has been continuously handed down from teacher to student for thousands of years. These techniques are universal and not restricted to the observance of a specific religion. I have personally practiced all the techniques presented in these pages and have thoroughly studied the theory behind them. Zen and Tibetan Buddhist philosophy and psychology have also influenced my meditation practice, especially in the application of mindfulness, compassion and simplicity to everyday life. Also, in my own practice I incorporate several Jewish meditation techniques, which I have discussed in this book. Tai chi is the meditation in movement that I most enjoy and often practice.

Over the years, I have experienced periods when my meditation practice has seemed stagnant and have had other moments of great inspiration and creative insight. I have had experiences when my body spontaneously assumed different yoga postures and other times when I would automatically do advanced breathing exercises, indicating the activation and release of the kundalini. I have had visual and auditory experiences that I can only describe as inspiring, joyful and at times blissful. I have also had to face conscious and unconscious anxieties and fears that sometimes arise during meditation. I have tried to be consistent with my practice, although at times I have felt discouraged or simply lazy. However, through it all, meditation has provided me with the strength and courage to understand my past, enjoy the present and prepare for the future.

My personal meditation practice varies depending on the intellectual or emotional issues I'm attending to, my mood, my intentions or even the time of day. I have different foci of concentration including the breath, the chakras, a personal mantra given by Swamiji and Swami Ajaya or more complex mantras. With respect to the chakras, I mentally move up the chakras from the lowest to the highest and focus on various aspects of each chakra such as its associated element, sense, seed (bija) mantra, color, Sanskrit letter, deity or yantra. I often use yogic locks and breath retention during my practice.

Many years ago, I had a very strong feeling I should incorporate some ancient and powerful Jewish prayers into my meditation practice. However, I also felt hesitant because Swamiji had given me specific practices. I wrote to him to ask him if I could use these Kabbalistic techniques in my yogic meditation practice. Swamiji wrote back a very kind letter, expressing his love for me and saying that I should always trust my intuition about such things, reminding me again that I should let my meditation be my guide.

In my practice, I sometimes use the ancient Hebrew prayer, the *Shema,* when focusing on the heart chakra. I visualize the individual letters and its spiritual meaning. I also often focus on the letters of the mystical, unspoken name of God in Judaism, *Yod Hey Vav Hey.* Besides the Jewish prayer and name of God, I also occasionally work with the Tibetan mantra: *OM Mani Padme Hum.* In Tibetan, this mantra is *Om Mani Peme Hung.* Again, the use of this mantra tends to be with a heart-centered, fourth chakra meditation. Another Sanskrit mantra I chant in association with the fourth chakra is *Om Hrim Ham Sa So Ham Svaha.*

PART V:

The Practice of Holistic Medicine

HOLISTIC MEDICINE IN GENERAL

Principles of Holistic Medicine

Holistic practitioners do not always use alternative methods and treatments to help their patients, as sometimes surgery or allopathic medicines are required. But the holistic doctor attempts to use the least invasive and most health promoting system possible. There are numerous approaches to holistic medicine that have been used over the years. While I have experimented with several of these, there are a few modern and ancient systems that I feel have had the most applicability in my holistic medical practice. And so in Part V I will focus on the therapeutic modalities I use to treat body, mind and spirit from a holistic viewpoint and will present these modalities within the paradigms of meditation and the yoga philosophy systems of raja yoga, chakras and koshas, as these ancient concepts represent a holistic perspective of the human being. The modalities are: diet and nutrition from the point of view of modern nutritional science as well as the principles of Ayurveda; hatha yoga and other forms of exercise such as tai chi; breathing and pranayama practices as described in yoga philosophy; psychotherapy; meditation (path of raja yoga); and homeopathy. At this point I would like to emphasize that sometimes treatment may be focused on a particular kosha or chakra. However, since the koshas represent a continuum of the different levels of consciousness, whatever influences one of these levels will of necessity also have an effect on the other levels to varying degrees.

Likewise, although each of the chakras may represent a particular level of consciousness, the chakras are also interconnected.

Initially, the study of ancient and other holistic systems seemed overwhelming and confusing and exposed such a multitude of available techniques that underlying perspectives were not immediately apparent. However, as my inquiry and experience progressed, commonalities surfaced to reveal unifying principles behind the fundamental teachings of different medical and philosophical systems, which includes the following ten principles.

1. A fundamental acceptance of the integrated nature of human beings as spiritual, mental, emotional and physical beings is of utmost importance when building a model of holistic medicine. The human being is multidimensional, not simply a physical entity that somehow develops a mind and intelligence as offshoots of the brain's biochemistry. It follows that health and disease can best be assessed with complete knowledge as to the degree of malfunctioning present on each of the levels of human consciousness. This view contrasts with the belief system of modern scientific medicine, which is Descartian in its assumption that there is a dualistic relationship between the separate and distinct entities of mind and body. Accordingly, diseases that manifest mostly on the physical level are diagnosed and treated with little or no consideration as to corresponding mental and emotional well-being.

Western medicine acknowledges several categories of disease causation. These include infectious diseases, genetic or inherited problems, deficiency disorders, such as nutritional or endocrine imbalances, neoplastic or tumor growths, inflammatory processes characterized by swelling and heat, allergies, autoimmune disorders, degenerative problems, accidents, emotional disorders and a large group of idiopathic or unknown causes.

Many of the above categories actually describe pathological or physiological manifestations rather than precipitating causes of disease. Disorders of the body are often classified after the disease process has already affected specific tissue damage, because then the disorder is easily measured and categorized. The process that has occurred within the person, the underlying predisposition that allowed the disease to progress in the first place, is usually ignored. Questions that are overlooked include: What allows the bacteria, virus or cancer cell to grow? What underlying factor is responsible for the system to become so overly sensitized that autoimmune diseases develop?

In orthodox Western medicine, the split between mind and body is reflected in the high degree of physician specialization. While specialists do a great service because of their highly focused knowledge, they are limited in function and scope by seeing only a particular organ system and not the whole person. A typical example of this situation can be found in a patient with chronic headaches who first consults an internist. If laboratory tests are found to be negative, the patient is then sent for evaluation to a neurologist who also might not find a cause of the headaches. The next step is to be sent to a psychiatrist who probes into the patient's present or past life circumstances that may have predisposed him to headaches. Even if the psychiatrist gains some useful insights, the headaches may remain. The patient may then be referred to another specialist such as a physical medicine physician for further evaluation, but again the problem may persist.

What is missing is a unified approach that looks at the headache from many different levels simultaneously and not just as an organ system malfunction or pathological phenomenon. Holistic medicine understands that the total human being includes the body, breath, energy level, conscious mind, many levels of the unconscious and the superconscious or Self. Because disease tends to occur simultaneously on various levels, the holistic doctor must have approaches available that correspond to all of them. Awareness that the causes of disease are multidimensional is essential.

For example, if a person's breathing is characterized by pauses or shallowness, and if in association with this they suffer nervousness, insomnia and headaches, then it makes no sense to prescribe only aspirin or xanax. A holistic doctor sees the abnormality to be a breathing problem and teaches breathing exercises to eliminate the irregularities and restore balance in the autonomic nervous system. In this way the suffering patient learns to minimize their anxiety and headaches as well as to recognize advance signals of distress and how to prevent the onset of symptoms. Or after careful observation, the patient may recognize that certain foods trigger the onset of a headache and the elimination of those nutritional culprits could prevent the headache from recurring.

2. A philosophic perspective of medicine is required to help facilitate the integration of spirituality and medicine. A vitalistic view of medicine and health is necessary, which implies that the processes of life cannot be explained by the laws of biology, physics and chemistry alone, but that life is endowed with underlying energy that gives it the power of continuation and self-determination. Since this energy cannot be readily measured by the physical sciences, it has been disregarded in modern scientific or evidence-based medicine. In holistic medicine systems, however, it is understood that this vitality forms the very foundation for sound mental, emotional and physical well-being. To increase the individual's resistance to disease, this vitality must be strengthened. In other words, this vitality underlies the body's defense mechanisms. It operates outside of everyday waking consciousness and is thus called the body's innate intelligence. In yoga this energy is called prana, in Chinese philosophy it is chi and in homeopathy it is the vital force.

3. A realization of the balance and unity that exists between humanity and nature arises in the quest for holistic approaches to health care. A human being is a part of nature and is subject to its laws. By eating natural foods and avoiding processed foods laden with chemicals and preservatives, by recycling plastics and by using renewable energy to shrink one's carbon footprint, one is following these laws, thus creating the experience of greater harmony between the individual and the surrounding world.

4. An understanding that health is not merely the absence of disease is essential. Being healthy implies that an individual is capable of positively adapting to changes in inner and outer environments. Health is not a static phenomenon but a dynamic process reflecting a positive physical and mental adjustment to varying stressful circumstances. These stresses can assume many different forms: emotional upheaval, climatic events, microbial infestation or enervating habits of one's everyday lifestyle.

5. Self-responsibility is a very important component in a holistic system of care. Although the therapist and the patient have an equally important role in a holistic medical care system, the patient must be highly motivated, sincere and willing to accept responsibility for his or her health. As long as one blames the outside world for one's ills, they will remain dependent. Such a person considers the weather, other people or tiny microbes to be the cause of disease and feels that treatment should be directed at eliminating those external conditions or organisms. Holistic medical systems also acknowledge that the environment is closely interconnected with human beings and may well contribute to ailments. Yet the holistic practitioner will go further in maintaining that it is the internal state of the body, breath, mind and habits that determines whether one is susceptible to illness. If one is balanced and living in harmony with respect to nutrition, exercise, breathing habits and emotions, then external factors will have less effect on general health. The immune system will respond appropriately to infectious agents and the nervous system will remain balanced. What this means is that a holistic practitioner should help guide the individual to realize that they are responsible for their well-being. Having recognized potentially harmful habits, the holistic doctor teaches the patient practical ways to change these habits and to replace them with positive, health-oriented ones.

6. Growth orientation is an offshoot of self-responsibility. An orientation towards personal growth is important as it leads the individual to take responsibility for maintaining health and overcoming susceptibility to disease. A holistic medical group should provide the stimulus and practical techniques for self-growth and enhanced self-knowledge. In order to guide the patient to new insights, the doctor or health professional should be a teacher as well as a healer. Both physician and patient should look at all life circumstances as potentially growth promoting and recognize that illness could provide an opportunity for the patient to learn about himself. Once a person becomes aware of harmful habits, negative modes of thought, emotional reactions and how they affect body and mind, they can slowly gain control over them. As a consequence, more energy is conserved and is available to be channeled into creativity. Then, as one's inner potential is gradually realized, growth and expansion of consciousness also occur.

Being healthy does not mean a person never feels mental or physical pain, but that they are able to put them in perspective and can learn from the experience and continue to grow. They are free to experience the full gamut of emotions but do not become enslaved to them. In accordance with this definition of health, symptoms represent the organism's attempt to reestablish homeostasis and well-being and are thus informative and protective.

Healthy people learn to view their symptomatology positively as a tool and as feedback that something is amiss internally. Many physical symptoms can be understood to be the body's attempt to eliminate wastes or toxins, as exemplified by skin eruptions or mucous membrane discharges. Mental and emotional symptoms can be viewed as the psyche's attempt to bring emotional repressions to the surface. A person who has chosen to be treated from the perspective of holistic medicine makes effort to live simply with awareness and is open to exploring the underlying causes of his or her illness. A curiosity about life's vicissitudes and unfolding circumstances, whether pleasant or painful, is ever present. The knowledge that is gained in this process helps one feel more powerful and less victimized by illness and is fundamental to understanding the basic universal phenomena of cause and effect.

7. **Nonsuppression** is an important aspect of holistic thinking. In a holistic system the techniques for establishing physical and mental homeostasis as well as the medicinal agents used are not designed to suppress symptoms. This can best be understood by using an analogy to psychotherapy. Thoughts and feelings that are repressed or suppressed are forced into deeper levels of the unconscious mind. Here they remain, causing the person either to act in unconscious ways and develop unconscious habits, or to erupt with uncontrolled and unpredictable force. In the psychotherapeutic process, the mental health practitioner helps the person uncover and reevaluate this unconscious material and then to diffuse and channel the built-up emotions.

Physical symptoms, similar to emotional ones, should not be forced deeper into the organism. It is not advisable to routinely and simply suppress skin eruptions with topical creams, inhibit fever with antipyretics or alleviate headaches with analgesics. All of these symptoms are reflections of inner imbalances, and even if the symptoms are ameliorated by drugs, the underlying process that caused the symptoms to occur may still persist. The therapeutic techniques of the holistic doctor lead to increased self-awareness and also strengthen the body's defenses. In the example of fever, the holistic doctor sees it as a signal that the body is actively at work defending itself. He or she may use natural herbs or homeopathic remedies that gently assist the body in the healing process, strengthen the immune system and at the same time minimize the concurrent suffering.

If drug or surgical intervention seems appropriate, the holistic practitioner will intelligently suggest these modalities. But after the crisis situation has ended, the physician commits to help the patient quickly recover and then to resolve the underlying imbalances that caused the illness. In essence, the holistic doctor respects the body's innate ability to heal itself and uses medicines and other methods that enhance the natural and inherent self-healing process.

8. Nontoxicity is an important concept in modern medical treatment. The idea of nontoxicity is the natural extension of nonsuppression. Since there are several million adverse reactions to medicinal prescription drugs yearly in the US, and because there were over 70,000 deaths in 2018 due to the recent opioid crisis, the question of medicinal toxicity becomes quite relevant. There are different remedies, herbs and drugs that can be matched carefully with individual problems and needs. The holistic doctor should study the various systems of medicine in order to determine the safest and most effective treatment possible. The holistic practitioner cautiously uses medicinal substances so as not to create more problems than the ailing person is already experiencing. In addition, the medicine or the remedy should cure or palliate the symptoms, while at the same time strengthen immunity.

9. Decreased cost is of major importance as hospital and drug costs are exorbitant and rising rapidly, and no way has been found to stem the inflation. Therefore, the most feasible alternative is to remain healthy. A holistic system should teach people how to sleep, eat, breathe and direct their emotions towards creativity. The initial financial output in learning these things may be slightly more than the quick interview and physical examination that is often given by one's allopathic physician. In the long run, however, the holistic system should save money for the patient and the community because one learns how to prevent illness before serious complications set in.

10. Access to care and insurance reform need to improve in the US. Due to poverty, lack of transportation and a dearth of funding in rural and inner-city areas, there are too many people who have little to no way to get their health care needs met. This includes areas such as routine primary care visits, emergency care and preventive services such as immunization and family planning. A more holistic approach to medicine could be helpful not only to encourage prevention but also to help bring down costs. The Affordable Care Act (Obama Care) offering everybody a free preventive medicine exam is a step in the right direction. And of course, national health care coverage for everyone is the ideal.

MY HOLISTIC PRACTICE

I am not a great risk taker; I would not attempt to parachute out of planes or climb dangerous rock faces, nor am I an intrepid world explorer. But some might consider it risky that I chose an unconventional career as a holistic physician, combining ancient Eastern transcendental and modern Western scientific approaches to health and healing. This does not mean I don't love modern Western medicine. From a personal health perspective, if not for excellent surgical intervention I might have died at age seven from a ruptured appendix. I would have lived my entire adult life completely blind if not for bilateral cataract surgery at age twenty-five. More recently, I might have been in kidney failure and possibly on dialysis if not for timely medical and surgical treatment. And most recently, a simple decompression surgery of my lower spine has allowed me to walk and stand without pain after many years of persistent discomfort.

And from a professional perspective, I have helped innumerable patients with the best of what the pharmaceutical industry and surgical referrals have to offer. However, throughout my professional career I have found that health and disease are multi-factorial and multi-dimensional and thus require multiple perspectives to complete the limited outlook of Western medicine that tends to focus mainly on the physical body.

My holistic practice is primarily based on yoga and meditation and the paradigms of the koshas and chakras because these philosophies recognize that humans exist on several levels. It naturally follows that disease also occurs on different levels, and that diagnosis and treatment should be focused at the appropriate level. Thus, the construct of the sheaths represents a model of preventive and holistic medicine that offers both conceptual theory and pragmatic treatment approaches into which various conventional and alternative therapeutic systems of health care could be organized and integrated. A therapeutic approach that incorporates the concepts of the koshas and the chakras provides very practical methods to analyze the problems that manifest on all levels: spiritual, philosophical, mental and emotional, energy and physical. There are various therapeutic modalities that fit well within these paradigms. This will become clearer when I examine how specific disorders or imbalances can be treated from this perspective when I describe different case histories towards the end of the book.

HOLISTIC THERAPEUTIC MODALITIES

I will be discussing only those therapeutic modalities that I use in my medical practice. These are: diet, nutrition and supplements; hatha yoga, tai chi and exercise; breathing and pranayama; psychotherapy; meditation as described in the practices of raja yoga; and homeopathy. I will describe each of these treatment modalities in relation to the different koshas and chakras in general and more specifically in the case histories.

Diet and Nutrition

The field of nutritional science is very complex biochemically and physiologically and well beyond the scope of this book. So I will discuss some general principles relevant to my holistic practice and how food plays an integral part in my approach to health within the paradigms of the koshas as well as raja yoga and Ayurveda. Based on the kosha paradigm, diet and nutrition are obviously of paramount importance in both the prevention and treatment of ailments of the outermost kosha. At this level, alternative approaches include more focus on natural foods and extensive supplementation with vitamins and minerals. This will be discussed in more detail under the topic of vegetarianism.

The types of foods a person eats and their attitude towards food is important in my medical practice as well as in the yoga tradition. In fact, many of my patients seek my advice on diet and nutrition. Fad diets and confusion about what to eat are commonplace. Obesity, hypertension, cancer, heart disease and diabetes all have some component of faulty nutrition. Everyone needs to eat healthy foods, therefore one of the first things I do when doing the initial assessment of a new patient is to have them fill out a four-day diet record. This gives me an idea not only of the quality of the foods they eat but also about their attitude towards their food selection. In addition, a blood test provides information about cholesterol and triglyceride levels and blood sugar. If elevated, we look at how to change their diet, often minimizing animal-based protein and encouraging whole foods. We also evaluate how weight loss could help normalize blood parameters.

How Food Affects Body and Mind

Fortunately, Western medicine has begun to broaden its understanding of how nutrition can affect the body, emotions, personality and mental states. For example, it is now recognized that foods that contain artificial colorings and preservatives can instigate hyperactivity in children and adults, and that allergic reactions to some foods can lead to irritability and confusion.

When strict attention is paid to what is being put into the mouth, it becomes evident that each food not only has a different taste, smell and consistency but also creates a unique subjective feeling. Eating a light salad leaves quite a different feeling from eating a big slice of roast beef. Similarly, eating an apple creates different feelings than consuming a banana split.

From the perspective of the Western scientist, these changes in the state of psychological functioning can be attributed to the pharmacological properties of food. Although food is primarily used for nutrients, many foods contain substances that have pharmacological effects on the mind and body. For example, milk and meat contain relatively high quantities of tryptophan, an amino acid that has a sedative property. This is one reason why a person feels sleepy after eating a large serving of meat or drinking a warm glass of milk at bedtime. Many other effects of food, however, cannot be as easily explained by simply using the laws of pharmacology.

However, by careful observation and especially through the clarity and receptivity developed through meditation, it is possible for the individual to determine which foods create a positive effect and which a negative one. For example, certain foods like grains and cooked vegetables are conducive to feelings of calmness. Other foods such as fruits have a lighter or more energetic feeling associated with them. Some foods like oatmeal have a warming quality or a stick-to-the-ribs feeling, whereas others like melons create a cooling effect. By paying attention to what foods in particular or what combinations of foods cause a bloated feeling, mental dullness or emotional lability, one can learn about one's particular reaction patterns and idiosyncrasies. The person can then intelligently alter the diet, eliminating problem foods and incorporating foods that lead to mental calmness and physical vigor. Coupled with a basic knowledge of nutritional requirements, one can experiment with the subjective qualities of food and formulate a personal checklist based on direct experience.

Unfortunately, most Americans grow up on a diet of processed foods saturated with sugar, trans fats and chemical additives and preservatives. They are accustomed to eating canned soups, frozen vegetables and white bread that stays "fresh" for weeks. To add to the problem, the sense of taste and smell are dulled by smoking cigarettes and air pollution. Eating on the run also prevents any appreciation of the taste or consistency of food, much less its subtle psychological influences. As a result, many people have lost the ability to discriminate for themselves which foods they really need to eat. Thus, the desire for food is often based on habit or easy availability rather than the nutritional needs of the body.

On a more positive note, the process of eating could be a means of self-expression and a vehicle for expanding awareness. The food an individual chooses reflects one's attitude towards oneself and the world. People who are always in a hurry will frequent fast food restaurants or pick foods that are pre-packaged or easy to prepare. They eat quickly and may suffer from digestive discomfort such as heartburn, flatulence, diarrhea or constipation. If a person is insensitive to their environment or their inner feelings and urges, they will have little appreciation for the subtle tastes and smells in their diet. However, anyone willing to make the effort, to let go of old habits and allow the inherent senses to take over, will find that by merely assessing how they feel after eating, the whole question of diet and nutrition becomes a simple matter.

There is a vast amount of information written about nutrition, including diet and weight loss, the types of vitamins, minerals and nutraceuticals needed for health and a growing interest in the specialty of functional medicine. Antioxidant foods such as broccoli and blueberries as well as natural anti-inflammatory foods like turmeric are described in great detail in both the scientific journals and the lay public social media. Because of easy availability of this information, I am not going to discuss these dietary issues in this book. Instead, I will offer just a bit in areas that greatly interest me and play an important role in my holistic medical practice.

The Microbiome

The microbiome is an example of how the physical body and mental functioning are interconnected. The word *microbiome* is defined as "the collection of microbes or microorganisms that inhabit an environment, creating a sort of mini-ecosystem." The human microbiome is made up of communities of symbiotic, commensal and pathogenic bacteria (along with fungi and viruses) all of which call our bodies their home. The microbiome also includes the collective genes of the microbes that live inside and on the human body. Within the individual there are about ten times as many microbial cells as human cells. The number of genes in the microbiome outnumbers the number of genes in the cellular genome by one hundred to one. In all, there are about 100 trillion microbes and 7 trillion microbial genes.

When a person is healthy, the plethora of bacteria, viruses and fungi work together and help to maintain the body's homeostasis. The microbiome is often referred to as an organ due to its importance in supporting and maintaining the health of both body and mind. Every person has a unique network of microbiota, which reflects such things as one's genetic inheritance, delivery through the vaginal canal and its microflora, exposure to mother's breast milk, the ecology of one's living conditions, types of food ingested, illnesses and antibiotic use. Generally, the microorganisms of the microbiome coexist, but if there is disruption of this symbiosis (mutually beneficial relationship), dysbiosis (microbial imbalance) can occur, leading to disease.

Besides being the organ system that digests food through absorption, assimilation and metabolism, the intestinal tract has other vital functions. There is an intimate connection among the microbiome, the intestinal tract and the brain. The intestinal tract, also referred to as the gut, has over 50 million nerve cells, about the same as the spinal cord. This is why it is called the enteric nervous system. In addition, taste and smell receptors lie within intestinal endocrine-secreting cells, which cause a release of hormones that affect brain functioning such as hunger, satiety, food cravings and food aversions. These cells secrete the protein ghrelin, which directly stimulates appetite.

Also, ninety percent of the body's serotonin, which is responsible for pain sensitivity and mood, is found in the gut cells. Serotonin is the chemical that acts as a neurotransmitter between nerve cells (neurons). Medication is often used to target serotonin when treating depression, including some of the well-known drugs: prozac, paxil, zoloft, celexa and lexapro. These are called selective serotonin reuptake inhibitors (SSRI) and work by blocking the reabsorption of serotonin back into neurons, allowing more to be available. The theory is that the more serotonin available, the better is the transmission of messages between neurons, which improves the mood and alleviates depression. Since so much serotonin is secreted in the intestinal tract, it is easy to understand how digestion and moods are so closely interrelated.

Located within the Peyer's patches of the small and large intestine are immune cells that not only kill unfriendly bacteria that may be present in our food but also help general immunological functioning. The major nerve that facilitates communication between the gut and the brain is the vagus nerve, and the vast majority of nerve signals travel from the gut to the brain rather than the opposite way, meaning that the intestinal tract is constantly sending messages to the brain.

To better understand why the microbiome affects so many organs, it is helpful to know how these connections have evolved. Single-celled microorganisms have lived in the murky and watery underworld here on earth for billions of years. Through trial and error and natural selection, these microbes learned how to communicate by sending signals through molecules to each other, affecting the behavior of one another. When marine animals began to evolve, these same microbes incorporated themselves into the rudimentary digestive systems of these minute ocean-dwelling animals. As this symbiotic relationship grew and animals continued to evolve, so did the sophistication of the communication. Simple nervous systems developed, and as this relationship became more sophisticated, more and more signaling chemicals helped to transmit information through the neuro-circuitry. This was the beginning of the gut-brain connection.25

As this relationship continued to evolve, the microbes helped the animal digest foods better and helped to synthesize important vitamins and to prevent damaging effects of food toxins and alien bacteria, viruses, parasites and fungi. An example of how the microbiome is helpful to the digestive process is seen when people eat whole grains. Since the GI system cannot fully break down all the fibers, there are resultant remnants called small chain fatty acids (SCFAs). The microbiome then will help further digest these SCFAs, allowing for an increase of available calories. A further breakdown product of these SCFAs is called butyrate, which helps the body to decrease inflammation and improve immune functioning. Not only does the human host benefit from these microbes, the microbes also benefit from this symbiosis by having a warm, safe environment to thrive and grow and to have abundant food to feast on.

Leaky Gut Syndrome

Leaky gut syndrome remains a bit of a medical mystery, and medical professionals are still trying to determine exactly what causes it. There are millions of bacteria in the gut, some beneficial and some harmful. When the balance between the two is disrupted, it can affect the barrier function of the intestinal wall. Similarly, yeast is naturally present in the gut, but an overgrowth of yeast may contribute to a leaky gut. A protein called zonulin is the only known regulator of intestinal permeability. When zonulin is activated in genetically susceptible people, it can lead to a leaky gut. Two factors that trigger the release of zonulin are specific types of bacteria in the intestines, and gluten, a protein found in wheat and other grains. However, some studies have shown that gluten only increases intestinal permeability in people with conditions like celiac disease or irritable bowel syndrome.

There are multiple contributing factors to leaky gut syndrome. A diet high in sugar, particularly fructose, harms the barrier function of the intestinal wall. The long-term use of NSAIDs like ibuprofen or aspirin can increase intestinal permeability and contribute to a leaky gut. Excessive alcohol intake may also increase intestinal permeability. Allergies to proteins in certain foods can damage the intestinal wall and cause increased permeability. Milk protein is an especially problematic allergen as well as wheat, eggs, soy and corn. Deficiencies in vitamin A, vitamin D and zinc have each been implicated in increased intestinal permeability. Chronic inflammation throughout the body can contribute to leaky gut syndrome. In addition, fatty foods, simple sugars, food additives and stress can cause a thinning of the thick and thin mucus intestinal barrier, allowing it to become more permeable. As a result, less friendly gut microbiota can come too close to the blood and lymphatic systems and release proteins that can penetrate the normally intact intestinal cell membranes. This causes release of an overabundance of signaling inflammatory molecules like cytokines, which can cause a cascade of other inflammatory reactions to occur, leading to systemic inflammatory disorders. If these cytokines bind to receptors on the vagus nerve, inflammation can occur in any part of the body that receives vagal stimulation like the brain, joints, cardiac tissue or the intestinal wall itself.

When the brain is affected by these cytokines, research has shown that certain neurological and neuropsychiatric illnesses can occur, including Parkinsonism, Alzheimer's disease, autism as well as obsessive-compulsive disorder, attention deficit hyperactivity disorder and chronic fatigue syndrome. Stress disorders like anxiety, depression and hypertension have been associated with changes in the gut microbiome. Disorders of the gut-brain connection affect the functioning of the hypothalamus, causing impaired levels of cortical releasing factors, which in turn cause disordered release of cortisol and norepinephrine, leading to abnormal stress responses. Meditation can help with chronic stress, which is a contributing factor to multiple gastrointestinal disorders, including leaky gut.

There is evidence that there is a difference in the intestinal microbiota between lean and obese people. The typical American diet of high calorie sugar and animal fat may adversely affect the intestinal tract by allowing more calories to be extracted and absorbed from food, contributing to increased weight gain. In fact, when lean mice have a fecal transplant from obese mice, the lean mice gain weight more easily. More obese mice have a fifty percent decrease in the microbial organisms called bacteriodetes and an increase in firmicutes, both of which are associated with weight gain. A plant-based diet, on the other hand, seems to result in a wider range of healthy lean-associated bacteria.

A recent study found statistically significant differences in the microbiome between healthy donors and people with multiple sclerosis (MS). Differences were also found between people with relatively stable MS and those with more progressive disease. Also, animal models have demonstrated that gut bacteria can initiate the immune-meditated demyelination that is typical of MS. There were also helpful species of bacteria that were more abundant in healthy controls compared to patients with relapsing-remitting, active and stable multiple sclerosis.26

For a healthier microbiome, one should eliminate sugar and processed foods from their diet. Refined carbohydrates, sugar and processed foods get absorbed quickly into the small intestine without any help from the microbes, which makes efficient and complete digestion more difficult. Because of this, it is best to get carbohydrates from vegetables and low-sugar fruits. Eating certain foods will help replenish the gut with healthy and diverse bacteria, including green leafy vegetables, radishes, Jerusalem artichokes, leeks, jicama, asparagus, carrots, garlic and turmeric.

It is good to include fermented foods that have helpful types of bacteria, such as sauerkraut, pickles, kimchi, kefir, yogurt (not processed) and kombucha. These foods are all rich in prebiotics, which include many healthy forms of bacteria. Glutamine, an amino acid (a building block of protein), can also help to rebuild and maintain the digestive tract and support proper digestion through improving the microbiome balance. In addition to eating the right foods, it is helpful to get into a meditative or relaxed state prior to eating. People who practice yoga and meditation believe that if you are eating in the company of other persons, you should try not to speak excessively or talk about negative subjects. Silence during meals is a yogic practice.

Gastric Esophageal Reflux Disorder (GERD)

Meditation, yoga postures and a sattvic type of diet can help prevent and alleviate hyperacidity, also called GERD. In this condition the esophagus becomes irritated or inflamed because of acid backing up from the stomach. When food is swallowed, it travels down the esophagus. The stomach produces hydrochloric acid after a meal to aid in the digestion of food, especially proteins. The cells of the inner lining of the stomach secrete large amounts of protective mucus to resist corrosion by this acid. Because the lining of the esophagus does not share these resistant features, stomach acid can damage it. The esophagus lies just behind the heart, so the term "heartburn" was coined to describe the burning sensation of excess acid. A ring of muscle at the bottom of the esophagus, the lower esophageal sphincter, prevents reflux (backing up) of acid. This sphincter relaxes during swallowing to allow food to pass and then tightens to prevent flow in the opposite direction.

With GERD, however, the sphincter relaxes between swallows, allowing stomach contents (gastric reflux) and corrosive acid to well up and damage the lining of the esophagus. GERD affects about twenty percent of the US population. Not just adults are affected; even infants and children can have GERD. To prevent GERD, it is best to maintain a healthy weight, eat less and slowly. Good sattvic foods to eat are dairy, oats, low-fat foods, vegetables, ginger, whole grains, egg whites, noncitrus fruits like bananas and apples and healthy fats like avocados, olive oil, flaxseeds and walnuts. Foods to avoid when GERD is problematic are tomato sauce and other tomato-based products, high-fat foods, such as fast food products and greasy foods, fried foods, citrus fruit juices, sodas, caffeine, chocolate, raw garlic, raw onions, mint and alcohol.

Ayurvedic Approach to Holistic Nutritional Medicine

Yoga and meditation philosophy are closely associated with the science of Ayurveda. Ayurveda was the dominant form of medicine in India for several thousand years, but only in the last 200 years has the Ayurvedic physician (*vaidya*) come to share responsibilities with homeopathic and allopathic practitioners. Today, Ayurveda still remains the primary treatment system in many villages of India, where the availability of modern medicine may be limited. Besides the focus on medicinal herbs, therapeutic massages and individualized dietary prescriptions, Ayurveda encompasses a variety of other therapeutic approaches, including hatha yoga, pranayama and meditation.

Over many centuries, Ayurvedic practitioners have determined which foods best suit a person's particular health needs. From this experimentation an empirical science of nutrition has evolved, which has revealed the most efficient ways to cultivate, prepare and combine foods as well as how to use food medicinally. In other words, food itself, not just the extracted and concentrated vitamin and mineral fractions, is medicine. Nutrition forms the very foundation of health.

I do not consider myself an Ayurvedic physician because the study of Ayurveda requires many years of formal training. But I do use the basic principles of Ayurveda that correlate with commonsense approaches to nutrition. Rudolph Ballentine and Swami Rama taught me how to approach a patient with Ayurvedic principles and perspectives, especially with respect to a person's constitutional and nutritional tendencies. What I present in this book is a synopsis of this very practical approach to understanding people's individual constitutional tendencies.

While dietary manipulation serves as a foundation for treatment, the Ayurvedic physician is also trained in other types of intervention. Often the approach used may be designed for specific locales, as in the mountains of northern India. Here, where a great variety of different herbs are available because of the wide range of climatic conditions in a small geographic area, botanicals are used to a large extent. For example, the ancient Ayurvedic doctors (vaidyas) used a preparation made from a fungus to treat certain infections, as is done today in the case of penicillin. Furthermore, they had knowledge of the use of a potent drug used in the preparation of the antihypertensive drug reserpine as well as many herbs to induce or reduce nausea, vomiting or urination.

In southern India, emphasis has been placed on massage, steam baths and the use of emetics and enemas. Furthermore, vaidyas prepare medicines from minerals, some of which are toxic in their native state, such as arsenic and mercury. Through proper preparation, the toxicity of the metal is removed, rendering a valuable therapeutic agent. It is interesting that some of the remedies take decades to prepare, and it is common practice for a physician to begin the preparation of a remedy so that his or her grandson can eventually use it. Many other traditional Ayurvedic remedies and concepts have found usage in modem medicine.

For example, garlic and onions have been used by Ayurvedic practitioners to prevent platelet aggregations and therefore may be effective to prevent blood clots.

It is noteworthy that thousands of years ago Ayurveda had a degree of surgical sophistication, especially in the field of plastic surgery. The Indian physicians, using simple yet sophisticated equipment, were able to sew back anatomical parts such as noses and ears severed in battle, and showed a deftness that made them famous in their lifetime. It is only recently, with the advent of new instrumentation and technology, that modem surgeons have been able to do comparable work.

Ayurvedic Clinical Applications: The Five Elements and Three Doshas

To understand the philosophic perspective of Ayurveda in more pragmatic terms, one needs to more fully explore the concept of the five elements. In the *Caraka Samhita,* an ancient Indian treatise on medicine, Vol. 2. p. 44, it is stated that all that we call life is composed of combinations of the five basic elements: ether (space), air, fire, water and earth.

Ayurveda has interesting advantages over conventional Western medical systems when evaluating some diseases. In orthodox Western diagnosis, there is no underlying principle that integrates mind and body. For instance, there is no explanation why a person may be troubled with constipation, have cracked nails and fluctuating appetite, and at the same time have reoccurring dreams of flying and insomnia as well as being anxious and fearful. A Western physician would pose several different reasons for these problems and may suggest many different drugs and therapies.

An Ayurvedic practitioner would evaluate the above person by recognizing that all humans in health and disease are composed of the three doshas that have distinct qualities with respect to foods and constitutions. These include *vata* (air and space), *pitta* (fire) and *kapha* (water and earth) and represent the *tridosha* theory in Ayurveda. In this vein of thought, an Ayurvedic practitioner would perceive the above problems as being related to an underlying predominance in the air element (vata). In this sense, Ayurvedic "physiology" transects the dichotomy of mind and body by showing that certain tendencies or ailments have their roots in an elemental imbalance that pervades both the physical and mental levels. It follows that foods should be prescribed that are low in the air quality and higher in the fire and water elements.

If one dosha becomes too predominant, it drives the person towards illnesses that reflect the qualities of that dosha. The tridosha system is strikingly similar to the five element theory in Chinese medicine and restates the principle of unity and balance that prevails between a human's existence and the natural world. This balance and unity in nature is recognized as a basic concept in ancient medical models.

In terms of diet, heavy foods such as dairy products and meat are considered kaphic. People that demonstrate a kaphic constitution tend to be large, overweight and perspire easily. Kapha also implies the quality of psychological heaviness, as exemplified by depression and apathy. In terms of eating, kaphic foods tend to make one feel heavy and lethargic and stimulate mucus production. After eating a very heavy and rich meal, a person often feels phlegmatic and torpid. Physiologically, the seat of kapha is considered to be in the lungs and the upper stomach. Thus, in kaphic diseases like asthma and upper respiratory infections, there is often an increased production of mucus. Abstinence from kaphic food would be recommended to a patient with a cold who is producing a lot of mucus, to an overweight patient or to someone who complains of lethargy and fatigue. Also, pittic foods that "burn off" kapha, might be prescribed.

Pittic foods include cooked foods, hot peppers and spicy foods. Pittic personalities are intense, energetic, fiery and hot blooded types. The duodenum and solar plexus are considered to be the location of the fire element. Pitta allows the body to burn food and transform it into energy. It is pitta that gives gastric fire its power, and it is no wonder that a person who exemplifies a pittic personality and is easily angered and hot tempered, often develops ulcers and stomach pain. The problem is that there is too much fire (pitta), and, he is in a sense burning himself up. The treatment would obviously be to reduce the fire by first cutting down on fuel and then to cool it off with water. Thus, the Ayurvedic physician would suggest eliminating foods that create excessive quantities of pitta, like hot or spicy foods, stimulants and alcohol. Raw foods such as nuts and salads would also be eliminated because these foods are very complex structurally and require more digestive fire in order to be broken down. A suitable diet would consist of foods that have a cooling or kaphic effect, such as milk and yogurt, vegetables and grains that have been well cooked. Cooked foods are more digestible and stimulate less pitta to insure their assimilation.

Vatic foods include many fruits and raw vegetables. A vatic type of personality might be seen as intellectual, heady or even spacy in an extreme sense. Many mental disorders are often considered to be vatic in nature. Eating only raw fruits and vegetables tends to make one feel lighter and psychologically less grounded. Too much vata can create an air of unreality as well as lack of concern for others and a tendency towards irresponsibility. The center for vata is the colon, and many intestinal diseases such as diarrhea and constipation result from vatic imbalances. Vata is the energy principle that conveys motion and its dynamic quality is apparent in the fact that constipation often leads to headaches.

Vata, which normally moves downwards in the body to cause the expulsion of solid wastes, can on occasion move upwards. When this happens, the stool tends to remain in the intestines, and as vata reverses course and moves upwards, this can manifest itself as a disturbance in the upper part of the body, resulting in conditions such as headache. One possible effective treatment for constipation is to drink a glass of hot water to which have been added the juice from half a lemon, a pinch of salt and honey to taste. This traditional folk remedy is a very effective natural laxative and is very mild. It restores the normal movement of vata downwards, reestablishing elimination and thus the disappearance of the headache.

A concrete example of using the tridosha principle in illness is found in the case of diarrhea that occurs in the summer months. Because diarrhea is considered to be a fire (hot) ailment and because the summer is a hot season, then it follows that eating hot foods could further increase heat and cause or aggravate diarrhea. The

Ayurvedic practitioner would discourage the eating of hot foods — those foods that interact with the body to create heat. According to Ayurvedic understanding, a food is hot because, when it is ingested, its chemical components induce secretion of digestive products of a particular composition appropriate to digest the food, and these in turn affect parts of the endocrine system that govern digestion. Hormones are then secreted that produce the effect of the "heat" of the food by strengthening the fire element. In the above case, examples of hot foods are mangos, walnuts and spicy foods. Cooling foods like yogurt and cooling drinks would be recommended to treat the diarrhea. By taking a preventive approach of avoiding fire-inducing foods during the summer months or by simply changing food choices if diarrhea does occur, the use of drugs could be avoided.

Another example of the Ayurvedic tridosha concept can be verified by Western common sense. When a person has a mucus condition (kapha) such as an allergy or upper respiratory infection, seasoning food with cayenne pepper or ginger to make it hot (pitta) will heat up the body's mucous membranes, which has the effect of decreasing the mucus-forming properties and clearing out the sinuses.

Much of Ayurveda revolves around the medicinal use of foods and spices to prevent and treat illness. Ayurveda also recognizes properties of foods in categories of dry or rough, oily or smooth, and heavy or light. These properties also have therapeutic applications. For example, if a person has a runny nose, their discomfort could be helped by using more drying foods like millet, buckwheat, chickpea, honey or black pepper. On the other hand, constipation is a dry condition. There is not enough water in the stool, which is therefore hard or crumbling. This can be treated by oily foods such as coconut, fats or overly ripe bananas. However, bananas that are greenish and not yet ripe would aggravate constipation.

Related to this is the idea of taste that is expounded upon in Ayurveda. According to the science of Ayurvedic nutrition, taste is not only a function of a particular food but, more importantly, a function of the person eating the food. This can be easily verified by observing that when a person gets the flu, or in more extreme cases like hepatitis, food no longer tastes the same. Here the food hasn't really changed but the person eating the food has. Curiously, one of the more unusual symptoms of the current Covid-19 pandemic is a loss of smell and taste.

Another way to appreciate the idea of taste is by looking at how spices can be used. While Western science maintains that spices have little nutritional value and only add flavor, Ayurveda goes much further to maintain that spices can change a food's properties and affect the way the food interacts with the body. The subtle tastes of foods and spices have important effects on each of the doshas. The six tastes are: bitter, astringent, pungent, salty, sour, and sweet. Honey is sweet according to this classification, but unlike most sweet foods that enhance kapha and increase weight, honey is converted upon digestion to a pungent substance that stimulates fire (pitta). Thus, honey in moderate amounts will not increase body fat but actually stimulates the body's heat and metabolism, having the effect of drying up mucus.

In a particularly interesting section of the Ayurvedic medical text, the Caraka, diet and proper eating habits are discussed. An explanation is given of how to regulate the measure of food in proportion to the strength of the "gastric fire," or the body's capacity to digest what is put into it. Changes in diet should take into consideration physical constitution and exercise habits as well as digestive abilities. As in Chinese medicine, the type of diet to be recommended varies with the seasons of the year. Diet should be adjusted to the climate and the alternation of seasons, for as each season has a different physiologic effect, an appropriate dietary modification is required. During the winter, for example, it is suggested that the diet consist mostly of heavier (kaphic) foods like grains and legumes, whereas the summer diet should be lighter, including more foods such as raw fruits and vegetables (vatic).

In Ayurveda as well as with practitioners of holistic medicine the trend is to reevaluate the relationship between humans and food and to observe the qualitative effects of food on consciousness. This careful observation of the subtle and gross properties of food with which ancient systems were concerned, combined with the contributions of modern clinical nutrition, provide the framework for nutritional therapy in modern holistic medicine. Defining the essence or the effects of each food as being yin or yang (Chinese), or vata, pitta or kapha (Ayurveda), or tamasic, rajasic or sattvic (yoga), helps to create a workable model for establishing criteria to describe the properties of all foods. Combining foods according to these constructs ensures a balanced diet. Within this context, many people are now eating less fatty and heavy foods such as red meat and turning towards a plant-based diet that emphasizes natural, clean-burning, lighter foods such as fresh vegetables, fruits, legumes and whole grains. Nutrition highlights many of the principles of holism that ancient medical systems support. Good food nourishes the mind and emotions as clearly as it strengthens the body.

Also, as people maintain a higher quality of nutrition, they become more conscious of the subjective effects of different foods, which serves as a vehicle for growth. In addition, nutrition is a vitalistic science as it strengthens resistance to disease by providing high quality fuel for increasing vitality. Furthermore, the subject of nutrition deals with the holistic principles of balance and unity in nature as they influence the greater community welfare. Nutritional considerations force us to struggle to feed the human life on the planet by using the most productive and ecologically safe means available, so that all can share in the bounty that nature can potentially provide. The principles of nutrition indicate the synergistic potential that exists between modern scientific knowledge and the intuitive wisdom of ancient systems.

In Ayurveda, knowledge of different health practices provides sound physical health, which in turn sets the stage for spiritual growth. Ayurveda is not concerned with lengthening life simply for the purpose of increasing longevity, but to increase the depth and quality of one's existence. It is the duty of the Ayurvedic physician to provide the tools and to teach the proper habits, attitudes and lifestyle that will lead an individual to a healthy body, a clear unfettered mind and a reverence for his or her spiritual nature.

Yoga Philosophy, the Gunas and Nutrition

In yoga science, food is one of the vehicles through which prana is taken into the body. The physical, mental and spiritual attributes of food are described by the gunas (rajas, tamas and sattva), the three qualities of all manifestation. These qualities as taught in yoga philosophy are comparable to the three doshas of Ayurveda and to the yin-yang theory of Chinese medicine.

In Ayurveda, stimulating foods such as spices are qualified as pittic. This stimulating quality of food is referred to as rajasic in yoga. Kaphic foods such as meat and dairy, which have a sedative effect, are categorized in yoga as tamasic. The right combination of fruits, vegetables, legumes and grains helps to create a sattvic state of body and mind that is characterized by alertness and tranquility. Each person has the ability to observe the effect that food is having on their state of mind. Irritability and lightheadedness are indications that too much rajasic food is being eaten, whereas the qualities of lethargy and apathy result from an excess of tamasic foods. This knowledge of the subjective qualities produced by food increases the depth and scope of therapeutic nutrition, establishing nutrition as a major modality in the maintenance of health.

Vegetarianism

Practitioners of yoga and people who meditate often gravitate towards a plant-based diet. Vegetarianism has been a very important part of my spiritual path. Being a vegetarian is certainly a life choice and in my medical practice I don't discuss my personal thoughts about vegetarianism unless asked directly by a patient. But I also recognize that not consuming meat and animal products is not for everyone. Some people really like the taste of meat or fish and say they would be unhappy if they didn't eat meat. There are others who don't feel they have enough energy unless meat is included in their diet. Still others have medical conditions where eating some meat might be helpful, such as in certain types of anemia. I do, however, generally encourage a more plant-based and natural food diet because, as explained below, there are many health benefits to eating a diet with less red meat.

I remember the day, forty-six years ago, when I became a vegetarian. I had been thinking about changing my diet for a few months as I explored meditation and the path of raja yoga. I was traveling on a train across Canada, from Montreal to British Columbia. My friend Alain and I had stopped off in the Canadian Rockies and were camping high in the mountains. Some young men were cooking fish at a campsite near ours. The smell overwhelmed me, and the fish looked greenish. At that moment, I knew I wouldn't eat flesh again.

Another odd influence on my spiritual path occurred later on this train trip across Canada. We met and traveled for a while with a young vegetarian man who had recently returned from traveling in Afghanistan and India. He seemed inwardly at peace. He mentioned that he had been practicing a form of Indian meditation and this had transformed his life. His calmness and travel experiences intrigued and inspired me, and I decided I wanted to learn more on my own. He and I parted after arriving at his home in Vancouver. I often wonder what happened to him.

Before delving further into vegetarianism, it is important to discuss some basic nutritional ideas. There are several ways to understand the principles of vegetarianism. For example, a person who eats no red meat, poultry, fish, dairy or eggs is a vegan. People who eat no flesh foods but eat dairy are lacto-vegetarians, and those who eat eggs but no dairy are ovo-vegetarians. A person who eats no animal meat but does take milk products and eggs is an ovo-lacto-vegetarian, which characterizes my personal approach to diet. While those who eat no red meat or poultry, but eat fish, call themselves pescatarian. In a strict sense of the word, they are not really vegetarian.

Importance of Proteins and Amino Acids

Plant-based foods contain plenty of the major components needed to sustain life, including proteins, carbohydrates, fats, vitamins and minerals. One of the most important aspects of vegetarianism is to pay close attention to the types of amino acids, the building blocks of proteins that are present in plant foods. Twenty amino acids make up the protein structures that build and maintain healthy tissues and organs of the body. While amino acids have similar structures, their side chains are different. After eating a meal, pancreatic enzymes, sent from the pancreas to the small intestine, break down the proteins in food into amino acids, which in turn are built back up in the body to become the proteins needed to form muscles and other tissues in the body.

Proteins are essential to maintain tissue and organ structures and underlie many bodily functions and the regulation of cellular activity. The three-dimensional structures of proteins are made up of the amino acids described above. Examples of the functions of proteins are: antibody production for immunological activity, enzyme production that is essential for cellular chemical reactions and formation of molecules by reading the genetic information encoded in DNA, messenger molecules like hormones that transmit signals for biological processes (growth hormone), giving structural support so the body can move (myosin and actin) and for binding and transporting molecules throughout the body (ferritin).

Animal-based foods, such as meat, fish, eggs, dairy and most seeds and nuts have all twenty amino acids. In addition, the body can make many amino acids by salvaging old bits of amino acids and combining them with other raw materials. There are, however, several amino acids that are called essential because the body cannot make them. Therefore, essential amino acids have to be consumed in the diet. The essential amino acids are: histidine, isoleucine, leucine, lysine, methionine, threonine, tryptophan and valine. Animal proteins contain all essential amino acids. As a result, people who eat meat or those who consume eggs and/ dairy products, get complete proteins in their diet. Since plant-based foods are deficient in a few essential amino acids, vegans do not consume all the necessary amino acids in sufficient amounts. However, plant-based foods can be combined with other foods to give a complete set of essential amino acids, thereby providing a complete protein. For example, grains and cereals are deficient in lysine. Peanuts, peas and beans, however, contain plenty of lysine. Since these legumes are deficient in cystine, tryptophan and methionine but are found in grains and cereals, they can be consumed together, and one receives the full complement of amino acids. Thus, legumes and grains contain complementary proteins. Seeds and nuts are also considered complementary to legumes because they contain tryptophan, methionine and cystine.

Examples of complementary proteins that one can eat are: corn tortillas combined with pinto beans, mung dahl and wheat chapattis, pasta and peas, peanut butter and whole wheat bread, peanuts and nuts and seeds in trail mix, black beans and brown rice, and hummus and whole wheat flat bread (pita bread). There are a few exceptions to the above descriptions. Soybeans are a legume that contains all nine essential amino acids. Soymilk, tempeh, tofu and edamame are forms of soy that can be eaten as a singular food. Amaranth and quinoa are grains that lack asparagine and glutamic acid, but these nonessential amino acids can be produced by the body so these are considered complete proteins.

Reasons for Vegetarianism

Vegetarians often sight four reasons for not eating meat. From a meditation and raja yoga perspective, the role of vegetarianism helps to reinforce the idea of ahimsa (nonviolence) and sattva (calmness and joy) as well as to maintain good health and have less problematic environmental impact.

Nonviolence (Ahimsa)

People often choose to follow vegetarianism when practicing the raja yoga concept of ahimsa, nonviolence. Peacefulness and gentleness in thought, speech and action towards others are often cited as a reason to not eat meat. Why eat a conscious and intelligent sentient being for sustenance when one could eat foods from plants? To some vegetarians, eating plant-based foods seems more commensurate with living nonviolently. When vegetarians eat dairy and nonfertilized eggs, they say this is fine as no life need be taken.

As described in the section on ahimsa, many raja yoga practitioners are vegetarian as they believe this diet creates the least amount of harm to other higher evolutionary forms of sentient beings. Yoga philosophy believes it is very important to not take any life unnecessarily. Nonviolence is the most important of the yamas and sets the stage for the other yamas and for the inner meditative work of this yogic path. Avoiding animal cruelty is an important aspect of ahimsa since the animals people eat are usually kept in crowded and unsanitary conditions. Avoiding the negative karma of killing is important from an evolutionary and spiritual perspective. From the yogic perspective, humans have conscious free will to decide to not kill and keep the endless cycle of the survival of the fittest going.

Some branches of yoga advocates, especially those of the Jain religion, believe in a lacto-vegetarian diet. In this diet not only does a person not eat red meat, pork, ham, veal, fish, poultry or eggs, but also avoids alcohol, onions, garlic, mushrooms and vinegar (rajasic and tamasic foods). Strict Jains even avoid root vegetables because when they are picked for consumption the plant dies. This includes potatoes, onions and other tubers. Because from a nutritional perspective, proteins in animal and plant foods per calorie are equal, people committed to the yoga path eat in moderation to maintain good weight control.

Sattvic Reasons for Vegetarianism

Yoga and meditation philosophy teach that it is important to act with gentleness in all aspects of life. To follow the ancient Indian philosophical principle of sattva in all aspects of life means to try to cultivate a peaceful demeanor, have regular spiritual practices and try to be truthful, generous and moderate in life habits.

From the perspective of the three doshas, vegetarian diets are considered to be sattvic. A sattvic diet helps to increase vitality, joy, clarity of mind, calmness and strength and helps quiet the mind for meditation. Sattvic foods include legumes and whole grains, vegetables, fresh fruit, seeds and nuts, herbal teas, natural sweeteners and dairy products.

Rajasic foods, on the other hand, create activity of the mind and body, and if consumed in great quantities, can sometimes contribute to restlessness and agitation. From the yogic perspective, active states of mind and body associated with rajasic foods, which may be important for being effective in the world, can interfere with times of reflection and meditation. Foods that are considered rajasic are raw onions and garlic, radishes, caffeinated tea, coffee, heavily spiced foods, soft drinks, heavily salted foods, overly hot and spicy foods as well as the Ayurvedic classified foods that are bitter, sour or saline in taste.

Tamasic foods make people sluggish and heavy and can dull the mind. These include meat, fish, alcohol, overripe or underripe fruit, vinegar, mushrooms as well as fermented, burned, fried, barbecued, reheated or deep-fried foods.

The practice of fasting often accompanies a vegetarian approach to diet and nutrition. Fasting helps the body stay healthy and the mind stay calm. It allows the digestive system a break from its constant activity of digestion, assimilation and absorption. Fasting also helps eliminate toxins from the body, increases a person's energy level and lets the mind focus on sattvic and spiritual practices.

Fasting once weekly or monthly for thirty-six hours is often recommended for students of meditation. Longer supervised fasts are also possible. Generally, in the yogic tradition, people do a juice fast using the juice of three fruits. Drinking plenty of water with lemon juice is encouraged. Certain herbal teas are used at times and one can take an enema the morning of the fast. When breaking a fast, a fruit diet is advised for twenty-four hours, or coconut water and vegetable soup are also acceptable. In the Himalayan tradition, it is strongly suggested to only do extended fasts in the mild and dry weather of early fall or late springtime.

Health Reasons for Vegetarianism

Many people who practice meditation, pranayama and yoga do so to help prevent and treat many illnesses. It is common for such people to gravitate towards plant-based diets, as vegetarianism has been shown to help maintain good health. For example, much medical research has demonstrated that vegetarians have lower rates of cancer, diabetes, arthritis and heart disease. A vegetarian diet has more fiber, folic acid, magnesium, potassium, calcium, vitamin C, beta carotene, phytochemicals and less saturated fat and cholesterol than meat-based diets, all of which have positive effects on health. Other health related reasons to be a vegetarian are that there is less hypertension, strokes, gastric ulcers, arthritis, gout and migraines in those who eat a plant-based diet.

Because there is less cholesterol in meatless diets, vegetarians tend to have fewer occurrences of blood clots and heart attacks. Other medical reasons for avoiding meat are that vegetarian foods tend to raise the PH of the blood and urine, which helps to decrease the tendency to form kidney and bladder stones. Less osteoarthritis is seen in vegetarians and women tend to have less estrogen in their bodies. This is important as too much estrogen can predispose women to breast cancer. There is less uric acid in plant-based foods and therefore there is less gout. Less calories from fat are often consumed as plant-based diets tend to have less fat than animal products, and this can be important to prevent obesity and diabetes.

Studies have consistently concurred that cancer incidence is lower in persons who do not eat meat. This includes colorectal, pancreatic, prostate, esophagus, liver and lung cancers, which are more common with diets that include processed meats like hot dogs, ham, bacon, deli meats and other red meat. The IARC, the cancer agency of the WHO, has recently even classified meat as a carcinogen. A recent study from Loma Linda Public Health School found that vegetarians have less type 2 diabetes and those who ate five or less eggs weekly had even lower rates.27

Animals are often bred on antibiotics and because of this, resistance to antibiotics can occur in both the animal receiving the medicine as well as in the people who eat the flesh of such animals. Animals are also fed hormones to help them grow more rapidly and to attain larger bodies.

From a human anatomical and physiological perspective, vegetarianism makes sense. For example, the intestines of humans and vegetarian animals are ten times the length of their bodies, a design that is not conducive to the process of elimination of flesh foods. On the other hand, carniverous animals have digestive tracts that are only three times the length of their bodies, which allows for quick elimination of fast-decaying foods like raw meats. In addition, humans do not have enlarged canine teeth like carnivores, which are essential for ripping apart flesh. In fact, humans have well developed molars like other vegetarian animals. Also, carnivores sleep during the day and herbivores sleep during the night, like humans.

One problem that can arise with vegans is that there is no way to get Vitamin B12 because only animal-based foods have this essential vitamin. A vegan, who avoids all animal meat as well as dairy and eggs, needs to take a supplement fortified with vitamin B12 or they can get it from eating plant-based fermented foods, like sauerkraut, kimchi or tempeh. A vegan diet also may be deficient in long chain fatty acids (omega-3) so supplementation with fatty acids like flaxseed and evening primrose oil can be helpful. The bioavailability of zinc may be less than optimal due to high levels of phytic acid in whole grains, which can bind to zinc. Vegans are advised to supplement with zinc or eat plenty of foods like sunflower seeds that are rich in this element.

Environmental Reasons for Vegetarianism

Ahimsa also implies nonviolence with respect to our communities and environment. From this perspective, a person should create the smallest possible environmental footprint, cause little disruption to our planet and work to preserve land, water and sea for the betterment of all sentient beings.

From environmental and ecological perspectives, it takes four to ten times as much land to raise animal versus vegetarian protein. Large areas of land are required to raise cattle, leaving less land to grow food to feed people. Plant-based protein needs less water to grow, creates less greenhouse gases (cow flatulence is made of the green gas methane), creates less water pollution (animal feces runoff into streams and rivers is a major source of water pollution) and there are fewer animal carcasses (which creates less need for resources for waste disposal).

From the perspective of greenhouse emissions, the production of meat creates many times more greenhouse gases than the cultivation of dried beans. Even the process of making cheese creates more greenhouse gases than growing legumes. Giving up meat once a week for a year is like not driving for three months with respect to production of greenhouse gas.28

Environmentally, manure from animals that are raised for meat, generates more than 500 million tons of feces yearly, which is three times human amounts. Manure can leach into storage containers, can cause odor pollution and can increase nitrogen and phosphorus levels that are air pollutants. Since cows are often fed antibiotics to stave off infection and are fed hormones to initiate faster growth, these substances can get into groundwater. And as manure decomposes, there can be increased dust and toxic gases from the outgassing.

Slaughterhouse waste creates another ecological problem. Carcasses that are discarded into landfills take up valuable space, and bone meal that is used to supplement animal feed can cause mad cow disease in humans. Also, when carcasses decompose in a group, it can lead to groundwater dead zones.

Hatha Yoga

Hatha yoga is generally considered to be part of the third rung of raja yoga, asanas. The word *hatha* is composed of two smaller words. *Ha* means "sun" and *tha* means "moon;" the word *yoga* means "to unite." Thus, *hatha yoga* means "to unite the sun and moon." The goal of the practice of hatha yoga is to unite the qualities associated with the sun: the right side, warmth, activity and masculinity, with the qualities associated with the moon: the left side, coolness, passivity and femininity. This merging of two polar opposites results in the birth of a higher consciousness.

Hatha yoga practices include a series of physical stretches and postures (asanas), body cleansings (kriyas), certain anatomical locks (bandhas) and hand positions that affect energy flow (mudras). The physical locks involve compressing and stimulating various glands, nerves and energy centers (chakras).

Hatha yoga, along with other forms of exercise such as aerobic exercise, martial arts and tai chi, can be used to treat ailments of annamaya kosha, the physical body. In addition, physical therapy and massage therapies are also focused on this level. Hatha yoga helps bring about greater body awareness, relaxation, flexibility, balance, strength and concentration. As a person works with hatha yoga, they become aware of bodily tension and where it is held. Yogic cleansing techniques help to cleanse the body of excess waste from the eyes, skin, upper respiratory mucus membranes, lungs, stomach, liver, colon, kidneys and bladder. Cell metabolism operates more efficiently since there are less waste and excretory by-products to interfere with normal tissue physiology. These yoga approaches can be used to both prevent and treat such diseases as upper respiratory infections, allergies, colitis and cystitis.

Hatha yoga techniques offer a systematic method of purifying and strengthening the body through the practice of various stretching postures that enable a person to become graceful, relaxed and supple. Hatha yoga postures also work to enhance balance and symmetry of the left and right sides of our body and to promote equilibrium between the sympathetic and parasympathetic nervous systems. This is accomplished by alternating standing postures with inverted postures, forward bending asanas with backward bending poses as well as practicing twisting postures first on one side and then on the other side. Because the poses cause gentle compression of the internal organs, digestive functioning often improves, and underactive endocrine glands are stimulated. Large and small muscles relax as a result of practicing hatha yoga asanas, and this can be of benefit for illnesses that are associated with abnormal muscular contraction such as high blood pressure, headaches and asthma.

On a deeper and subtler level, the practice of hatha yoga helps to prepare for meditation as follows: the body is strengthened and made stronger and more flexible to allow for the undisturbed sitting required for meditation; the pranic sheath is cleansed and the nadis purified so the flow of energy is unobstructed. By coordinating the movements of the body with breath awareness and mind awareness, one develops an awareness of the subtler energy level, the mind becomes clearer and one is able to concentrate for longer periods of time.

To understand how the practices of hatha yoga affect the body and mind and prepare the student for meditation, it is important to first describe the interconnection between the brain and the musculoskeletal system. The areas of the brain responsible for maintaining muscle tone are located deep within the brain. These areas, such as the cerebellum, are referred to as the lower primitive brain centers. They were the first to develop as the brain evolved. These reflexes are modified by input from the conscious part of the brain, the cerebral cortex. The cortex is the latest part of the brain to evolve and is considered to be the higher brain center.

As the body ages, not only do tendons become less supple and muscles become weaker, but also one's conscious concerns and desires begin to interfere with the normal maintenance of relaxed muscle tone. The proper practice of hatha yoga allows the primitive unconscious lower brain centers to adjust muscle tone unimpeded by inhibiting thoughts and thus helps maintain a relaxed supple body. This is done by assuming different postures, which leads to the activation of certain reflexes that are integrated in the lower brain centers that normally function without conscious awareness. It is through these reflexes that normal tone is reestablished. The postures used are, in a sense, also primitive in that they mimic the positions of animals, as is reflected in their names: the butterfly, lion, scorpion, dog, peacock, cobra and locust. Perhaps these postures facilitate a regression to the evolutionary roots of human beings, where posture was not distorted by conflicts of the conscious mind. To ensure that the lower brain centers are free from conscious cerebral inhibitory control, the mind is focused on the breath. Then the lower brain centers can reestablish proper muscle tone through natural reflexes as initiated by the hatha yoga postures.

To gain the maximum benefit from hatha yoga it is best to relax while doing the postures, to breathe evenly and slowly and to focus on the area of stretch. The postures should be held with little movement and coming out of the postures should be done slowly and gently. When hatha yoga postures are done for health purposes or in preparation for meditation, following a consistent sequence is recommended. The teachers at the Himalayan Institute recommended the following sequence: preliminary stretching exercises, standing postures, backward bending postures, forward bending postures, twisting postures, inverted postures, relaxation techniques and breathing exercises. In the Sivananda tradition, we practiced the following postures in a different sequence: relaxation, general leg stretches, sun salutation, headstand, child's pose, shoulderstand, plow, bridge, wheel, sitting forward bend, inclined plane, cobra, locust, bow, spinal twist, crow, standing forward bend and triangle.

When beginning to practice the asanas, one should be receptive, patient and calm. It is good to attempt to practice regularly and at the same time daily. It is also recommended to practice early morning after emptying the bowels and bladder and taking a warm shower. However, if early morning is not convenient, doing hatha yoga at night helps to reduce the tension accumulated during the day and is conducive to a restful sleep. When practicing asanas, pranayama or meditation, it is best to wear loose fitting cotton clothes and to practice in a quiet, draft free room. One should wait at least two hours after a light meal and four hours after a heavy meal, and should always relieve the bladder and bowels before commencing the postures.

It is recommended that women who are menstruating refrain from doing the more strenuous postures and inverted postures, but meditation can always be practiced. While some mild discomfort may occur when stretching tense muscles, there should be awareness not to stretch beyond one's comfortable capacity to avoid injury. Easing up on the poses is important when feeling burning pains or involuntary shaking.

The manner of practicing hatha yoga determines the quality of the benefits experienced. A systematic program should be followed, allowing for gradual perfecting of the postures while incorporating the progressive development of the following qualities: flexibility, balance, strength and stillness. In general, the beginner should endeavor to develop each of these qualities in this order, achieving a certain level of proficiency in each one before attempting the next. For example, if one is just starting to practice hatha, they should initially practice gentle stretching exercises, which are designed to increase flexibility and mobility of the body, thus laying the foundation for the development of balance. A stretch in one direction should be balanced by a similar stretch in the opposite direction.

Only after having attained a certain degree of flexibility and balance, should one attempt postures that involve greater strength and power. While working to enhance flexibility, balance and strength, it is essential to establish a smooth and even rhythm to the flow of the breath and to coordinate the breath with the movements. As muscle tension is released, the flow of energy and prana are also unblocked. As sensitivity increases, a person learns to sense energy flows within the body and mind, and by careful observation and analysis, can learn to locate energy blocks that underlie physical muscular tension. By mentally sending messages to the body and by observing the breath and energy flow, one can learn to relax muscular tension and help better regulate tension related diseases such as high blood pressure and migraine headaches. Sensitive individuals can even predict oncoming physical ailments by experiencing alterations in energy flow or changes in the breath, the main vehicle for energy transmission. Continued practice of coordination of the breath with the postures helps to balance the two branches of the autonomic nervous system, which leads to a state of relaxation, calmness and inner stillness.

Because of these relaxing effects, hatha yoga is also helpful on an emotional level. While doing the physical postures, the release of muscle tension not only results in increased flexibility but also helps to liberate pent-up emotions and conflicts that created or underlie the original body tension. Working through or letting go of physical resistance can trigger a concomitant response on the emotional level, helping to liberate the person from the subjective feeling of restriction.

Hatha yoga also has important benefits on the mental and spiritual levels. As one increases the capacity to hold a posture for an extended period of time, not only is physical strength enhanced, but also psychological endurance and will power are strengthened. Through the cultivation of self-discipline and will power, you will become able to assume a posture effortlessly and to hold it without discomfort. This leads to the quality of stillness, when all movement of the body and mind is quieted.

As the depth and degree of concentration and relaxation are increased, the breath becomes very subtle. As a result, one can learn to let go of body consciousness and become aware of the energy flowing within. At this point, the mind can be allowed to flow with the breath and a mantra can be repeated, with the result that the body, breath, mind and mantra become one. This coordinated effort leads to deeper levels of concentration and meditation.

While asanas should ensure physical well-being, strength and flexibility and have many positive health benefits, the eventual goal is to develop a strong and flexible spine, which is needed for increasing the length of time one can sit comfortably for meditative practices. Yogis say asanas make a person like a mountain. The ultimate goal of practicing asanas is to transcend body consciousness so mind is no longer attached to the body, and one can go deeply within.

The Kriyas

There are six cleansings *(kriyas)* that are part of hatha yoga practices. Not only do these cleansings prepare the body for hatha, they also have important therapeutic benefits. Some of the kriyas help prepare for meditation by enhancing the power of concentration. The six kriyas are as follows:

Neti is the nasal wash and is a simple and frequently used technique where lukewarm saltwater is poured into one nostril and allowed to pass out through the other nostril or out the mouth. This cleans the nose, back of the throat and sinus cavities and helps to prevent or relieve the tendency to sinusitis, allergies and upper respiratory infections.

Trataka is a gazing technique that involves focusing the open eyes on an external object such as a candle flame. The eyes can also be directed upwards to stare at the ajna chakra (third eye) or downwards at the tip of the nose. This has the effect of improving both eyesight and mental concentration.

Kapalabhati is a vigorous breathing technique that flushes out the respiratory system. It is especially helpful for people who have asthma, sinusitis and digestive problems.

Nauli is a technique in which the two central abdominal muscles are rolled in a wave-like manner. This promotes better digestion and bowel function. The third chakra area is also stimulated and activated by this kriya.

Dhauti is an unusual technique practiced only by advanced hatha yoga practitioners. A strip of cloth is carefully swallowed and then gently pulled back out to aid in cleansing the throat, esophagus and stomach.

Basti is another complicated procedure that is used to cleanse the lower colon, where the practitioner drinks very warm lemon water very quickly before the lower esophagus valve has a chance to close. A related technique, the upper wash, is yet another type of cleansing that involves swallowing a large amount of salty or lemon-flavored water and then quickly regurgitating the contents of the stomach. This has a great therapeutic benefit for stomach problems and asthma. These cleansing techniques should only be attempted under the supervision of a very experienced practitioner.

Bandhas

Bandhas are physical locks that are used during hatha yoga as well as during pranayama and meditation to enhance and intensify certain practices. There is a more thorough discussion of the bandhas in the section on kundalini and pranayama.

Jalandhara bandha is the chin lock where the practitioner places his or her chin onto the chest. In *mula bandha* (anal lock) the practitioner contracts the perineum and anal muscles. *Uddiyana bandha* is the stomach lift or lock in which the abdominal muscles are pulled towards the back while retaining the breath on exhalation.

Mudras

Mudras are hand, arm and finger positions and movements used in the yoga tradition. One usually associates the hands and fingers as tools to feed oneself or others, to make things, to write or to express oneself. For example, one uses the hands to express joy or may throw the hands up in exasperation or gesticulate with the hands when feeling upset or excited. People often communicate with each other with the hands. In fact, a relatively small amount of all human communication is verbal, while the majority is nonverbal, including facial expressions and hand movements. For instance, one touches a friend or loved one to console them or as a way to express affection; or one may touch an old friend on the back to get their attention or wave a hand to someone when leaving them. People clap their hands for something enjoyable or shake hands when they meet a colleague or greet a person they are meeting for the first time. The hands are also very important to communicate words through sign language with the deaf.

Functionally, humans use the hands and fingers to build things such as skyscrapers, nanosized computers or to create art or drama. From an anthropological perspective, the dexterity of the human hand, and especially the opposition capacity of the thumb, has enabled human beings to stand upright and learn to use tools. This advancement set the stage for the evolution and development of the cerebral cortex of the brain.

The hand movements that represent mudras, however, have a very different purpose in that they help direct energy to enhance meditation practice. Certain hand positions create a seal of energy that has the power to lead an individual to experience different states of consciousness. In many spiritual and religious traditions, deities such as those in the yogic tradition hold their hands in ways to express particular spiritual qualities such as fearlessness, piety or reverence.

In the Ayurvedic medical tradition, each finger is associated with a different element and chakra: small finger (water and second chakra), ring finger (earth and first chakra) middle finger (ether and fifth chakra), index finger (air and heart chakra) and thumb (fire and third chakra). When the fingers are placed in certain positions, they can affect certain health parameters, emotional qualities and subtle energies of the associated elements and chakras. Some mudras are used to heal illnesses like asthma, bronchitis and back pain; some are used in the morning and some at night.

Chin mudra is one of the most important mudras in the raja yoga system. This mudra is often used when sitting in the meditation posture. Here one touches the thumb and index finger together lightly, with palms up or down and hands placed on the thighs or knees. In this mudra, the thumb symbolizes universal consciousness and the index finger represents individual consciousness. The connection between the tips of the thumbs and fingers symbolically creates a union between the two. When the breath is deep and smooth and the body straight in alignment, the chin mudra enhances the meditative process.

Dhyana mudra is another important meditation related mudra. This is the classic hand position that Zen practitioners use in meditation. Here the right hand is placed inside the left palm and the thumbs gently touch, forming what is called the mystic triangle in Buddhism. As the hands form a bowl, representing the void, one remains empty and open to receive all knowledge that there is in the cosmos to help one on the spiritual path. It is also representative of wisdom, peace and forgiveness. The Buddha had used this mudra when he attained enlightenment while meditating under the Bodhi tree.

Atman mudra is used in prayer, where the hands are placed together with the fingers pointed upwards and in front of the heart.

Anatomy and Physiology of Hatha Yoga

In order to understand how asanas affect the body and mind, I will present some basic information about yoga anatomy and physiology. Some of the information here is adapted from an excellent teaching guide called *Sivananda Yoga Teacher Training Manual*.29 Two other very good sources that I've studied on this subject are: *Anatomy of Hatha Yoga* by David Coulter 30 and *Yoga Anatomy* by Leslie Kaminoff and Amy Matthews.31

This chapter will describe the parts of the body most involved with hatha yoga postures, which are the skeleton, muscles, joints and ligaments. Asanas closely affect certain organ systems as well, and these are described later.

The Skeletal System

The skeletal system components include 206 bones, ligaments to hold the bones together, and tendons that bind muscle to bone and joints where two or more bones meet. The five major functions of the skeletal system are: to provide structural framework, to protect the internal organs, to produce red and white blood cells in the bone marrow, to store minerals like calcium and phosphorus that are released in response to parathyroid hormone and to allow movement. Bones make up eighteen percent of total body weight (about twenty-five pounds), are hard on the outside, spongy inside and are coated by a fibrous material called the periosteum. Upright movements and active walking help to stimulate the minerals and cells within the bones. This promotes calcium mobilization from the blood to the bones.

The structures with the greatest number of bones are the skull with twenty-three, the vertebral column of the spine with thirty-three and the rib cage with twenty-four. The thirty-three vertebrae in the spinal column that allow movement and flexibility include the seven cervical bones that curve forwards, the twelve thoracic bones that bend backwards, the five lumbar bones that curve forwards, the five fused sacral bones that curve backwards and the four fused coccygeal bones that curve forwards.

Ligaments bind bone to bone, as opposed to tendons that bind muscle to bone. There are two types of ligaments: non-elastic white and elastic yellow. White ligaments bind the bones of the foot so that it curves into an arch to act like a spring and a cushion. The yellow ligaments bind joints that have movement such as the spine. If ligaments rupture, surgery may often be required and they take a long time to heal.

A joint is where two bones come together. They are mobile and allow the bones to move. Cartilage covers the surface of bones at the joint. Examples of movements allowed in the spine and associated asanas are: flexion (forward sitting pose), extension (cobra), rotation (spinal twist) and lateral flexion (triangle).

The spinal discs are fluid filled, soft and compressible structures located between the bony vertebrae. They have no blood supply in them and therefore need compression and expansion for circulation of interstitial fluid through them. With age and lack of adequate stimulation, discs tend to dry out and lose their suppleness. Herniated or slipped discs occur when there is damage to the disc, vertebrae, postural muscles, spinal ligaments or the disc itself dries out. This mostly occurs in the cervical and lumbar areas of the spine. If a desiccated disc moves backward and presses on one of the spinal nerves, it causes great pain and can lead to loss of motor and/or sensory functions. Asanas are very helpful as they help to gently compress the discs, allowing more fluid to bath the disc as well as help to make the support muscles and ligaments suppler and stronger.

The Muscular System

The muscular system includes 600 muscles, making up half the weight of the body. The skeletal muscles make movement possible and keep the organs in place. Muscles can be ribbon, spindle or flat sheet shaped and each muscle has an origin, an insertion (attachment) and a fleshy middle belly. They are often present in pairs to work in opposition and are attached to bones by tendons or by cartilage.

Three types of muscles:
- *Voluntary* or striated muscles that cover the skeleton of the body. These are controlled by the voluntary nervous system and allow the extremities to move in response to a thought or command.
- *Involuntary smooth* muscles are controlled by the autonomic (involuntary) nervous system and control the muscles of the digestive tract, blood vessels, bronchial tubes and iris and
- *Cardiac muscle* is striated but has an electrical system that creates a coordinated contraction without outside stimulation.

Movement of muscles:
- Nervous system activity controls the operation of skeletal muscles.
- Connective tissue restricts or facilitates muscular movements, which depend on the health of the bones, cartilage, tendons, ligaments, joints, joint capsule, fascia, touch and inner ear for balance.
- Muscles have to move against gravity, therefore, gravity dominates the hatha yoga practice. In the cobra and bow, the body is lifted against the force of gravity. In the shoulderstand, gravity holds the shoulders against the floor, but the inversion works against gravity.

Types of movement of muscles:

Muscles can move in several different ways. It is important to remember that flexion and extension occur at joints and that muscles help facilitate these movements.
- *Flexion* decreases the angle of joint, bringing two bones closer together.
- *Extension* increases the angle of the joint.
- *Abduction* takes the muscle and bone away from the midline of the body.
- *Adduction* brings the muscle and bone towards the middle of the body.
- *Rotation* increases the range of motion on a longitudinal axis.
- *Elevation* raises a body part.
- *Depression* lowers a body part.
- In *pronation* the palms are turned downwards; in supination the palms are turned upwards.

Underlying the movement of muscles as well as all bodily functioning is the process of cellular respiration. The efficiency of this process depends on the availability of two molecules — glucose and oxygen. Glucose is the sugar molecule that is the breakdown product of all carbohydrates; oxygen is the gas present in the air that sustains life on this planet.

With respect to muscular activity, aerobic (oxygen-dependent) exercise can be facilitated by regulating the breath. Breathing that is slow, smooth, even, deep and continuous encourages efficient energy utilization. The classical practice of doing asanas with slow and controlled movements along with deep breathing and breath awareness promotes efficient aerobic energy metabolism and delays the onset of fatigue.

However, during strenuous exercise when oxygen availability becomes limited, muscles switch to anaerobic metabolism, which yields low energy and produces lactic acid instead of carbon dioxide. Contrary to popular belief, lactic acid is not the cause of muscle soreness but instead it is caused by the release of inflammatory molecules like cytokines. Muscle fatigue also results when impaired contractile function leads to reduced force or power production. Biochemical changes during anaerobic muscle activity also lead to fatigue by inhibiting biochemical reactions that support muscle contraction. Muscle fatigue also results from a drop in energy stores when oxygen is not available, such as after vigorous exercise or in high altitudes where there is less oxygen available. This fatigue actually acts as a protective mechanism against injury as a person has to slow down to avoid damage to the muscles.

Relaxation and contraction

Muscles can be relaxed or contracted during movement. If a muscle is held steady and there is no resistance, the muscle will be in *relaxation.* If a muscle is held steady and there is resistance, it is in contraction. Sphincter contraction reduces the size of a body opening. *Tension* is contraction of a muscle and makes it more rigid.

Muscles provide an important source of heat to maintain body temperature as muscle contraction creates the friction that heats the blood flowing in nearby vessels. An example of this is the phenomenon of shivering, which happens when the brain sends messages to the muscles to increase contractions. This results in warming up the body.

There are three types of muscle contractions: *isometric, isotonic concentric* and *isotonic eccentric contraction.*

- During *isometric* contraction, muscles remain the same length. The muscle contracts against a load but doesn't shorten. Continued contraction increases the tension. This is seen when pushing against an object or holding a yoga posture.
- *Isotonic concentric* contraction means to contract muscles while keeping the same tension. An example of this is seen when lifting a dumbbell by flexing the elbow, which causes shortening of the biceps tendon.
- *Isotonic eccentric* contraction occurs when the muscle elongates while holding the same tension. This can be seen when lowering a dumbbell by extending the elbow, which causes lengthening of the biceps.

From a molecular perspective, the proteins actin and myosin that make up specialized tissues called sarcomeres slide towards each other in contracted movements. *Extension* causes a sliding of the sarcomere proteins away from each other. Muscle soreness is the result of inflammation of the sarcomeres that have been overstretched.

Yoga postures emphasize elasticity and flexibility, especially of the muscles, spine and joints:
- Muscle *flexibility* represents the range of motion in a joint. It reflects the ability of the muscle and tendon structures to elongate within the mechanical limitations of the joint. Flexibility is enhanced through the practice of yoga postures that create static pressure and prolonged, nondamaging elongation. Tissues change with aging. There is loss of the elastic component of muscle and of hydration. The surrounding matrix (glycosaminoglycans) becomes rigid (crystalline) and more interlocked, leading to a loss of mobility. Exercise, stretching, nutrition and hydration delay this loss of flexibility. It is important to drink plenty of water to keep muscles and connective tissue hydrated and supple.
- *Stretching* is the elongation of muscle structures.
- *Elasticity* represents the ability to elongate and return to

original length. A muscle sprain happens when a muscle has been stretched beyond its elastic limits.
- *Plasticity* is the ability to elongate and hold a particular shape.

There are yoga correlations to differing types of stretching:
- *Ballistic elastic* stretching, such as doing vigorous exercise without warm-up, stretches cold muscles with high force for short duration. This increases the risk of injury and leads to post-exercise soreness.
- *Plastic stretching,* as seen in yoga, uses warm muscles and achieves permanent lengthening. It is associated with low force and is of long duration. This allows the tissue to cool before releasing, which helps to minimize the possibilitly of injury and to reduce post-exercise soreness.

With its emphasis on relaxation and breath awareness, yoga places importance on slow and controlled movements and the regulation of oxygen exchange. Yoga also helps to gain control of normally involuntary muscles and creates balance of the sympathetic and parasympathetic nervous systems, allowing for better regulation of hormonal release. Whereas people are often unconscious of their posture, which reinforces problematic spinal posture, yoga emphasizes awareness of posture and leads to improved structural and body alignment over a period of time.

Twelve Major Postures

Traditional schools of hatha yoga often teach twelve major asanas along with their variations. The order in which the postures are taught varies, but generally asanas focus on forward bends, backward bends, side bends, twists, and inversions. In this book, I will discuss the practices of hatha yoga that the Himalayan Institute tradition teaches (where I first learned yoga) as well as the practices of the Sivananda organization (where I received my more formal yoga teacher training). My intention is to focus on the therapeutic and health-related aspects of these twelve postures as there are several very good books that describe how to do the postures themselves. The specific therapeutic effects of these asanas have come from studies done observing hatha practitioners, common sense, and commentaries and self-observation by advanced practitioners.

The *seated forward bend* stretches the lower and mid back, increasing flexibility of these areas, and opens up the disc space between the vertebrae, which allows the facet joints to open up and relieve pressure on the sciatic nerve. It also helps to decrease excessive lordosis of the lumbar spine area and stretches the hamstring muscles to improve leg strength and flexibility. The seated forward bend stimulates intestinal peristalsis, pancreatic functioning and adrenal activity. If practiced for longer periods of time, this posture helps to increase concentration and promotes relaxation and mental calmness. It is to be done cautiously by persons who have sciatica, especially when there are herniated discs or facet joint impingement. This posture stimulates the first, second, third and fourth chakras.

The *standing forward bend* promotes balance and hamstring and calf flexibility. Blood moves to the head as the upper part of the body bends forward to bring the head to the knees. The abdominal organs are compressed to help release necessary hormones and enzymes and to improve bowel functioning. Since the head is placed forward, some of the same precautions should be attended to as with the headstand described below.

The *side bend* (triangle) promotes balance and stretches the spine in a lateral direction, helping the muscles and ligaments of the back to remain supple. Hip and leg flexibility are improved, and one learns to balance oneself on each side. The liver and spleen are compressed and massaged because these organs are on the side of the body where the stretch occurs.

The *cobra* provides extension to the spine, which promotes spinal flexibility and increases circulation to the discs. The extension of the cervical region is helpful to relieve tension and pain in this area. It is useful for increasing lumbar lordosis in people who have a flat back and can also help to gently reverse thoracic kyphosis. The cobra may also help to relieve mid and lower back pain. By opening up the chest, the cobra is helpful to decrease the symptoms of asthma. The pressure on the abdomen provides a massage to the abdominal organs and pelvic organs in women. There is third and fourth chakra stimulation.

The *locust* helps increase flexibility of the back as this puts the back into extension, especially the lumbar area. The neck, biceps, deltoids and triceps are contracted and strengthened. The chest is opened up slightly. The abdominal muscles are contracted and strengthened and the pressure on the abdominal organs helps to improve digestion, metabolism and excretion. The lower pelvis is stimulated, thus helping bladder and female reproductive system functioning. Energetically, the locust stimulates the lower three chakras.

The *bow* combines the benefits of the cobra and locust as it gives a full backward stretch in extension to all areas of the spine. The back muscles are massaged and stretched as well. The abdominal muscles are stretched and since all of the weight rests on the abdomen, the pressure on the abdominal organs helps improve functioning of the pancreas, stomach, spleen and intestines as well as the pelvic organs in women. This posture is also helpful for kyphosis of the thoracic spine. The practitioner can sway and move in many directions while lying on the abdomen creating an even greater massage of the inner organs. This has a beneficial effect on the second, third and fourth chakras.

The *spinal twist* helps to keep the spine flexible since the twisting motion rotates the spine in both directions. Fluids can circulate more freely through the discs as this posture works like a pump. In addition, the spinal ligaments are twisted, lengthened and strengthened. Because the abdominal and pelvic organs are compressed and massaged by the twisting motion, there is a stimulating effect on all abdominal organs. Yogis feel that the spinal twist is the best posture to enhance the digestive fire. The spinal twist is good for balancing the second, third and fourth chakras.

The *plow* stretches the entire spine, loosens up the hamstring muscles, increases spinal circulation and relaxes the shoulder and neck muscles. The plow also strengthens core abdominal muscles and puts pressure on the abdominal muscles to improve digestive functioning. It is to be avoided with hyperthyroidism, asthma, heart disease and cervical disc conditions. The plow stimulates the fourth and fifth chakras.

The *shoulderstand* stretches the deltoid, rotator cuff muscles and other shoulder muscles and ligaments. It is helpful for hypothyroidism, Hashimoto's thyroiditis, low parathyroid conditions, chronic laryngitis or sore throats as well as various cognitive functioning problems such as difficulty communicating, writer's block and loss of creative drive. There is increased blood supply to the upper regions of the body, including the thoracic and cervical spinal nerves and it is also good for improving kidney and adrenal functioning. The shoulderstand increases venous circulation back to the heart so it is useful for hemorrhoids and varicose veins. It enhances deep abdominal breathing as the posture limits upper lung breathing since the chin is compressed into the chest. The shoulderstand is to be avoided if there is history of cervical spine injury or pain, severe headaches, hyperthyroidism, hyperparathyroidism, eye disorders or a history of eye surgery and during menstruation. This posture primarily stimulates the fifth chakra.

The *fish* stretches and relieves neck, cervical spine and shoulder stiffness, helps reduce kyphosis (rounded shoulders and back), strengthens the arms and expands the chest by releasing tight chest muscles. It is helpful in such conditions as hypothyroidism and asthma but is to be avoided if there is hyperthyroidism or cervical disc disease. It activates the fourth and fifth chakras.

The *tree* is a balancing posture that involves standing on one leg and stretching the arms overhead. As one leg is bent at the knee and placed on the inside of the opposite thigh, it improves flexibility of the hip joint. It also stretches the groin and shoulder joint. It is an excellent asana for improving leg strength, coordination of arms and legs moving in different directions and mental concentration. The legs correspond to the roots of the tree, the abdomen and chest to the trunk, the upward placed arms to the branches and the hands to the leaves.

The *headstand* is helpful to increase neck and core abdominal strength. It takes the pressure off the lower spine, especially the lumbar and sacral areas, and can help with chronic back pain. It improves circulation to the brain, head, eyes and ears and helps relieve varicose veins, hemorrhoids and constipation. Recurrent practice can slow the heart rate over time. It can help improve concentration and meditation. The headstand should be avoided if one is pregnant, during menstruation, if there is high or very low blood pressure, recent nerve or spine surgery, neck pain, glaucoma or other eye problems such as recent eye surgery, detached retina, vitreous tears or macular degeneration. From an energetic perspective, the headstand stimulates sixth and seventh chakra activity.

Three Relaxation Postures

Also included in the pictures below are three yoga postures for relaxation: the child's pose, the crocodile pose and the corpse pose. The child's pose is often done after the headstand to relax the upper and lower back and to allow the blood to reequilibrate after the reversing of the blood from the headstand. The crocodile pose is often practiced as a relaxation before doing the yoga postures that begin lying on the abdomen. The corpse pose is often done throughout the hatha yoga practice to allow the body and mind to relax after more strenuous poses. This is also done after completing the full set of hatha postures, as a means to reengage in normal activities.

Breath and Pranayama

Breathing is the first thing a human being does at birth and the last thing during the process of death. Even the connotations of the words that refer to the process of breathing are important: The word inspiration means "to take in air and also to be motivated and excited," while the word expiration means "to let out air, and also to die." Yogis refer to their age not by the number of years they have been alive but by the number and the quality of the breaths they have taken.

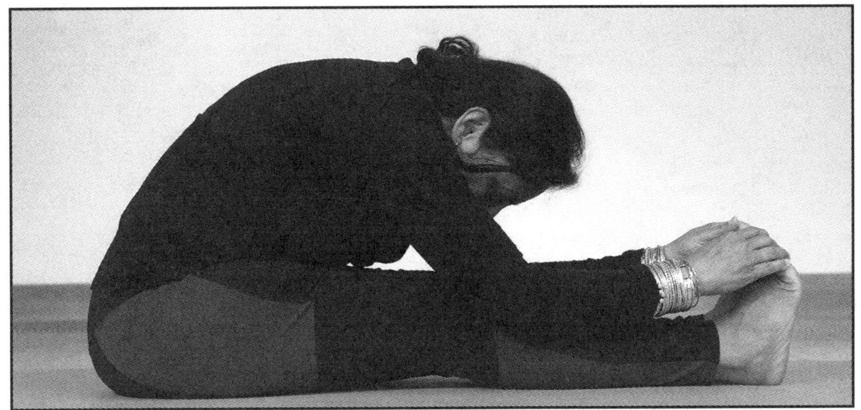

Seated Forward Bend (above)

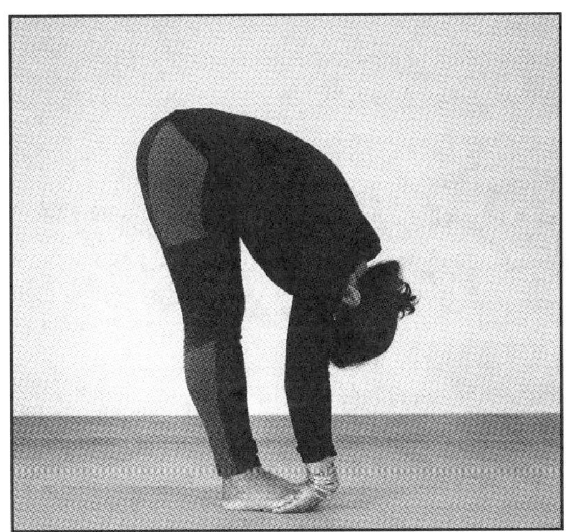

Standing Forward Bend

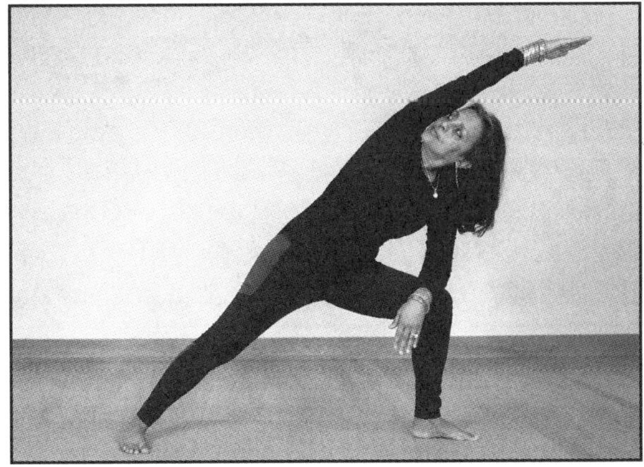

Side Bend

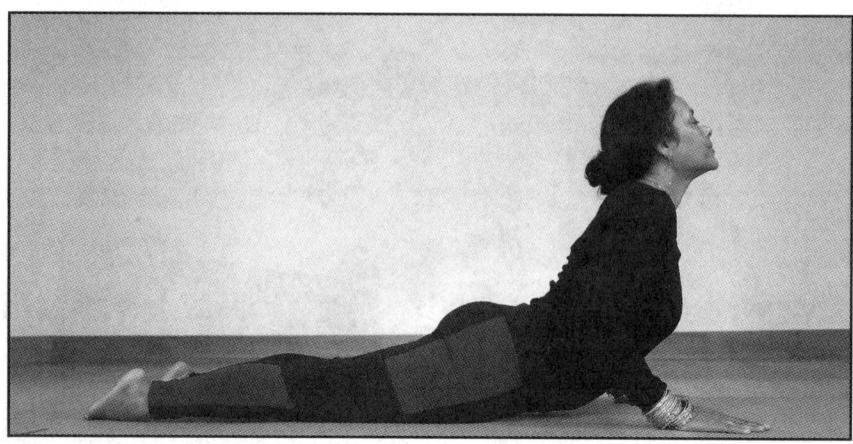

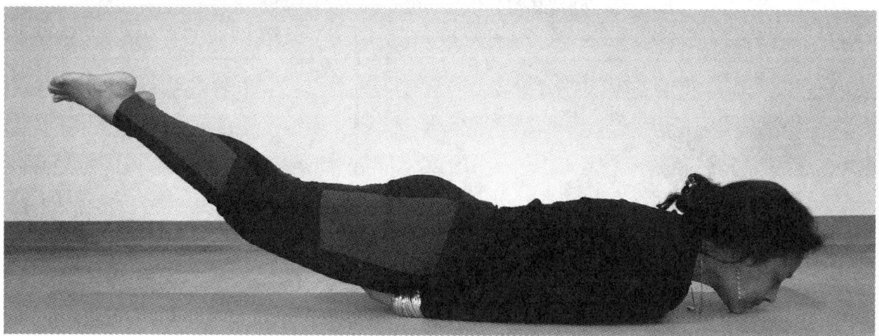

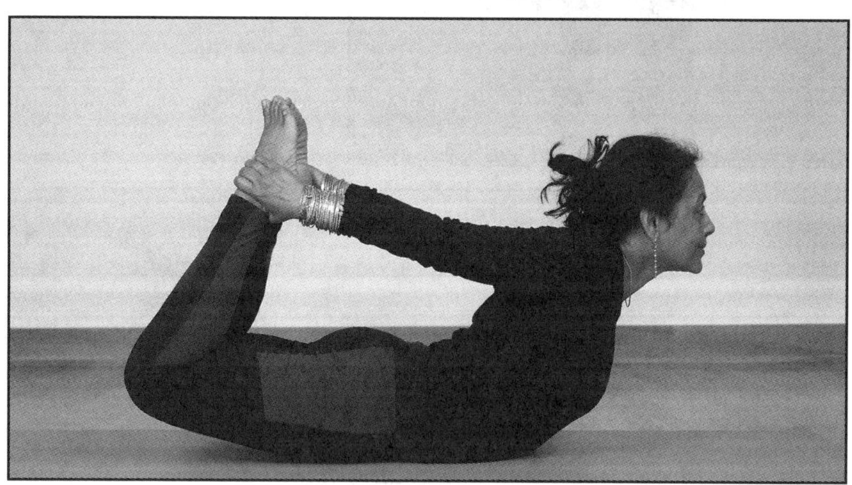

Cobra (top)
Locust (middle)
Bow (below)

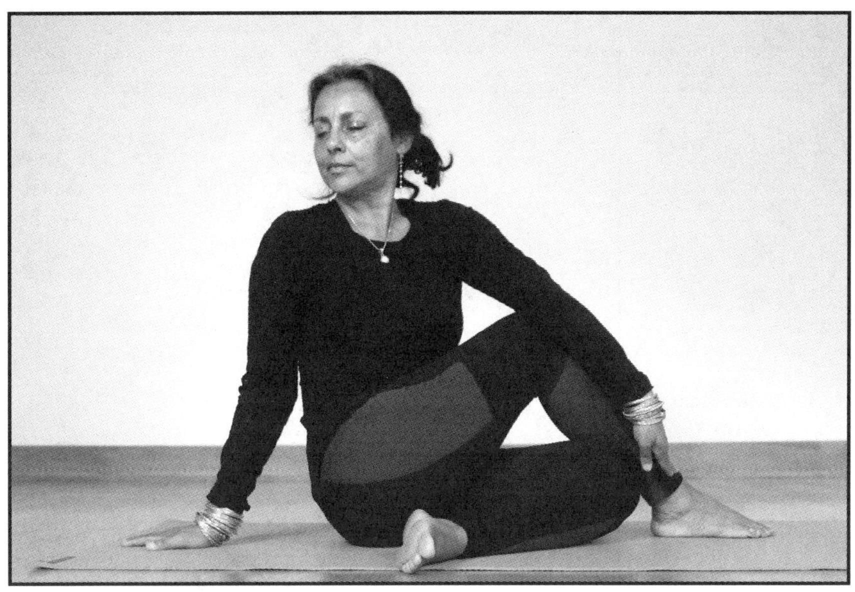

Spinal twist

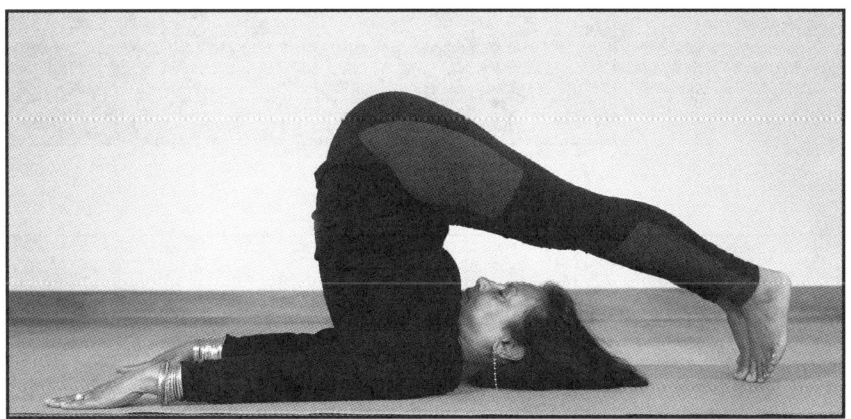

Plow

Shoulderstand
(right)

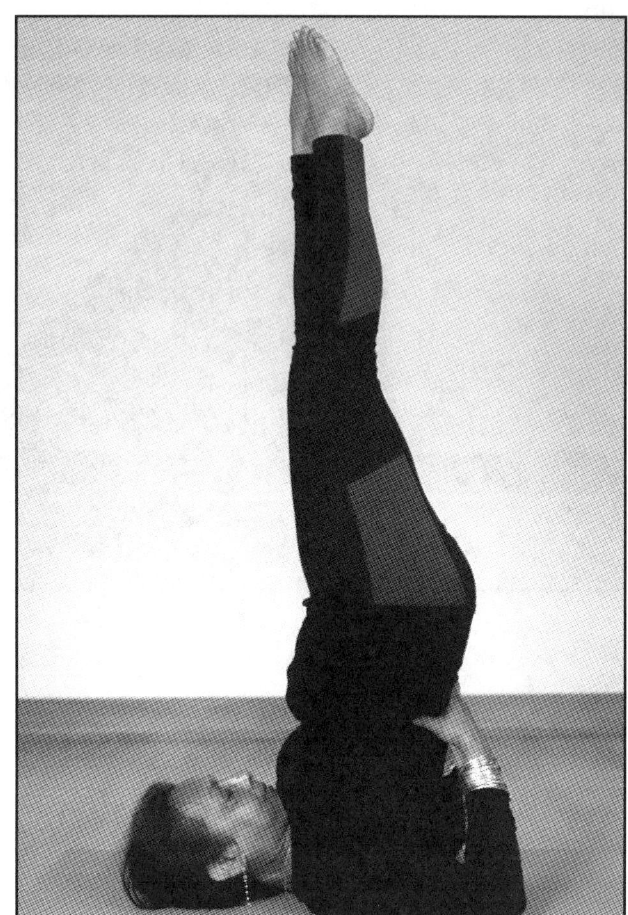

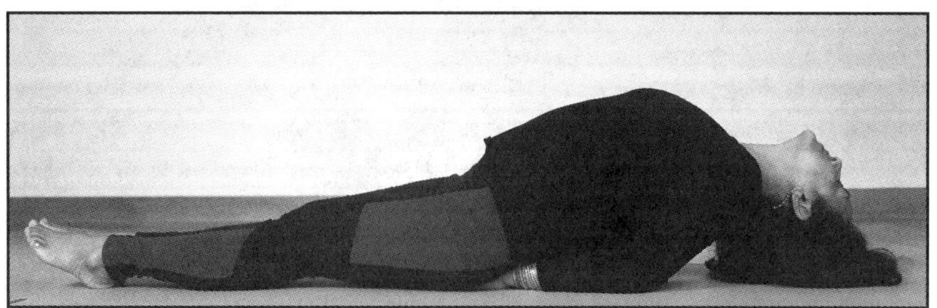

Fish

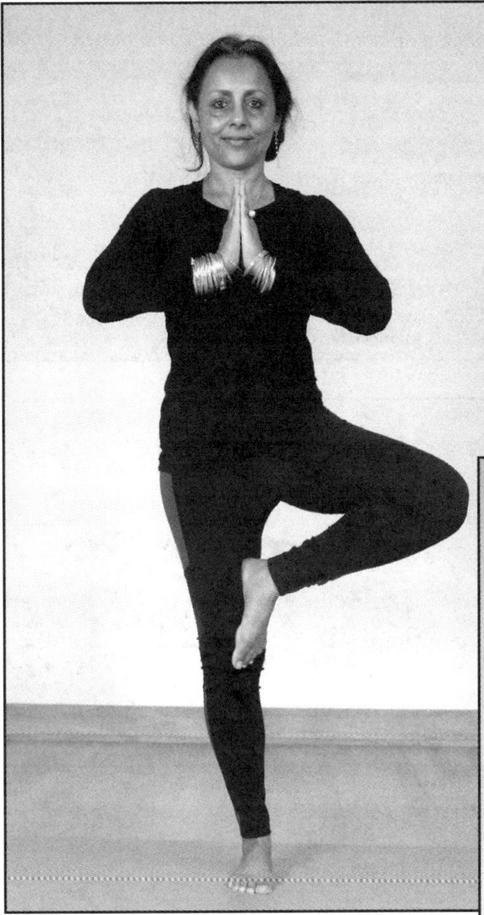

Tree (left)

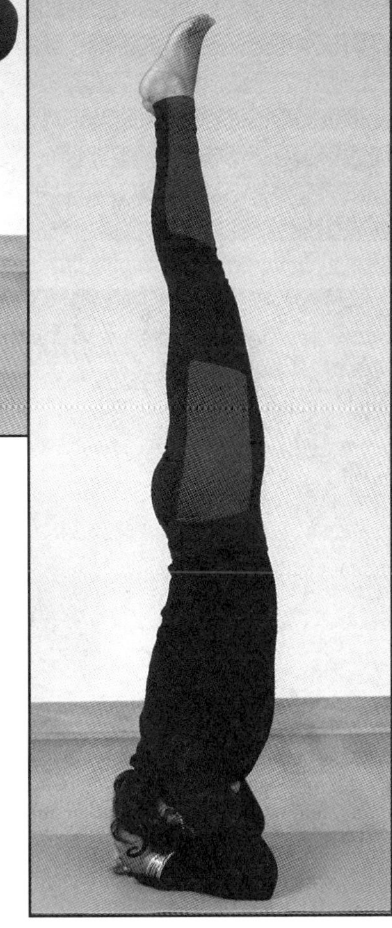

Headstand (right)

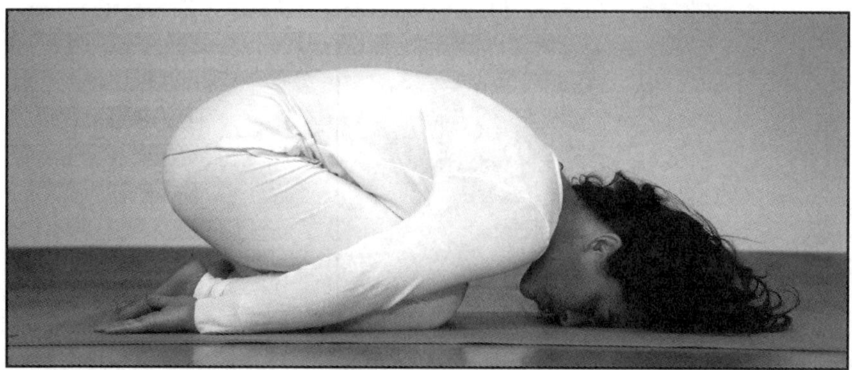

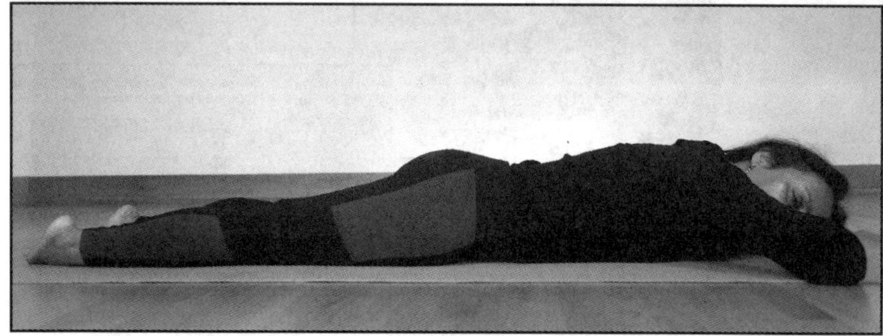

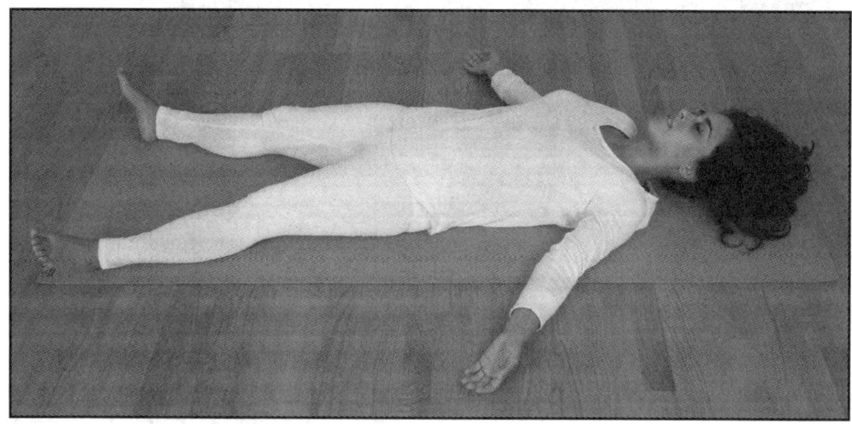

Child's pose (top)
Crocodile pose (middle)
Corpse pose (bottom)

Anatomy and Physiology of Breathing

It is important to know the anatomy and physiology of breathing in order to understand how the body, breath, emotions and mind interconnect and interact. The lower respiratory tract includes the bronchi, bronchioles and alveoli. There are rings of smooth muscle in the bronchi and bronchioles. The respiratory tract ends in clusters of alveoli where gas exchange takes place. Asthma and COPD are diseases that involve the bronchi and alveoli.

Lungs

There are two lungs, the right having three lobes and the left having only two lobes to allow room for the heart. The apices of the lungs sit under the clavicles (collar bones) and the lower, broader parts rest on the diaphragm. Pleural membranes cover the lungs to protect and support the lung tissue. The cilia that line the inside of the respiratory track produce sticky mucus that acts like a filter to trap particles. Cilia also move mucus up towards the pharynx to be coughed out.

The lungs interact with the heart to bring life-giving oxygen to the cells of the body and to eliminate the cellular waste product, carbon dioxide (CO_2). The lungs receive oxygen (O_2) from the outside world, which mixes with blood from the heart to oxygenate it. A general summary of the interaction of the heart and the lungs is as follows. Bright red blood rich with oxygen is pumped out of the left side of the heart to circulate through the body. The tissues take up O_2 and release CO_2 into the blood that is carried by the veins back to the right side of the heart. Because this blood has been deoxygenated it is bluish in color. From here, the blood moves into the lungs where CO_2 is exhaled from the lungs and the blood picks up oxygen that the lungs have inhaled.

Anatomically, this flow and exchange is as follows. The inferior and superior vena cava, which drain the lower and upper parts of the body carry deoxygenated blood to the right atrium of the heart. The blood then flows through the tricuspid valve to the right ventricle, which sends blood to the lungs through the pulmonary valve to the pulmonary artery. The blood picks up oxygen from the lungs as it gives off carbon dioxide. The oxygenated blood now is red in color. It enters the pulmonary vein where it goes to the left atrium. Next the blood goes through the bicuspid mitral valve to the left ventricle from where it is pumped through the main aorta to all areas of the body.

Arteries are defined as the blood vessels that leave the heart and carry red blood replete with oxygen to the body, and veins are the vessels that carry bluish blood full of carbon dioxide, the result of cellular respiration, back to the heart. The only exception to this is the pulmonary artery that leaves the heart but carries deoxygenated blood from the right ventricle to the lungs and the pulmonary vein, which then carries oxygenated blood from the lung to the left atrium of the heart. Venous circulation is more sluggish than the arterial system as the heart's strong contraction propels the arterial blood out of the heart into the body circulation, while the circulatory system relies on the weaker closing action of the values of the veins to return the blood back to the heart. To help move the blood back to the heart through the venous system, the contraction and relaxation of the diaphragm creates a partial vacuum in the thoracic cavity. This suction effect helps to pull up the venous blood into the inferior vena cava. Venous return is also aided by the movement and muscle contraction of the legs. Because this is a closed system, the heart's contraction also helps the venous circulation.

Nose

The nose is much more than an ornament in the center of the face. There are several very important functions that the nose serves. For instance, the nose warms and humidifies the air so that cold or very dry air does not injure the lower respiratory tract. Anatomically, the nose has both a prominent mucous membrane layer and a layer of erectile tissue. The only other organ with erectile tissue is the genitals. Thus, these two layers share the common property of expansion when emotionally excited, leading to nasal changes such as a stuffy nose. There are also three turbinates on both sides of the nose that swell and shrink to direct air and control the amount of pressure that flows into the lungs. The small hairs (cilia) in the nose capture foreign particles and microorganisms to protect the lower respiratory tract from injury and infection. The mucus that lines the inside of the nostrils is also protective in that it helps move dirt, dust and microorganisms out of the body. The yoga cleansing technique, neti (nasal wash), helps clear the nose of mucus, shrinks swollen membranes and allows for better air and prana flow. This can be performed either from one nostril to the other and out the nose or into the nose and out the mouth.

For all the above reasons, yoga teaches that people should always try to breathe and do breathing exercises through the nose rather than the mouth. Mouth breathing should be used only during special situations such as vigorous exercise, where a maximum amount of inhaled air is necessary due to increased bodily demands. There are also a few pranayama techniques that promote inhaling through the mouth for specialized effects.

There are three nerves in the nose that play a role in breathing: the olfactory nerve (first cranial nerve), the sympathetic nerve and the parasympathetic nerve. The olfactory nerve is responsible for the sense of smell. It is located high up in the nose, which is why one sniffs deeply to take air into the higher parts of the nose to appreciate certain smells. This nerve also sends fibers to the rhinencephalon (smell brain), an ancient part of the mammalian brain responsible for instinct and intuitive thought. This nerve tract also has interconnections with the hypothalamus (hormone control), the preoptic centers and the motor tracks of the vagus nerve. The sympathetic and parasympathetic nervous systems have fibers in the nose, and these affect the autonomic nervous system in a myriad of ways. These autonomic nerve fibers are partly responsible for maintaining a two-and–a-half-hour natural cycling when one or the other side of the nose is more open. This rhythm affects the body, emotions and mental functioning, as described below.

Breathing has interactions with the autonomic nervous system and the immune system. When there is stimulation of the nasal portion of the vagus nerve (the tenth cranial nerve), sensory fibers in the nose send transmission signals to inhibit a molecule called tumor necrosis factor. This inhibition has the effect of stopping the production of cytokines that can lead to inflammation. Also, vagal stimulation directly enhances natural killer cell activity. This can have the effect of helping the immune system be more effective.

The vagus nerve is the nerve that is most closely involved with the parasympathetic nervous system and the release of acetylcholine, which has the effect of relaxing the body and mind. There is a paradox, however, in that stimulation of the parasympathetic nervous system, especially when practicing certain breathing exercises, usually has a relaxation effect. On the other hand, overstimulation results in bronchial constriction, which can lead to asthma. Similarly, oversecretion of stomach acid, can lead to gastroesophageal reflux and ulcers. More on this subject can be found later in the discussions about asthma and ulcers.

Generally, overstimulation can be modified and counteracted by the relaxation effects associated with certain yogic breathing techniques. Gently activating the parasympathetic nervous system promotes the release of brain endorphins and natural brain opioid neuropeptides, neurochemicals that act to modulate pain and relax bronchial smooth muscle.

In addition, when the vagus nerve is stimulated through breathing techniques, there can be a reduction in inflammation. Inflammation stimulates the sensory part of the vagus nerve, which then sends messages to the medulla. From here neural messages stimulate the motor fibers of the vagus, resulting in messages being sent back to the inflamed areas with release of acetylcholine. Acetylcholine then suppresses the release of tumor necrosis factor from the macrophages. The overall effect of this mechanism is decreased inflammation.

Three Phases of Breathing

With respect to the lungs, there are three phases of breathing: diaphragmatic, chest and clavicular (collar bones). Since blood tends to pool low in the lungs, it is important to bring the air down low and deep into the lungs so the blood can mix efficiently with the inhaled air.

Diaphragmatic breathing is extremely important, not only for efficient normal breathing but also for its relaxation effect that is necessary for more advanced pranayama techniques. The abdomen should move out when inhaling and inwards towards the back when exhaling. However, many people breathe paradoxically, meaning they push the belly in when inhaling and out when exhaling. This is inefficient and can create feelings of anxiety. The optimal qualities of normal breathing are as follows: The breath should be taken in and out through the nose, not the mouth; and, it should be quiet, slow, smooth, even and deep, but not forced. There should be no pauses after inhalation ends and exhalation begins or after exhalation ends and inhalation begins. I recommend visualizing a circle or a sine wave to help with the process of smooth and uninterrupted breathing. In general, slow breathing causes a slight shift to hypercapnia (increased carbon dioxide), which promotes the parasympathetic relaxing effects.

Yoga teaches us that uneven breath results in an erratic flow of prana. Physiologically, irregular breathing influences every cell of the body by its effect on oxygenation and blood flow and on the central and peripheral (autonomic) nervous systems as well as on the emotions and thought processes. With conscious control of the breath, a person can learn to observe and direct the amount and quality of energy entering the body. Through slow, deliberate practice of simple breathing techniques such as diaphragmatic breathing, one learns to discern which irregularities of the breath flow are associated with particular illnesses, how certain states of mind adversely affect breathing patterns and also how to redirect and guide the breath to create harmony between mind and body.

Diaphragmatic breathing is the most efficient and relaxing method of breathing. It is most effectively learned in stages as the person who is just beginning to do breathing exercises usually experiences difficulty identifying with or experiencing the movement of the diaphragm. In the initial stage, focus is on breath awareness and becoming aware of the qualities of the breath. Through breath awareness one can become sensitive to their normal way of breathing and how it makes them feel. The qualities of the breath to observe are as follows: is your breath fast or slow, smooth or jerky, noisy or silent, even or irregular and are you creating a pause between the two phases of breathing, inhalation and exhalation. During the practice of breath awareness, the movement of the breath can be observed wherever it is taking place—chest, lower abdomen, upper abdomen. The point is just to become aware of your breathing habits without judging them or making your breathing forced or unnatural.

The diaphragm is the flat, horizontal musculotendinous structure that divides the chest cavity and the abdominal cavity. It is attached in the front to the xyphoid process of the sternum, posteriorly to the lumbar spine and laterally to the intercostal muscles that lie between the eleventh and twelfth ribs. In diaphragmatic breathing the movement is in the upper abdomen just below the rib cage. Inhalation is initiated by contraction and flattening of the diaphragm. Exhalation is passive with relaxation and doming upwards of the diaphragm. The abdomen's connection to the diaphragm creates a coordinated mechanism, whereby the upper abdomen moves away from the body and the lower rib cage expands as the diaphragm drops on inhalation and flattens when the diaphragmatic dome moves upwards on exhalation.

With respect to the mechanism of the lower respiratory muscles, inhalation causes contraction of the respiratory muscles, which enlarges the chest cavity; then, air with abundant O_2 moves in as the diaphragm lowers and flattens out. These muscles contract to bring the ribs closer together, lifting the chest slightly and increasing lung capacity. During exhalation, the respiratory muscles relax, causing the lungs to deflate and push out the stale air; simultaneously the diaphragm domes upwards against the base of the lungs to assist in the release of breath and CO_2 from the lungs.

Chest breathing involves contraction of the intercostal muscles, which expands the chest on inhalation and contracts the chest on exhalation. This is more stimulating in general and is necessary during strenuous exercise. However, if one habitually breathes only with the chest and locks up the abdomen and diaphragm, this results in an inefficient exchange of air and makes pranayama practices difficult.

Clavicular breathing is characterized by slightly raising the collar bones to get a bit more air into the lungs, especially if exercise is extremely vigorous. This is also seen in people who are struggling to breathe in such illnesses as asthma and COPD.

The Breath and Health

Breathing helps to control the autonomic nervous system, which is responsible for the stress response, the physiological reaction to emotional upheaval, and aspects of normal functioning of the immune system. The autonomic nervous system regulates the involuntary physiologic functions of various internal organ systems such as respiration, pulse rate, blood pressure, reproductive functioning and digestion. The word *autonomic* implies that these systems work automatically, without the need for conscious volition to direct their functioning. This is in contrast to the musculoskeletal, or voluntary, nervous system, which regulates voluntary muscle movement. Breathing stimulates the parasympathetic system by activating the vagus nerve through nerve endings in the nose and stretch receptors in the lungs, and by activating the carotid bulb within the carotid artery. This brings about a relaxing effect via the nerve endings along the spine and also helps decrease pressure on the adrenal glands. It seems reasonable to assume that part of the control afforded by breathing exercises and yoga in general may be due to the pacification of the sympathetic system. This control is accomplished through correct upright posture, which removes tension from the two sympathetic cords along the spinal canal as well as decreases pressure on the adrenal glands, both of which are the main sources of adrenaline (epinephrine), which triggers the body's fight-or-flight response. Also the relaxation effect is facilitated through activation of the opposing parasympathetic system by diaphragmatic breathing and control of the nerve plexuses associated with the chakras. For example, special control of the solar plexus, which is mainly supplied by the vagus nerve, seems essential to achieve parasympathetic control. The conscious relaxation that results from diaphragmatic breathing also effects the pacification of the large sympathetic glands, the adrenals, which are located in the area of the solar plexus. Parasympathetic nerves (found in the nose, pharynx, stretch receptors of the lungs, and chemoreceptors of the carotid body) are stimulated by pranayama techniques. Parasympathetic nerve plexuses are also found in the major centers in the body that correspond with the chakras.

In fact, many yoga practitioners who are versed in anatomy and physiology state that it is the essential control and stimulation of the parasympathetic system, primarily through the right vagus nerve, that is actively promoted through breathing exercises. Activation of the parasympathetic system through breathing exercises and deep concentration is generally associated with relaxation and slowing down of physiological processes. After learning to consciously regulate the parasympathetic nervous system, the practitioner who advances in breathing exercises may gain greater control of the hypothalamus, where the parasympathetic nervous system finally sends its sensory nerve impulses.

From the central controlling station of the hypothalamus, control of the connecting limbic system (emotions), cerebral cortex (thoughts and intellectual ideas), pituitary gland (endocrine gland activities), rhinencephalon (instinct), appetite center and body temperature center may be gained. This may explain how pranayama may lead the advanced practitioner of yoga to control of body, mind and senses.

It is important to not confuse these physiological mechanisms with those of the subtler pranic energy pathways. They are separate parallel systems, operating simultaneously, yet at different vibratory levels. Prana underlies all physical functioning, for yoga philosophy states that without prana there would be no physiology or life. By controlling the parasympathetic system, sympathetic nervous system, spinal and cerebral centers, the physical body is calmed and, in a sense, purified, allowing the subtler, underlying parallel pranic forces to be observed, directed and regulated. By controlling these various nerve systems, unconscious aspects of a person's mind come into conscious awareness. With the control of pranic forces through pranayama and more advanced breathing exercises, one can experience expanded states of consciousness.32

Breath Control and the Mind and Emotions

The breath is the link between body and mind. Prana is transmitted through the breath and is thus the bridge between the different levels of consciousness (koshas). Specifically, the physical sheath (annamaya kosha) and the mental sheath (manomaya kosha) are linked by the pranic sheath (pranamaya kosha), which is mediated through the breath. Meditation theory suggests that because energy links the body and mind, imbalances on the energy level often reflect or predate physical disorders or emotional problems. Before mental disease can produce physiologic changes, the disharmony first may pass through the intermediary energy level. Conversely, physical illnesses may manifest as changes in energy patterns before affecting the mind or emotions.

Disruptions in concentration are often associated with pauses and hesitations in breathing. Practicing simple techniques to regulate the rhythm of the breath brings about greater mental clarity and continuity of thought. Emotional states are often accompanied by altered breathing patterns. Examples of such alterations are the sobbing sounds of grief, the sighs of disappointment and sadness, the trembling breath of anger, gasping when surprised, rapid breathing when frightened, holding the breath when worried and irregular breathing when anxious. Breath control helps slow and regulate these altered patterns of breathing and results in greater calm and control of emotions.

Breathing Exercises and Pranayama Techniques

Breathing exercises are essential for integrating body, emotions and mind. They are useful in the treatment of many physical illnesses such as asthma, sinus conditions, digestive problems and thyroid disorders. They are also helpful for controlling stressful situations and treating emotional problems including anxiety, obsessive-compulsive disorder and depression. The ability of breathing exercises to affect the mind and emotions can be explained by the fact there are direct nerve connections from the nose and lungs to the brain with important relays to the nervous and endocrine

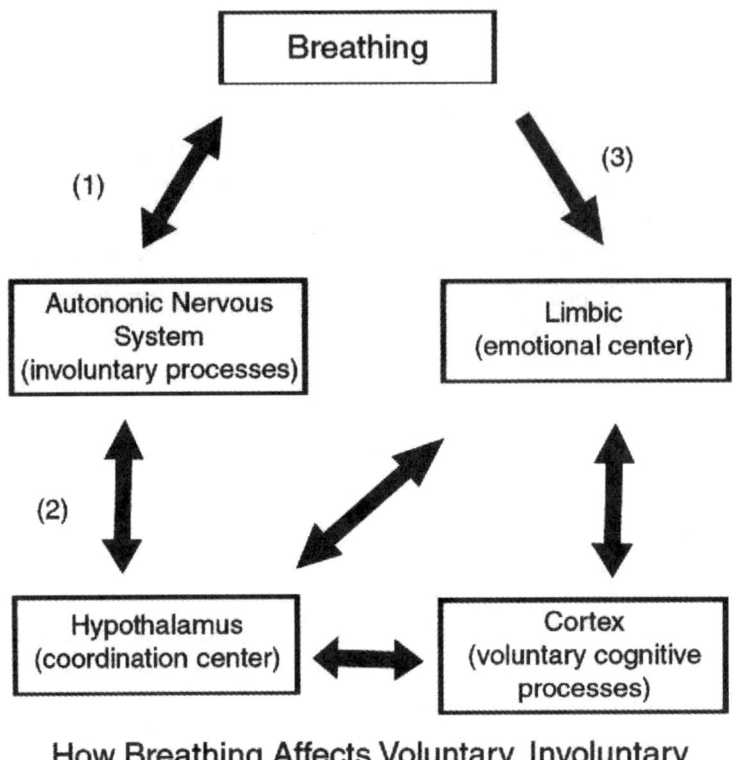

How Breathing Affects Voluntary, Involuntary and Emotional Processes

(1) through vagus-parasympathetic nerves (nose receptors, lung stretch receptors, cardiac-celiac plexus, carotid sinuses)
(2) nose (olfactory nerve to rhinencephalon)
(3) parasympathetic nerve

(hormone) systems. Pranayama techniques are also essential in the practice of meditation.

Breathing exercises have many beneficial effects on all the levels of consciousness. Over a lifetime people develop bad habits and do not breathe with maximum efficiency. Shallow and irregular respiration, accompanied by the pollution in the air, precipitates and exacerbates such diseases as asthma, pneumonia and bronchitis. Breath cleansing techniques can contribute to the prevention of such common disorders as allergies, sinusitis, tonsillitis and laryngitis. Deep, smooth breathing assures that a sufficient amount of oxygen is supplied to all the tissues, including brain, heart and muscles, reestablishing homeostasis and physiological equilibrium.

Breathing exercises also induce memory processing as the vagus nerve's ascending fibers stimulate nerve fibers in the brain stem (nucleus of the solitary tract), which causes release of norepinephrine into areas of the brain that process memory (amygdala and hippocampus).

Breathing is considered to be the link between the conscious and unconscious mind. Unlike heart, kidney or gastrointestinal functioning, breathing is the only physiologic function that can either be voluntarily controlled by the mind or, if one chooses not to pay attention to the flow of the breath, the body can involuntarily and automatically control the breathing process. Therefore, in the conscious act of doing certain types of breathing exercises, one gains greater awareness and control of involuntary physical functions as well as of the unconscious mind.

The following breathing and pranayama exercises should only be practiced under the guidance of an experienced yoga teacher.

Breath Awareness

While it may seem as though many thoughts are occurring in the mind simultaneously, in reality the mind is rapidly moving from thought to thought. When the mind follows the inflow and outflow of the breath, the mind becomes more focused, does not wander or rapidly change, and thus it becomes a more potent tool to appreciate and experience both the inner and outer worlds. Awareness of the breath flow in and out of the nose can also help quiet and focus the mind to deepen meditation. This can be further amplified by simultaneous silent repetition of a mantra.

By cultivating the skill of breath awareness, "standing back" for a few moments to impartially view the nature, direction and rhythm of the breath flow, a person can begin to transform their consciousness. They will come to understand that certain emotional stimuli or thought patterns alter the inspiratory and expiratory cycle. For instance, the consequences of holding the breath while studying for exams may be tiredness and weakness. If someone breathes rapidly with short bursts while driving in heavy traffic, they may become fidgety and nervous. Or if anger is suppressed, there may be activation of the sympathetic nervous system, associated with chest breathing, constriction of arteries and possible hypertension.

A person who has practiced and experienced the benefits of smooth, effortless breathing can adapt this fluidity to times of stress that are usually associated with breathing irregularity. Irrational feelings or scattered thinking can then be brought under more conscious control. Slowly one learns to watch the respiratory cycle with such efficiency that emotional extremes are minimized or prevented.

Breathing and Pranayama Techniques	
Complete yoga breath	abdomen, chest, and clavicles
Nadi shodhanam	alternate nostril breathing
Ujjayi	sobbing breath
Kapalabhati	shining skull breath
Bhastrika	bellows breath
Bhramari	bee breath
Sitali	hissing breath
Sitkari	cooling breath
Surya bheda kumbhaka	alternate nostril breathing with retention

The *complete yoga breath* brings a great deal of oxygen to the body and so feels quite energizing. It is a specific technique to energize the nadis and the nervous system. It involves exaggerating the three phases of breathing in a continuous, slow and deep manner. To begin with, the abdomen slowly moves out on inhalation, followed by rising of the chest, and finishing with the collarbones moving upwards towards the neck. Exhalation follows in the reverse order. The complete yoga breath is therapeutic for asthma and chronic bronchial conditions because there is stretching of the thoracic muscles, which decreases stiffness and increases vital capacity. Similarly, because of its stimulation of the abdominal muscles and internal organs, it is also helpful in gastritis and irritable bowel syndrome.

Nadi shodhanam (alternate nostril breathing), also called *anuloma viloma*, involves breathing through alternate nostrils. After a full and relaxed inhalation and exhalation through both nostrils, the practitioner uses the tip of the right thumb to block off airflow to the right nostril and then inhales through the left nostril. After slowly taking a full breath, the left nostril is blocked off with the tip of the ring finger and air is eliminated through the right nostril. After completely exhaling through the right nostril, the breath is drawn in again through the right nostril. Then the right thumb blocks the right nostril and breath is exhaled through the left nostril. This completes one cycle. The process then repeats itself and, in the beginning, it is practiced three to seven cycles, with increasing numbers reserved for more experienced practitioners. As a pranayama technique, the airflow is shifted with the mind rather than using the fingers to open and close the nostrils.

Breathing affects brain laterality and the functions in the various areas of the brain. There is a crossover of the nerve pathways from the nose to the brain. Therefore, stimulating the right nostril affects the left structures of the brain and vice versa. Alternate nostril breathing uses the above principle by alternately breathing gently through one nostril and then the other.

A person can open a blocked side of the nose by lying on the opposite side while leaning on the elbow with the palm of the hand placed on the side of the head or by placing the opposite arm pit from the blocked side of the nose over a chair. According to yogis, applications of having specific sides of the nose open are: it is best to have the left nostril open during deep sleep, the right side for men and the left side for women during sex, right side for better digestion, left side for creative endeavors and right side for intellectual discourse.

It is sometimes helpful to focus on the sixth chakra (ajna chakra) while repeating the mantra *OM* during alternate nostril breathing.

This technique is often done before beginning meditation because it purifies the nadis and brings clarity to the mind. Alternate nostril breathing has also been shown to be very useful in the treatment of psychological problems such as anxiety, obsessive thought disorders and depression.

Ujjayi (sobbing breath) is practiced by breathing in slowly through both nostrils and feeling the inspired air on the roof of the soft palate. A soft, continuous sobbing sound is made because the glottis remains partially closed. Mental repetition of the mantra *SO* can accompany inhalation. Without any pause, exhalation begins with the outflowing air also being felt on the roof of the mouth. Mentally, the mantra *Ham* (rhymes with the word "rum" and "numb") can be repeated. Seven to twenty-one repetitions can be practiced. Ujjayi helps to calm the mind and is useful in physical conditions such as sore throats, nasal congestion and sinusitis.

Kapalabhati (shining skull breath) consists of rapid, vigorous and forceful expulsion of air using the abdominal muscles and diaphragm. This is followed by a relaxation of the abdominal muscles and a passive, gentle, spontaneous inhalation. Seven to twenty-one repetitions can be done, followed by a brief rest. Three to seven cycles can be practiced in the beginning. Kapalabhati is both a breathing exercise and a kriya (cleansing) and is helpful for sinus infections, nasal obstruction, asthma, and for stimulating the digestive organs and exercising the abdominal muscles.

Bhastrika (bellows breath) involves forcefully moving the abdominal muscles in and out so that exhalation and inhalation are vigorous and rapid. One in-and-out breath is one cycle. Between seven and twenty-one cycles are generally practiced and then repeated three to seven times. Alternatively, the practitioner can close off one nostril and do both inhalation and exhalation out of the same side for several repetitions and then switch sides. The benefits of bhastrika are similar to kapalabhati.

Bhramari (bee breath) is a technique that involves partially closing off the throat and glottis and bringing air in through the nose. A sound is produced on both inhalation and exhalation that resembles the sound of bees in flight. When several people practice this exercise simultaneously it makes a beautiful, melodious sound.

This breathing exercise can be practiced from seven to twenty-one times. Bhramari can be used for thyroid conditions, throat problems and sinus congestion. It also helps bring about mental clarity before meditation.

Sitali (hissing breath) is practiced by breathing in through the mouth and out through the nose. Two methods of inhalation are possible. The student can turn the tongue backwards so that the tip is resting on the soft palate. Breath is then taken in through the pressure of the combined resistance of the tongue and soft palate. The other more common approach is to roll the tongue lengthwise into a tube-like structure and protrude the tongue a little beyond the lips. Exhalation in both instances is slowly out through the nose. This technique is useful for cooling the body, which is helpful for conditions that involve excess body heat including fever, menopausal hot flashes or being overheated from exercise or hot weather.

Sitkari (cooling breath) involves breathing in through the mouth and out through the nose. The teeth are closed, and the tongue is placed so that it does not touch the teeth, palate or bottom of the mouth. Air is drawn in making a loud noise. The breath is deep and slow. Exhalation is done quietly. This can be practiced from seven to twenty-one times. Benefits include cooling the body, helping insomnia, and controlling the appetite.33

Pranayama Techniques and Bandhas

When physical locks and breath retention are added to the techniques described above, simple breathing exercises become important pranayama exercises. This should only be done, however, under the guidance of a teacher who is skilled in the science of breath and who knows the student's general health and formal meditation practice. Except for a few techniques, pranayama exercises involve sitting with an erect spine, breathing only through the nose, and allowing the upper abdomen to move away from the body on inhalation and towards the body on exhalation (diaphragmatic breathing). The rhythm and rate may vary but it is deep, though not overly forced, and smooth without pauses or jerkiness. If breath retention is not practiced, there should be no hesitation after exhalation or inhalation.

Pranayama cleanses the nadis of obstructions to the flow of energy and increases one's capacity to tolerate and channel the great amount of energy associated with the highest stages of consciousness. Specific yoga pranayama or breathing techniques in association with stress reduction techniques and relaxation exercises help to facilitate smooth and efficient transmission of pranic energy between the outer and inner worlds as well as within the subtler levels of the practitioner.

The Science of Meditation

As a physician trained in a traditional medical school, the University of Michigan, I strongly believe in science and experimental design. My life partner, Ruma, who is a professor of biochemistry at the University of Michigan, and I have had many interesting discussions about the interface between science and Eastern philosophy. We both acknowledge that the scientific method, inquiry and proof are of absolute importance for such things as the development of drugs and vaccines and the epidemiology of public health issues. We can especially see the importance of this during our current battle with COVID-19.

Yet, personal experimentation and experience provide another time-tested method to prove efficacy and validity. People have been practicing yoga and meditation for thousands of years and have had insights and experiences that have been similar over these many years. In the following section, I try to bring these two methodologies together by discussing the science behind meditation and its effects on the brain and nervous system, heart, lung and digestive functioning along with immunity. Some of the research articles may be a bit technical, but I thought a more thorough discussion would be interesting to those readers who would appreciate a scientific approach to understanding how meditation affects body and mind.

Overview of Meditation and the Brain

The practice of meditation directly affects brain wave patterns. The EEG, which captures these brain wave patterns, often shows several types of changes that reflect less anxiety and a calmer mental and emotional state during and after sitting for meditation. There are reports of lower amplitudes of all brain wave patterns, reflecting less intense responses to stressful stimuli. Beta activity is reduced, indicating less activation of the frontal brain region, which is the area responsible for emotional reactivity. There are more frontal alpha waves upon exposure to loud noise, which is associated with less anxiety. This alpha activity is not easily blocked, even by the sensory stimuli of heat, cold, sound, light or vibration.

The Menninger Foundation's research with Swami Rama in the early 1970s found that he was able to produce delta brain wave patterns on EEG while remaining totally conscious and aware. This is highly significant, because delta waves are found only in deep sleep, the most restful of all human states, in which there are no dreams or rapid eye movements. Remaining wakeful during this relaxed state results in extremely pleasurable and calm experiences. In meditation philosophy, the state of sleepless sleep (turiya) is considered to be an evolved and expanded state of consciousness.34

Attention to the rhythms of mantra recitation and breathing patterns during meditation creates an anti-anxiety and calming effect and, in a sense, acts as a natural tranquilizer. The act of observing and letting go of disturbing thoughts and feelings has a desensitization effect, similar to behavioral therapy. This helps one to become less reactive to hidden fears and anxiety and thus can be helpful for conditions like generalized panic disorder. Consistent practice results in an increase in feelings of self-confidence, optimism, fewer guilt feelings and a decrease in unreasonable internal expectations. Improved self-esteem, less intense grief reactions and diminished separation anxiety are also mentioned as benefits of meditation.

The yoga breathing technique of alternate nostril breathing (described above) can be modified so that both inhalation and exhalation take place through the left nostril. This technique has

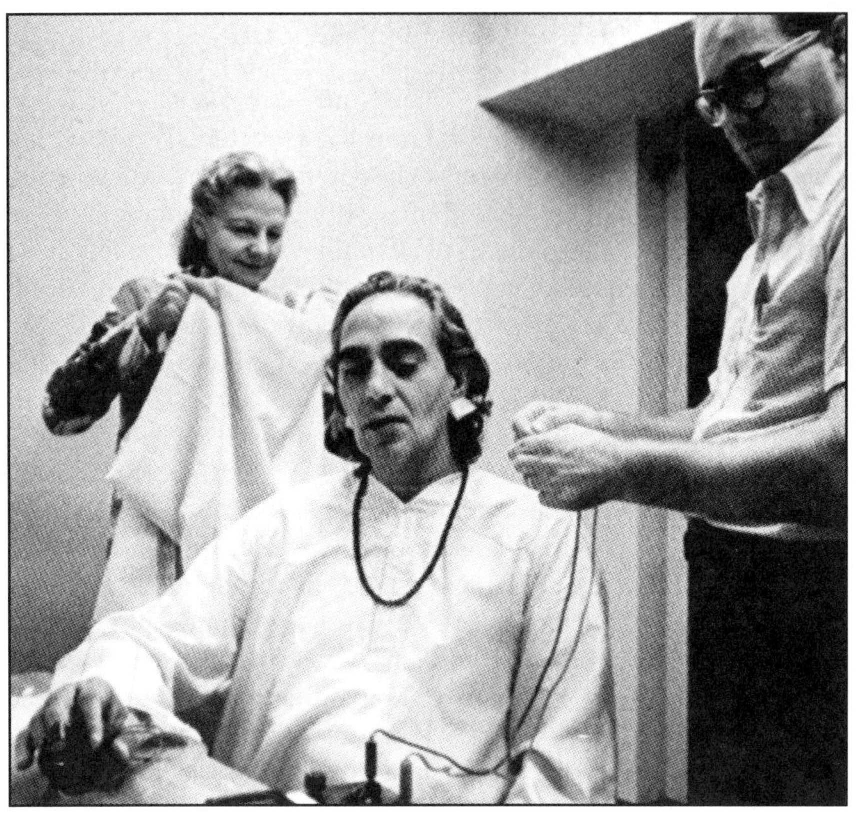

Swami Rama at the Menninger Foundation

been shown to be effective in obsessive-compulsive disorder. The explanation for this is that this disorder seems to be associated with less activity in the right side of the brain. By stimulating the left nerve endings in the nose that then cross over to the right side of the brain, there is increased stimulation on the right side of the brain, resulting in the blocking of some obsessive-compulsive urges.35

During meditation, there is a shift to a greater balancing of activity between the two hemispheres of the brain. The left hemisphere, which is dominant in most people, is responsible for linear, time-oriented and verbal thought. The right brain is more involved with creative, intuitive and abstract thinking. Since meditation and breathing exercises create more of a balanced effect, there is greater integration between reasoning abilities and creativity. The practice of visualization-based meditative techniques also leads to a more creative use of the imagination.

Repetition of the mantra or uninterrupted focus of the mind on an image causes a blanking out of all thought and decreases responses to internal and external stimulation. The result is a renewed enthusiasm for new stimuli and thought patterns, reminiscent of a young child's excitement when presented with new experiences. This is similar to the concept of the "beginner's mind" described in the Zen Buddhist meditative tradition.

Meditation and the Stress Response

The practice of meditation can be of great therapeutic benefit when dealing with stress. Stress can be a disrupting influence affecting physical, emotional and mental well-being. Symptoms that can occur as a result of stress are anxiety, nervousness, rapid heartbeat, cold and clammy hands and muscle tension. External events such as bright lights, loud noises or environmental pollution as well as internal concerns such as fearful thoughts, troublesome memories or emotional traumas can cause stress. By its effects on the autonomic nervous system and on the endocrine glands, stress literally affects every cell in the body. A wide variety of diseases are attributed to the influence of stress, including hypertension, ulcers, migraine headaches, arthritis, heart disease and cancer.

In actuality, it is not the stressful event that causes problems, but one's response to stress that leads to illness or unhappiness. The physiological stress response itself is a vital and necessary adaptation for survival because it is one of the body's inherent mechanisms for protection. The act of pulling one's hands away from a fire, generating enough strength to beat off an attacker, or activating the immune system to increase the number of white blood cells to kill off invading virulent viruses or bacteria are all examples of healthy stress reactions. In normal circumstances, confrontation with a stressor (the agent or factor causing stress) is a self-limited experience because there is a finite period of time when the attack is taking place. The stress response has three stages: alarm (or recognition), resistance (or dealing with the stressor) and exhaustion (or recovery, when the organism rests to recuperate from the trauma of the stress). This mechanism works well in sudden and self-limited situations.

Problems occur with the normal stress reaction when the stressors are chronic, as is often the case in crowded urban living conditions where there is constant noise, congestion and pollution. The chronic stress response also occurs when a person is plagued by ongoing fear or anxiety. In this situation, the third phase of the normal stress response cannot be completed. Without the time for rest and recovery from the exertion of stress, one becomes exhausted and overwhelmed by a habituated stress response. As a result, there is a feeling of being run-down and weak, with lowered stamina, and eventually resistance is lowered to a point where one becomes vulnerable to serious disease. Again, the problem is not the stress itself but the prolonged or chronic stress response.

Whether or not a situation is stressful varies in individuals. For some, a traffic jam, preparing for a party or concerns about the welfare of one's children are major sources of stress, while for others these situations are not stressful at all. A person's psychological and emotional state of mind is crucial in determining how severe a disruptive challenge has to be before it is experienced as stressful.

Meditation can help us to develop resilience, inner strength, balance and adaptability so that the stress threshold is raised. This implies that the stress response is controllable and can be moderated when a person is faced with challenges. The goal of meditation is to learn how to observe one's thoughts and feelings with an objective awareness and to create a calm inner center. By applying what is experienced in the meditative state to life's everyday events, one can prevent the stress response from becoming chronic, habitual or exaggerated.

Breathing techniques, such as diaphragmatic breathing, alternate nostril breathing, and bhramari (bee breath) can also be of great benefit to diminish the stress response. To understand how these exercises are helpful, it is important to understand the physiology of the stress response. This is complex and involves interactions between the central nervous system (brain and spinal cord), autonomic (involuntary) nervous system, endocrine glands (hormones), and the organs, tissues and cells of the body.36

Meditation, the Brain and the Autonomic Nervous System

One experiences a stressful event through one of the five senses (hearing, touch, vision, taste and smell) or from a thought or feeling. Signals from the organ that receives the stimuli travel via nerves or nerve cells to the brain. The cerebral cortex then interprets the event and sends messages to various parts of the body to respond to the stressful thought or occurrence. If signals go to the frontal lobe or the limbic system in the brain, emotions will be experienced. The cerebellar response to activation would be to affect balance and movement. If the hypothalamus, amygdala or pituitary gland are stimulated, hormones are secreted that travel to different glands of the body. The endocrine glands (adrenal, thyroid, parathyroid, and sex glands) also respond by releasing various hormones, which in turn affect the metabolism and the immune system of the body.

Another system that is often stimulated by the pituitary gland is the autonomic nervous system, which is subdivided into the sympathetic and parasympathetic systems. While these subsystems often work in opposition to each other, the net result of their interaction is to create harmonious regulation (homeostasis). If one of the systems is chronically overstimulated or understimulated, physical illness or emotional problems related to the stress response may occur.

The sympathetic system controls the active internal processes and is the predominant system in dangerous situations. Activation of the sympathetic nervous system induces the following reactions: pupil dilation, increased blood flow to the heart and brain and constriction of blood vessels that supply digestion, kidney function and small muscles. This response is called the fight-or-flight mechanism. When dealing with an emergency, it makes sense for the following things to occur: pupils dilate so a person can see better, the heart speeds up to increase circulation and the blood vessels constrict so that a larger flow of blood may be directed

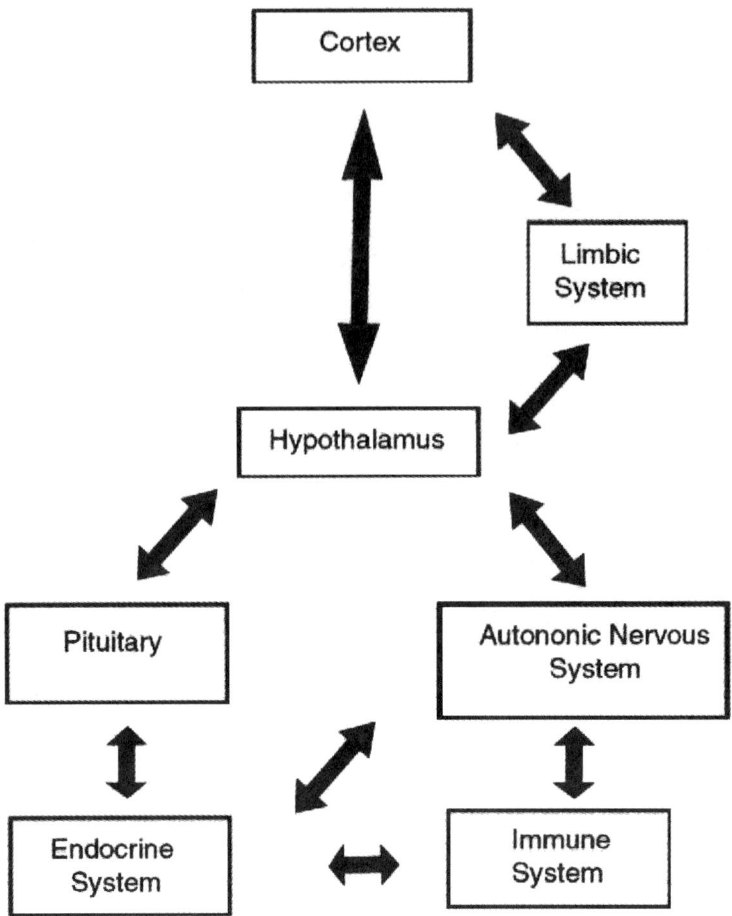

Relationship Between the Brain, Nervous System, Immune System, and the Glands

away from less vital structures to the larger muscles and the brain. This allows for more active responses and clearer thinking. Other changes that occur during activation of the sympathetic nervous system include: tensing of the muscles in the hands, feet, shoulders and neck; tightening of the throat; and changes in breathing from diaphragmatic to chest breathing or the holding of one's breath.

Organ	Sympathetic Nervous System Action	Parasympathetic Nervous System Action
Salivary gland	Stop secretion	Secrete
Heart	Accelerate	Decelerate
Bronchial tubes	Dilate	Constrict
Stomach	Stop secretion of acid	Secrete acid
Intestines	Decreases activity	Increases activity
Bladder	Relax	Contract
Blood vessels	Constrict	Dilate
Pupils of eyes	Dilate	Constrict
Skin temperature	Cooler	Warmer
Muscles	Tense	Relax

There are also important interconnections between the sympathetic nervous system and immunity. It is known that sympathetic nerve fibers have contact with and stimulate lymph glands, the spleen and the thymus gland. These tissues are responsible for producing certain biochemicals (cytokines) and lymphocytes (natural killer cells) that regulate the body's ability to fight infection. Increased sympathetic activity causes a marked reduction in the function of these natural killer cells, resulting in increased susceptibility to infectious diseases. The cytokines also communicate with other endocrine glands as well as with the brain cells of the hypothalamus, thereby affecting the function of these organs. All these interactions illustrate how stress can affect the body's ability to maintain hormonal balance and fight off infection.

These sympathetic nervous system responses are primitive instinctual reactions to danger and are required in an emergency. But if these reactions occur on a regular basis in the absence of a real threat, then one will experience the symptoms that characterize the stress response, such as heart pounding, sweaty hands, mind racing and general muscle tension.

The sympathetic nervous system is responsible for stimulating the glands that secrete adrenaline (also called epinephrine), which is the active hormone that causes the aforementioned responses. The two large sympathetic nerves running along each side of the spine stimulate the adrenal glands to secrete adrenaline. It seems reasonable that part of the control afforded by meditation, breathing exercises and yoga postures in general may be due to the pacification of the sympathetic nervous system. There are several techniques that regulate and pacify this system. During meditation the mind remains calm and emotions are brought under more conscious control, which has the effect of decreasing the release of adrenaline from the nerve endings and glands. Breathing exercises and meditation encourage a strong upright posture that takes the pressure off the sympathetic nerve chains that run alongside the spine. By efficient diaphragmatic breathing during meditation, the smooth and efficient movement of the abdominal and back muscles puts less pressure on the adrenal glands, located in the area of the solar plexus, so they produce a more regulated release of adrenaline.

The other way to balance the sympathetic reactions is to gently stimulate the parasympathetic nervous system. This system is responsible for opposing the reactions initiated by the sympathetic system and is generally associated with relaxation and feelings of well-being. The heart slows, the skin feels mildly flushed because the blood vessels relax, and the mind becomes calm as blood is no longer being hurriedly shunted to the brain. The kidneys and digestive organs become active and the muscles relax.

The main nerves associated with the parasympathetic nervous system are the paired cranial nerves, the vagus nerves. These wandering nerves leave the right and left sides of the brain, cross over to the other side of the body and have connections to many organs and tissues of the body. Meditation techniques that bring about a calm inner state allow the individual to gain greater control of the activity of the vagus nerves. When the vagus nerves are gently activated, this inhibits secretion of the hormones associated with the sympathetic nervous system, resulting in a state of relaxation.

Parasympathetic nerve endings that emanate from and travel to the vagus nerves are also found in the nose, throat, stretch receptors in the lungs and the chemoreceptors of the carotid artery (carotid bulb). Because these nerves are so closely associated with the organs of respiration and breathing, certain breathing techniques directly stimulate the parasympathetic system. Parasympathetic nerve endings are also found in the nerve plexuses located in the major gland centers in the body that correspond to the subtle chakras. Advanced practitioners of meditation who are versed in anatomy and physiology believe it is control and systematic stimulation of the parasympathetic nervous system, primarily through the right vagus nerve and its nerve endings, that is actively promoted through advanced breathing exercises. Activation of this system through breathing exercises and certain concentration techniques is generally associated with relaxation, the slowing of physiological processes and deeper meditative states.

Alternate nostril breathing is a particular breathing technique that is said to stimulate the vagus nerve endings in the nose and lungs, which has the effect of enhancing voluntary control of the parasympathetic nervous system. Diaphragmatic breathing, along with methods of concentration on the solar plexus area (third chakra), also helps bring about voluntary control of the parasympathetic nervous system.

After mastering the above-mentioned techniques to con-sciously stimulate and control parasympathetic nervous system activity, it is then possible to gain greater voluntary control of the hypothalamus located deep within the mid-brain. It is in the hypothalamus where the parasympathetic nervous system sends many of its signals and nerve impulses. From the central controlling center of the hypothalamus, control of the other interconnecting organs and body systems may be gained. This includes the limbic system (emotional center), cerebral cortex (thought and intellectual center), pituitary gland (endocrine gland activity), rhinencephalon (instincts), appetite center and body temperature center. These close connections may explain how breathing exercises and other meditative techniques allow a person who is more advanced in meditation, to control body, mind and senses.

As in all of life, balance is of utmost importance when dealing with the autonomic nervous system responses. When the sympathetic system is chronically activated, one experiences the symptoms of stress that lead to illness. If the parasympathetic system is over activated, one may not react quickly enough to situations that require immediate responses. One may become inappropriately relaxed to the point of being inactive or lazy. The path of meditation, as a complete system, enables us to balance and have greater control over the autonomic nervous system to create physical and mental harmony.37

Medical Research on the Health Benefits of Meditation and Yoga

Most of the medical research into the health benefits of meditation has focused on one of the following forms of meditation: meditation based on Zen philosophy uses breath awareness as its object of concentration; Transcendental Meditation (TM), a system practiced by followers of Maharishi Mahesh Yogi, uses specific mantras as its focus; Clinically Standardized Meditation is an unstructured Western-derived practice that uses various nonmantra sounds without breath awareness as a focus of concentration; and, Kundalini Yogic Meditation uses breathing techniques and mantra as a focus of concentration and has contributed to medical research. In addition, Herbert Benson, a physician who has done research on the relaxation response, developed a meditative system called Respiratory One Method, which uses repetition of the word *one* coordinated with the breath.

Mindfulness Meditation (Vipassana), also called Insight Meditation, is a Buddhist-derived system that encourages observation of thoughts and images with a nonjudgmental attitude and has no specific object of concentration. The Tibetan Buddhist approaches to meditation that use more abstract visualization, as promoted by the Dalai Lama and his associates and students, have also been studied in some depth.

The Tantric/Samkhya/Vedantic form of meditation, based on the eight principles of raja yoga, that is described in this book, uses an integrated method of breath, mantras, yantras and chakras as its objects of concentration. It is a system practiced in the Himalayan Mountains of India, Nepal and Tibet and its tenets and techniques have been handed down from teacher to student for thousands of years. I have studied this approach to meditation with Swami Rama. There are many documented health benefits associated with this form of meditation. However, the ultimate goal of this meditative tradition goes beyond its positive health effects and involves the desire to experience more expanded states of awareness. These more comprehensive states are often difficult to quantify because they tend to be nonverbal, experiential and anecdotal.

The following information on the various physiologic and psychological benefits of the above-mentioned forms of meditation is primarily based on two excellent books that summarize many research studies in clear and comprehensive ways: *Zen and the Brain* by J. Austin and *Complementary & Alternative Medicine* by L. Freeman and G. F. Lawlis.38

These research studies have shown that the practice of meditation is beneficial in the treatment of many diseases. On the physical level, people with heart disease have fewer palpitations and abnormal rhythms, including premature ventricular contractions and supraventricular contractions. In general, heart and respiratory rates decrease. Meditation is also effective in alleviating the symptoms of chronic medical conditions such as hypertension, chronic pain, insomnia, chronic fatigue syndrome, irritable bowel syndrome, menopausal symptoms, hot flashes and seizures.

In chronic stress syndrome a regular practice of meditation slows the release of hormones in response to stress, including cortisol from the adrenal glands, thyroid stimulating hormone (TSH) and growth hormone (GH) from the pituitary gland in the brain. There are increased levels of the hormone DHEA-S from the adrenals, which are generally lower as people age. The hypothalamus in the brain secretes less corticotrophin-releasing hormone (CRH), which has the effect of slowing the physiological responses to stressful events. Other important physiologic changes include a decline in the blood lactate level, which indicates the body is reacting less to stressful situations. Oxygen consumption is lowered to a level generally only seen after many hours of sleep. There is less suppression of immunity in response to stressful events, and there are lower amounts of the CD8+ cells, which are inhibitors of the important immune enhancing T cells.

Meditation also has important benefits on the emotional and psychological levels. In the treatment of depression, meditation is helpful because it increases the availability of serotonin and tryptophan in the central nervous system, both of which are important for mood elevation. Substance abuse problems, such as alcoholism, cigarette smoking and drug abuse have also been helped by meditation.

Over the years, I've been accumulating research articles about the effects of yoga and meditation on the body and mind. There have been some excellent journal articles that have provided further research on the positive effects of yoga and meditation. I will summarize the findings of this research, and at the end of the book you will find the credits and footnotes for these articles.

One study from a recently published research article demonstrated that a three-month training program in yoga and meditation positively affected the signaling pathway of brain derived neurotropic factor (BDNF), cortisol awakening response (CAR) and other immune markers.[39]

Another study comparing the effects of yoga and exercise found an improvement in a number of health-related outcome measures including blood glucose, blood lipids, salivary cortisol and oxidative stress. Furthermore, yoga appears to improve subjective measures of fatigue, pain and sleep in both healthy and ill populations.[40]

With respect to depression, anxiety and overall stress symptoms in women were reduced by a regular twelve-week hatha yoga practice. This included women with multiple sclerosis, on hemodialysis and who were pregnant.[41]

Recently I also came across an article that was an excellent summary of many other studies. This meta-analysis refers to seventy-four articles on the various effects of yoga and meditation on such conditions as diabetes, other endocrine abnormalities, immune and inflammatory cell dysfunction, depression and anxiety. Although this study details rather specific hormonal and biochemical changes, I encourage any student of yoga who is interested in the beneficial physiological and emotional changes associated with yoga and meditation to carefully read this article. Below is a summary of some of the major findings in this article.42

Diabetes is a growing problem in the world, especially in the developing world. It estimated that by the year 2030 there will be 330 million people in the world with type 2 diabetes, including 30 million in the US. Obesity and stress play a big role in the development of type 2 diabetes, which generally develops in adulthood. With respect to stress, the following hormones that are related to the stress response and are mediated in a positive direction by yoga, pranayama and meditation are: corticotrophin-releasing hormone (CRH), melatonin, growth hormone, prolactin, luteinizing hormone, thyroid hormone, cortisol, aldosterone, testosterone, adrenaline and other neurotransmitters like endorphins, serotonin, 5HIAA, VMA and GABA. Insulin secretion and cellular sensitivity to insulin have improved during these practices as well.

As discussed before, stress induces activation of the hypothalamus, pituitary, autonomic nervous system and sympathetic nervous system, which in turn causes hypersecretion of the pro-inflammatory proteins interleukin (IL-1, IL-6, IL-10) and decreased interferon gamma, which is important to a healthy immune system. Increased levels of B endorphin are seen in individuals who practice yoga. Meditation is also associated with an increase in melatonin levels, which is important for normal sleep cycles.

Regular yoga practices help to decrease blood glucose and glycosylated hemoglobin level (HbA1C) and result in improvement in the glucose tolerance test (GTT). A decrease in fasting insulin level, along with a rise in insulin receptors with increased percentage of receptor binding (even before glycemic control), suggests decreased insulin resistance and improved sensitivity to insulin. Also beneficial for the diabetic condition is the weight loss that commonly occurs from regular yoga practice, the decrease in body mass index (BMI) and the improvement in mood and quality of life. Better cognitive functioning and enhanced nerve transmission in diabetics have also been noted. Measurement of cerebral blood flow using single photon emission computed tomography showed activation of the right frontal lobe, prefrontal cortex and right sensory motor cortex during meditation. In addition, the meditation of kundalini yoga practices may increase the hippocampal and right amygdala activation and the parasympathetic response through right ventromedial hypothalamic stimulation.

The joyful feeling that follows yoga practice could be due to increased lateral hypothalamic stimulation, while the experience of calmness may be due to increases of melatonin. With respect to some out of body experiences that some practitioners have described as having occurred during meditation, it is hypothesized there is reduction in the brain hormone GABA that causes decreased spatial orientation. Also associated with altered states of consciousness are both an increase in N-acetylaspartylglutamate (analogous to the anesthetic and sometimes hallucinogenic drug, ketamine) and 5-methoxydimethyl tryptamine that derives from pineal enzymes.

Another important article written by Woodyard suggests that yogic practices lead to increased ability to concentrate and tranquility of the mind. Yoga decreases the perceived response to stress through activation of the cerebral-hypothalamic or corticolimbic pathway, which influences cortical areas that affect neurotransmitter and hormonal release.43 In another article on the neurobiology of spirituality where neuroimaging techniques were used, it is reported there is activation of the prefrontal and inhibitory thalamic reticular nucleus and a decrease in parietal lobe overactivity.44

Muscles, Cellular Respiration, Mitochondria and Energy Metabolism

The biochemical equation of cellular respiration is: Glucose + Oxygen = Carbon Dioxide + Water + ATP (energy). The chemical equation with the number of molecules in parenthesis is: $C_6H_{12}O_6$ + (6)O_2 = (6)CO_2 + (6)H_2O + ATP + heat. The interpretation of this formula is: during aerobic metabolism, glucose added with oxygen is converted to carbon dioxide and water and this yields high energy. In biochemical terms, this represents a redox reaction where one molecule loses electrons (it is said to be oxidized) and one molecule gains electrons (it is said to be reduced). Thus, in cellular respiration, glucose is oxidized, having lost electrons (and protons) to become carbon dioxide, while oxygen is reduced, having gained electrons (and protons) to become water.

The glucose molecule represents the breakdown product of food. Oxygen is taken into the body through the air that is inhaled. The resulting carbon dioxide in this reaction is a waste product that has a very important function in its own right as it is taken up by trees and other green plants to reproduce oxygen through the action of photosynthesis. This equation is carbon dioxide + water + light energy = glucose + oxygen. The chemical equation with the number of atoms and molecules in parentheses is $(6)CO_2$ + (6) H_2O + light energy = $C_6H_{12}O_6$ + $(6)O_2$. So, when carbon dioxide and water are combined with the energy from light in the presence of chlorophyll from plants, this converts to a carbohydrate (glucose) and oxygen. In this case, CO_2 is reduced, and water is oxidized.

As a result of the cellular respiration reaction, the energy molecule ATP is produced, which serves many very important functions. It is used as fuel for other cellular functions such as to drive metabolic reactions that do not occur automatically, to transport chemicals across cellular membranes and to help do mechanical work for structures in the body, such as to move muscles. ATP is a limited energy store; the bulk of it is stored in fats and carbohydrates. ATP delivers energy to support various cellular functions.

ATP has three components: a nucleotide (adenine), a sugar molecule (ribose) and a chain of three phosphate groups, the latter attached to the ribose molecule. Energy is stored in the phosphate bonds and this energy is released when one of the phosphates is cleaved off. When water is added, energy is released through the process of hydrolysis and a new molecule called ADP, which has only two phosphates left, is produced. Another process called phosphorylation allows ATP to transfer one of its phosphate groups to another molecule to activate other cellular functions. While ATP is constantly being broken down to fuel cellular activity, it is also being synthesized from ADP through cellular respiration, similar to the charging of a rechargeable battery. An enzyme called ATP synthase, which is present in mitochondria, converts ADP back to ATP by adding another phosphate to the ADP.

Mitochondria are small organelles that exist within cells. They number in the many trillions in the body. One important function of mitochondria is to generate ATP from the carbohydrates and other foods that we eat and the oxygen that we breathe. Healthy mitochondria are needed to have efficient energy metabolism. This is why it is essential to avoid mitochondrial decay, membrane injury, oxidative stress and free radical damage. Free radicals are molecules that have a free electron and because of this, these substances are very reactive and can damage mitochondria, DNA, RNA, enzymes and cell membranes. When this happens, the aging process is quickened, inflammatory conditions increase and even cancerous changes may occur.

There is also evidence that mitochondrial DNA damage can lead to metabolic diseases, Alzheimer's disease and Parkinson's disease. In general, a primary source of oxidative stress in cells is leakage of high-energy electrons during the process of respiration. Mitochondria are protected from oxidative stress by manganese-dependent superoxide dismutase, catalase, CoQ10, Vitamin E and glutathione, which is produced in the cytoplasm and transported across the mitochondrial membrane. Resveratrol has been shown to increase mitochondrial ATP production.45

To maintain the body in a healthy state it makes sense to feed the body healthy foods that are nutrient rich, nonsteroidal and antibiotic-free whole foods that contain plenty of vitamins, minerals, healthy fats like omega three fatty acids, plant-based proteins and foods and nutraceuticals that are rich in anti-inflammatory molecules, antioxidants and phytonutrients. Specific foods that can protect the mitochondria include omega three fatty acids that help build mitochondrial membranes, CoQ10 that helps the mitochondria synthesize ATP and is important in transporting high energy electrons, pyrroloquinoline quinone that helps to protect the mitochondria from oxidative stress and the intake of healthy amounts of magnesium (through green leafy vegetables, fish, nuts and tubers) to help in the production and transfer of ATP. Acetyl-L-carnitine helps in the transport of fatty acids into brain mitochondria, which improves mood and memory. Mitochondria can produce reactive species of molecules that can contribute to vascular dysfunction and contribute to blood pressure problems. Since acetyl-L-carnitine and lipoic acid have been shown to reduce oxidative stress, these molecules can improve mitochondrial function.46 Antioxidants such as curcumin found in turmeric, quercetin found in broccoli and blueberries, green tea extracts, vitamin C and resveratrol are also important for mitochondrial health.

Meditation, pranayama and hatha yoga have also been shown to improve overall mitochondrial functioning. A very important study, "Relaxation Response Induces Temporal Transcriptome Changes in Energy Metabolism, Insulin Secretion and Inflammatory Pathways," reviewed the effects of the relaxation response (RR) on genes and mitochondria. The types of RR included in this study are from different forms of yoga and meditation including TM, Zen, Vipassana, Kundalini yoga, pranayama, Qi Gong and tai chi. The study included three groups of practitioners: long-term meditators, short-term meditators and novices at meditation. Various biochemical and molecular changes, gene expression changes and temporal gene expression changes were measured. This was the first known study to use genomic analysis methodology and systems biology analysis to examine temporal transcriptional and gene changes during one session of RR practice.

A very important result of this study was it revealed that people engaged in long-term practices had immediate and prolonged gene expression changes, such as upregulation of genes that support improved mitochondrial energy metabolism, including efficient electron transport and oxidative phosphorylation as well as lowering oxidative stress and cellular aging. RR was also shown to help upregulate mitochondrial ATP synthase, which is critical for ATP production.

RR practices were also linked to pathways that play critical roles in the inflammatory response, including lowering the amounts of the pro-inflammatory transcription factor, NF-kB. Downregulation (meaning suppressing its expression) of NF-kB inflammatory response genes leads to reductions in oxidative stress, insulin resistance and apoptosis (cell death). NF-kB has also been identified as a potential bridge between psychosocial stress and oxidative cellular activation. This has been demonstrated previously in other studies where meditators had NF-kB downregulation in response to stressful situations, such as caring for dementia patients and in dealing with their own serious types of illnesses. Not having an abundance of NF-kB in the body helps to avoid mitochondrial oxidative stress responses, which can lead to the production and rapid cascading of inflammatory molecules. Such inflammatory molecules can lead to many illnesses and especially to the metabolic syndrome, which is characterized by hypertension, obesity, insulin resistance and hyperlipidemia.

Since psychological stress can cause disruption of mitochondrial function, reduced telomere length and accelerated cell death, RR practices can play an integral part in mitochondrial health. Telomeres are tiny caps that are located at the ends of each twisted strand of the DNA molecule, kind of like the little plastic piece at the tip of a shoelace. Telomeres protect the ends of the chromosome from fraying or being damaged, thus protecting genetic data. Each time a cell divides the telomeres shorten a bit, so that is one reason why DNA gets damaged with aging. Telomerase is an enzyme that prevents the telomere from shortening and there has been some research to block telomerase to promote death of rapidly growing cancer cells. One stumbling block is that if telomerase is also blocked in healthy cells, it could accelerate aging.

Another cause of aging is oxidative stress caused by highly reactive substances that damage DNA, proteins and lipids (fats). Oxidants are naturally produced during respiration but are also found in foods and are generated during cigarette smoking or processing alcohol after it has been consumed. Oxidants are also used for self-defense during infections to ward off pathogens. The third major cause of aging is glycation, which occurs when glucose binds to DNA, protein and lipids, thereby preventing these molecules from doing their work efficiently.

In long-term RR practitioners, it was found that pathways associated with genomic stability, including normal telomere packing, improved telomere maintenance and good tight junction interaction were upregulated. Long-term RR practice helped stabilize histones, which are responsible for DNA structure as well as cytochrome C, which is needed for mitochondrial respiration. The calcium channel gene was also upregulated, which improves such calcium-mediated functions as muscle contraction, neurotransmitter release, gene expression and slows cell death.47

In summary, this study provides evidence that RR supports healthy mitochondrial functioning, which in turn, could help mitigate some of the negative effects of stress.

Muscles, Energy Metabolism and Yoga Philosophy

The relationship between ATP production and the yogic idea of regulating prana is quite interesting to me. In the yogic tradition, natural and healthy foods are consumed, and rhythmic breathing is practiced. This supports the efficient elimination of body fluids and waste, as prana flows through the nadis and the chakras. From yogic and Ayurvedic perspectives, a subtle underlying association that parallels the biochemical equation of cellular respiration (glucose + oxygen = carbon dioxide + water + energy) can be rewritten as healthy food (that breaks down to glucose) + regulated breath (oxygen smoothly flowing into the body) = mala (efficiently produced waste product in the form of carbon dioxide that is reused by plants in the process of photosynthesis) + ojas (subtle underlying principle and essence of the water element) + prana (subtle energy that underlies the energy of the ATP molecule).

Psychotherapy and Meditation

Personal History in Western Psychotherapy

My first residency after having completed medical school was in psychiatry at the University of Wisconsin. I chose Wisconsin because I had discovered there was a strong spiritual community in the city and two of my close friends from medical school were doing their residency there. It seemed to be a very good program with an emphasis on classical Freudian analysis, Rogerian empathic approaches, family systems and group therapy.

While I enjoyed the psychiatry program and learned a great deal about human behavior and psychopathology, I was disappointed that they hadn't developed an orientation on the integration of body and mind. Other aspects that interested me that were not part of the Wisconsin program were Jungian analysis and medical anthropology. I was also deeply immersed in yoga and Buddhist philosophy and was especially interested in the interface between Western psychology and Eastern thought and meditation. My final decision to leave the program occurred when I met Swami Rama and he asked me to study meditation, homeopathy and psychotherapy with him in Glenview, Illinois at his ashram.

In my work at the Himalayan Institute, I learned that according to ancient medical systems the treatment of suffering individuals must ultimately focus on the mind, from where disease largely originates. Psychological study categorizes the manifestations of mind, the characteristics of personality and the qualities of emotional experience. Although Western psychology has undoubtedly played an integral role in the understanding of mental illness, the split between man's psyche and soma has been widened by increased subspecialization in medicine and psychiatry. If the patient's problems are not viewed in totality, treatment can be fragmentary, and the patient may not really understand how to interrelate emotional problems and specific physical ills.

In addition, there are really no approaches in traditional allopathic medicine that can diagnose or treat a patient on the higher levels of consciousness, mainly because conventional perspectives do not adequately recognize the existence of these levels. Modern psychotherapy often lacks a perspective of a human being's spiritual nature, which is fundamental to psychological health. Yoga philosophy maintains that since disease manifests in the energy fields of human beings, treatment methods that are directly focused at these levels of existence can effectively eliminate suffering. Areas of health care associated with the subtler levels are hatha yoga, relaxation and concentration techniques, breathing and pranayama practices, meditation, homeopathy and Chinese acupuncture.

According to ancient medical systems, questions often left unanswered by psychological study are: What controls the mind? What are the underlying causes of emotion? What are thoughts and how can they be positively directed and controlled? What are the different levels of the unconscious? How does individual consciousness fit into the universal consciousness?

Western Approaches to Psychotherapy

Psychiatric inquiry and observation have described in great detail characteristics of emotional and personality disturbances. Psychology, however, may be limited in scope in explaining certain aspects of human mental processes and behavior because there tends to be an emphasis on the negative, pathological side of man. Balanced mental health is primarily considered to be an avoidance of conflict and the maintenance of a "steady state" (ego) between inner needs (id) and outer demands (superego).

Many Western psychotherapists deal with this level of ego reintegration, as do certain yogic concentration techniques. The most important purpose of these types of therapies is to strengthen the ego in the Freudian sense of conscious decision-making. More specifically, the models of psychosomatic medicine and the meditational therapies of yoga and Buddhist philosophies emphasize nonattached observation of the thought flow.

In psychotherapy prevention of emotional problems or mental illness often revolves around successful resolution of early infantile conflicts. Because of this disease orientation, the positively oriented issues of growth and expansion of consciousness are often neglected. Issues of a person's potential creative abilities and positive expression of their inner self tend to be neglected, though Jungian psychology and some humanistic and transpersonal schools are more growth-oriented in dimension.

Behavioral Psychology

From the perspective of cognitive behavioral psychology, a person's reactions and emotional character directly reflect the positive or negative rewards or punishments they receive. Behaviorism, in a general sense, represents a conditioning process. A behavior therapist might teach relaxation techniques or promote positive habits and positive self-aphorisms to substitute for habits that interfere with a person's well-being. Techniques that cognitive behavioral therapists use can help people who are suffering from such conditions as severe anxiety attacks or post-traumatic stress disorder.

Freudian Psychology

From a Freudian perspective, which is one of the most prominent schools of psychotherapy, underlying conflicts stemming from maladaptation in periods of infantile and childhood growth are analyzed in depth. The Freudian psychoanalytic therapists especially penetrate into repressed feelings associated with childhood and adolescence, so that the person can learn to identify these unconscious suppressions. Patterns of interaction with parents are discussed and sexual inhibitions and other types of frustrations identified. In the psychoanalytic framework, a person passes through specific stages of development: the oral, anal, phallic, latent, adolescent and adult periods. If conflict or inhibitions have occurred in any of these stages, certain predictable emotional patterns will arise. For example, if a young infant was not allowed enough time for suckling, certain types of neurosis could develop. The baby might suck his thumb for an inordinate amount of time, the adolescent might bite his nails, the adult might overeat when under stress or a businessman might develop a gastric ulcer in response to work pressures. In a similar vein, a toddler forced to toilet train before being emotionally mature may later develop severe constipation or diarrhea, anal compulsiveness or peculiar obsessions like frequent hand washing.

In Freudian psychiatry, libido is the energy that drives and motivates a person. According to psychoanalysis, the main form of libido is sexual energy, and it is believed that unfulfilled libidinal (sexual) desires lead to unconscious conflict. Repressed sexual feelings and desires are considered by Freudians to be a major source of emotional problems, and interpretations of conflict tend to be oriented around this issue.

Inherent in psychoanalysis is the theory that human life consists of a struggle to counteract childhood impulses and to uncover suppressed emotions and experiences. This system's major focus is on delineating the symptoms and signs of disorder. The real meaning of psychological health is not clearly established. Psychoanalysis describes positive health through inference by stating that "normal" people are able to maintain an intricate balance and identity (ego) between inner urges (id), and outer parental, environmental or social demands (superego). The ego in this scheme is constantly being pulled by the id and the superego. A person who is able to keep both these influences from greatly disturbing daily functions is considered to be in relatively good psychological health.

Psychosomatic Psychology

Psychosomatic medicine, an offshoot of classical Freudian psychology, was systematized by Franz Alexander in the 1940s. As a body of knowledge, it has had many adherents over the years, but with the upsurge of medication therapy for mental health, this approach to understanding human behavior (as well as many other schools of psychotherapy), is not discussed as often. While recognizing that emotional problems are related to internal conflicts, defenses and repressed feelings, psychosomatic medicine attempts to explain how these affect specific body parts and the nervous and endocrine systems, all of which contribute to certain physical diseases. Thus, psychosomatic medicine attempts to bridge the gap between mind and body. This model represents a prominent Western approach to holism through the synthesis of psychology and medicine. The appreciation of the interconnections between the dynamics of mental processes and the body's physiology leads to a greater understanding of the integrated nature of the human being.

Western-based medicine has defined the term psychosomatic to signify specific illnesses where there are no pathological changes, but instead seem to be linked to a disturbed emotional state. The term psychosomatic has been used colloquially to include those diseases for which no biochemical or X-ray abnormality can be found, but which still lead the patient to seek medical aid. And so many types of chest, stomach and back pains as well as complaints of numbness or ringing in the ears, which are enigmas in conventional diagnosis, are now labeled "psychosomatic." This latter usage of the term psychosomatic disorders is not the concept being defined in this section.

Psychosomatic medicine, as a distinct field of inquiry, uses psychological techniques and language to describe the linkage between emotions and physiology. This system incorporates psychoanalytical methodology to interpret how psychological conflict affects physical functioning as projected through the autonomic nervous system.

By combining the knowledge of ancient medical systems and holistic medical perspectives with modern medical theory and technology, mental and physical processes may be seen to be truly inseparable, and the practice of classifying disease as physical or mental becomes obsolete. To say that a disease is "only in the patient's mind" is to erroneously minimize the importance of the direct effect that thoughts and feelings have on body physiology. We can only speculate on the reason that some people react to emotional conflict and develop disease, while other people who are subjected to similar situations remain free of illness. Those who develop actual disease are in some way unable to adapt to the various problems that arise during life. They cannot let go of certain patterns of response and this leads to physical illness.

According to psychosomatic medicine, psychological conflicts can influence a person's physiology in a number of ways. There may be a modification of (1) satisfaction of basic needs, (2) emotional expression and (3) nervous system activity. Psychological imbalances can affect the voluntary activities that deal with the satisfaction of primary needs such as hunger, self-protection, sleep and sex. A person generally has voluntary control of when and how to satisfy these basic needs. Suppressed emotional conflicts can cause distortion or loss of this control, resulting in physical discomfort or disease. The malady anorexia nervosa exemplifies this problem. A person exhibiting symptoms of this disorder experiences complete loss of appetite, perhaps as a result of chronic depression, unresolved anger, anxiety or obsessive-compulsive tendencies. This leads to the obvious physical problem of severe malnutrition.

Psychological conflicts may affect the means of emotional self-expression such as laughing, crying or blushing. When these conflicts are repressed, certain physical problems arise. For example, suppression of anxiety may lead to an inappropriate affect such as hysterical, uncontrolled laughter. Also, if a person's feelings are inhibited, abnormal body posturing or tics may result. If maintained over a prolonged period of time, irregularities in posture can lead to structural deviation in the musculoskeletal system, resulting in such problems as chronic arthritis.

Psychological factors also affect the autonomic nervous system and the physiological functions under its control. It is here that psychosomatic medicine focuses most of its attention. In this context, psychosomatic medicine is concerned with specific illnesses or physiological processes that have psychological counterparts, perceived subjectively as emotions and desires.

Activation of the sympathetic system is associated with active responses in general, and activation of the parasympathetic nervous system is associated with more passive type responses. According to psychosomatic medicine, a person may respond actively to conflict by anger, hostility or self-assertiveness. If the outward expression, and hence release of these feelings, is inhibited by certain circumstances such as societal values that limit self-expression, the sympathetic nervous system, which is normally acutely activated by such feelings as anger, may remain chronically activated as a vent for expression of frustration. The sympathetic-like symptoms of anxiety and stress result, such as palpitations of the heart, increased perspiration, muscular tension, constricted pupils and decreased activity of the digestive organs.

Specifically, some chronic sympathetic nervous system responses are diabetes, which can result from ongoing increased mobilization of carbohydrates, arthritic conditions from increased muscle tension around joints, cardiovascular disease and high blood pressure and migraine headaches from increased blood vessel constriction. Thyroid hyperfunctioning may occur as a result of overstimulation of the thyroid gland or higher brain centers (pituitary or hypothalamus) that control the thyroid gland.

Similarly, a person may respond passively by running away (withdrawal). Again, if overt withdrawal is inhibited by societal standards or specific events, the parasympathetic nervous system may remain chronically stimulated as an expression of this passive withdrawal. This results in overactivation of digestion and bronchial tube constriction, which manifest as ulcerative colitis, peptic ulcer disease or asthma.

For example, according to psychosomatic medicine theory, the typical ulcerative colitis patient reacts to stress not by action but by withdrawing (physically, emotionally or mentally). If this withdrawal is inhibited (not allowed by emotional rejection or punishment), the parasympathetic nervous system is activated. Increased gastrointestinal activity, a parasympathetic dependent activity, can result in diarrhea. In psychoanalytic theory, the parasympathetic response that contributed to the diarrhea symbolically represents a regression or withdrawal to times of infancy when the mother or parent may have punished the child for not controlling their bowel movements during toilet training.

Another interesting example of mind-body interconnection, which is included in the study of psychosomatic medicine, is the inhibition of the central nervous system (CNS). The CNS is responsible for voluntary action, that which keeps a person consciously in communication with the external world. Inhibition of normal CNS responses can lead to a disorder called conversion hysteria. This illness is characterized by paralysis, loss of speech or loss of coordination, yet no physiological or pathological evidence can account for these symptoms. The symptoms of conversion hysteria are associated with the voluntary and sensory systems, both of which are necessary to communicate with the outer world.

Psychologically, the person withdraws into fantasy (also directly controlled by the CNS). Unlike the ANS type disorder, the CNS ailment has no observable physiological disturbances such as ulcer crater or joint swelling. As soon as the conflict is resolved, the symptoms disappear, leaving no lasting damage.

Jungian Psychology

The Jungian approach to psychotherapy, called analytical psychology, tends to be more positively oriented in that it recognizes one's inner potential and need for a creative outlet. It also describes the deeper aspects of the mind, the unconscious, as reflected in dreams and universal symbols, and the close association between religious or spiritual questions and psychology.

Dreams, symbols and myths are "observable" reflections of the deeper levels of the mind, representing the mind's attempt to handle stress and emotional conflict. Dreams often revolve around the day's unfinished business or represent attempts to express repressed fears of daily living. They also, through their symbolism, give glimpses of higher states of consciousness. Dreams are thus manifestations of those hidden dimensions of life that normally evade our conscious scrutiny.

Deeply rooted in the mind are specific images, fantasies and myths that are common to all mankind. These "archetypes" in a sense reflect primordial patterns of psychic energy that give all people an interrelatedness by virtue of this dynamic force. Jungian psychology recognizes the great power of the energy associated with these archetypes, which are stored and accessed in the unconscious mind. If misunderstood or misdirected, this energy forms into certain patterns called emotional complexes.

There are many similarities between this system and Freudian psychoanalysis, which is not surprising since Jung was originally a student and colleague of Freud. However, there are also important differences, especially with regard to interpretation of psychological conflicts and events. Besides the relevance of problem identification and resolution, Jungian psychotherapeutics maintains that inner mental unrest represents the person's attempt to integrate various unknown qualities of their being. In this sense, emotional conflicts can be viewed positively as reflections of deeper aspects of a person's mind. Releasing and understanding these hidden mental forces can lead to great creative insight and experiences.

For example, a Jungian analysis of a snake in a dream might be interpreted as representing primal energy and the potential power for spiritual enfoldment, rather than simply a penis, which a Freudian analyst might suggest. The Jungian analyst would point out that the myths and symbols of the most ancient cultures and of philosophical systems like yoga commonly identify the symbol of the snake with the force that uplifts people to a more evolved state of awareness. The Jungian therapist helps the patient understand that one's problems, dreams, images and emotions are all there to teach him, and that people throughout history have experienced the same joys, fears and tribulations in their journey through life. In Jungian theory every person has a male side (animus) and a female side (anima). These aspects play out in one's life in myriad and complex ways.

This approach has many therapeutic benefits in that it helps the patient to identify with other people and to feel less alienated, and it provides a model that exemplifies the universality of mankind. This common reservoir of experiences is called the collective unconscious. It also enables the patient to view their conflicts as untapped inner resources that are there to teach them the lessons of life. By learning these lessons, one can continue to evolve and expand their consciousness.

Dream Psychology

"Once upon a time, I dreamt I was a butterfly, fluttering hither and thither, to all intents and purposes a butterfly. I was conscious only of my happiness as a butterfly, unaware that I was myself… Soon I awaked, and there I was, veritably myself again. Now I do not know whether I was then a man dreaming I was a butterfly or whether I am now a butterfly dreaming I am a man.

"How do I know that enjoying life is not a delusion? How do I know that in hating death we are not like people who got lost in early childhood and do not know the way home? …How do I know that the dead do not regret their previous longing for life?

One who dreams of drinking wine may in the morning weep; one who dreams of weeping may in the morning go out to hunt. During the dream state a person does not know they are dreaming. One may even dream of interpreting a dream. Only on waking do they realize it was a dream. Only after the great awakening will all realize that this is the great dream."48

These famous statements come from Chuang Tzu, a great Chinese philosopher, who lived sometime between 369 BC and 286 BC. He, along with Lao Tzu, the author of the Tao Te Ching, is considered by many people to be the greatest of all Taoist spiritual masters. These two quotes reflect the mysteries of the dream space and the multiple layers of consciousness with respect to what is reality. One can see a great similarity with Vedantic thought of the oneness of Brahman and the illusory state of maya. In this philosophy, the analogy of consciousness is that when one dreams, they think the dream is real. When they awaken they realize it was only a dream. It is said that when one awakes to the understanding and experience that there is nothing but Brahman, then the person knows that daily existence and life are only another form of dream, which represents the illusion of maya.

Dreams are mysterious and represent another aspect of the manifestation of consciousness. With training and diligent effort, along with the help of someone skilled in dream analysis, the interpretation of dreams can unlock some of the mysteries of the unconscious mind.

Dreams and Modes of Consciousness

Dreams represent a mode of consciousness that has both interested and perplexed humans throughout the millennia. Dream interpretation spans the full gamut of human experience, having been associated with the diverse areas of culture, religion, psychology, mythology, philosophy, alchemy, mysticism and science. The interpretation of dreams and fantasies can lead to an understanding of the tendencies rooted deeply in the unconscious mind. Free association and dream analysis are techniques that allow a person to objectively perceive and analyze the mind's contents and to identify enervating and distracting thoughts. Growth and expansion of awareness take place as the patient learns to integrate more of the unknown into the conscious objective mind.

The symbolic relevance of dreams depends upon the dreamer's ability and desire to comprehend or observe its contents. Some tribal societies believe that the dreams of the common person are illogical and irrelevant. Only the dreams of the priest, shaman or wise man have significance because they are believed to be prophetic and concerned with overall tribal welfare.

In a surprisingly similar way, many modern people disregard their dreams generally because they lack understanding of their symbolism. Interpretation will only be of interest if the dream alters the dreamer's emotional state, mood, or if the dream is recurrent or exceedingly bizarre. Another way in which modern humanity reduces the importance of dreams is by simply looking at the dream picture as a composite of the previous few days' antecedent events thrown together in a haphazard manner.

It was in reaction to simplistic attitudes that psychologists like Sigmund Freud and Carl Jung developed techniques and theories of dream analysis. While their contributions to the understanding of the hidden psychic nature of dream phenomenology have been monumental, other great philosophies, psychologists and scientists have also explored the inner complexities and associations of dreams.

Scientific investigation has also recently attempted to explain dreams in a rational way. The level of mental awareness that corresponds to the dreaming state is associated with the alpha wave of the EEG machine. The eyes exhibit a specific type of motion called "rapid eye movement" (REM). Dreams are part of REM sleep. This is in contrast to deep sleep where no dreams are experienced, and which is associated with the delta frequency on EEG.

Between the working state (beta and some alpha waves) and the sleep state is the hypnogogic state (theta waves), which is associated with pre dreamlike images and sensations such as a feeling of falling, seeing clouds or people's faces. If a person can extend the theta period and recall the figments occurring in this state, they may be able to tap into unconscious ideas or concepts of a highly creative nature. For example, if a person were working on a math problem, scientific inquiry or an emotionally challenging concern, the answer might be revealed in an instantaneous flash in the theta wave state.

Freud believed that a dream represents a complex psychic creation that has its roots in antecedent associations. To him, dreaming has a logical meaning representing the competition between various tendencies. The incoherent images form a facade that hides the more important latent content of the dream thought. Because dreaming is a meaningful process, it is subject to systemic analysis.

Freud maintained that each dream represents the psychological fulfillment of a repressed desire. These wishes, which form the dream picture, are rarely openly admitted during the waking state because they usually are emotionally painful. As a result, these thoughts and feelings are suppressed into the unconscious mind through a mechanism called "the censor." This resistance often excludes the ability to consciously reflect upon an emotional issue, so the feelings get expressed indirectly in dreams. Dreaming as a process helps diffuse the underlying psychic pressure that has been accumulating through the act of repression.

Freud observed that if the dreamer is encouraged to verbalize dream images and the emotions and thoughts that these evoke, they will be able to understand the obscured unconscious background of their mental distress. This is a form of "free association," which is, in a sense, similar to the process of meditation where the meditator observes the flow of memories, images and feelings that emerge from the inner realms of consciousness.

While Freud was the first Western psychologist to systematically present both a theory of the dream mechanism and how to interpret unrecognizable images, it was Carl Jung who expanded the phenomenology and interpretation of dream analysis. He expounded on the underlying symbols that manifest themselves in the dream material and illustrated the universal nature of these images. He described how the symbolism in dreams is strikingly similar to the esoteric symbolism in the Abrahamic religions and Eastern philosophies such as Buddhism, Vedanta and Tantrism.

Jung disagreed with Freud's conception that dreams protected a person against the shock of disagreeable memories or feelings. He felt this type of interpretation inferred that the unconscious mind, from where dreams arise, is only a dumping ground into which disagreeable aspects of the conscious mind are deposited. He felt instead that some dream images correspond to primitive rites, allegories, myths and ideas that are living meaningful metaphors that exist to help us understand emotionally charged issues. He believed that the main function of dreams was to reestablish a psychological equilibrium and thus function in a "compensatory" role. For example, if a person has unrealistic or grandiose opinions of him or herself or attempts to live beyond their capacity, they may have dreams of falling or flying. These dreams compensate for emotional deficiencies and may actually alert the person to possible accidents if the present course of action were not altered. The symbols represent a natural mechanism to reunite opposite forces within the psyche. This conception is quite similar to the idea expressed in yoga philosophy as the word *yoga* itself means "to unite."

Jung believed that by recollecting and interpreting dream symbols, a person could expand their consciousness as they assimilated in the conscious mind mental contents that have been lost or repressed. He described another important function of dreaming as a way to integrate into conscious awareness symbols and ideas deeply rooted in the unconscious and soul of all human beings. Within this collective unconscious all people share common experiences, emotions and psychic patterns, which Jung referred to as archetypes. All people in all ages have dreamt about, ritualized, mythologized or created religious doctrine around these potent symbols. While the cultural motif may differ, these eternal symbols common to all of humanity are: the Hero figure, the Mother-Earth figure, the Father of All figure, the archetype of initiation into adulthood or spiritual discipline, the beauty and the beast conception, the Son of man conception and the symbolization of transcendence. As all human beings share physical and mental characteristics with a long evolutionary chain of human ancestors, the human psyche is an evolutionary composite of the primordial images of one's archaic human predecessors, and as a result, all humans have similar themes that reside in the collective unconscious of all cultures and peoples of the Earth.

However, modern industrialized people often have lost their inherent unconscious identity with all things and thus they no longer feel an affinity with nature. Unlike old world and more indigenous people who are connected to the planetary environment, humans no longer hear divine whispers in the wind, feel the spiritual flow of "old man" river, see the trees as intimately sharing the planet with human beings, recognize the latent potential energy of the snake symbol, speak or listen to the plants and stones nor understand that entering the cave is symbolic of journeying inwards into the caverns of the spiritual heart. Having lost this contact with nature also implies a loss of the latent and profound emotional energy that is supplied by this symbolic interconnection.

It is in this capacity that dream symbols compensate for the psychological split with the underlying forces of the universe. By using language to discuss dreams, dreams reconnect people with their instincts, primitive emotions and transcendent capacities. By understanding and integrating the energy behind these dream symbols, a person taps into deep creative forces. Thus, dream analysis can enhance the intuitive capacity like the process of meditation, which is also an inward journey. Even the symbols used in the visualizations practiced in yogic meditation are also found in dreams and mythology. The eternal truths embodied in cultural and religious symbols emerge during dreams and if inwardly experienced can lead the person closer to these ideals.

Dream Analysis

I ask some patients to keep a dream journal by their bedside and to write their dreams down with as much detail as possible as soon as they awaken. Once they get into the habit of writing dreams down on paper, it becomes easier to remember dreams. Just the suggestion or intention of trying to remember dreams before bed, will enable the dreamer to better recall their dreams in more detail. Usually, it's the recurrent or very unusual dream that is most amenable to deeper interpretation.

What the dreamer associates with the dream images forms the nucleus of the dream's interpretation. The psychotherapist only amplifies and clarifies the dreamer's observations and feelings. The dream is considered to be an important psychological experience, couched in symbolic language to help the person to better understand their feelings, motivations and concerns. Like the body that will continually attempt to rebalance itself to homeostatic equilibrium, the mind also has self-regulating mechanisms. In this context, dreams have potentially adaptive and growth-promoting functions.

Each dream has many levels of interpretation. Every character or object in the dream is not only associated with the obvious external person or object, but also represents an internal quality or feeling within the dreamer. For example, if a person dreams of their mother, this can be analyzed from many perspectives and in great detail. The dream may reflect one's relationship with one's real mother, the feminine and nurturing side of one's personality, the passive or receptive side of one's psyche, the energy of Mother Nature, the creative force of one's spiritual side or latent shakti power or kundalini forces.

A dream of a doctor about to deliver a baby may be interpreted concretely if the dreamer is soon to have a baby or even get pregnant, but it also can signify an archetypical figure. The "inner midwife" is a universal symbol in mythology, fairy tales and religious thought that heralds an internal rebirth of spiritual urgings or of experiencing the purity and innocence of the newborn baby or inner child.

Dreams can also presage events that may happen in the future, or past events may be felt in dreams to be in the future. The dimension of time is nonexistent in the dream world, so past, present and future do not occur in a continuum as they do in the waking state. Time needs the dimension of space to have any reality, since there needs to be at least two points with space between them so that time can exist in its normal linear fashion. Since the mind's images and dreams occupy no space, time becomes irrelevant.

Dreams, Vedanta and Yoga Philosophy

Vedantic philosophy, as espoused through Mandukya Upanishad, describes the manifestation of the universe as having emanated from a single source, the Self or Brahman. Because all existence is one, all external manifestation is illusion. Thus, dreams as well as waking consciousness are not considered "real" when analyzed from the profound unitary perspective. The subject of dream interpretation would create identification with unreality, whereas the goal in Vedanta is identification with universal consciousness, not with its innumerable and infinite manifestations.

Yogis say that dreams do not occur once a person has merged into the evolved state of more expanded states of consciousness and samadhi. This can be understood from the perspective that dreams function to reunite aspects of the unconscious mind with the conscious mind. In Self-realization all opposites are unified, all questions answered, and all unconscious aspects of the mind are available for conscious scrutiny.

According to Mandukya Upanishad, there are four levels of consciousness: waking, dreaming, deep sleep and sleepless sleep, or turiya. The fourth level is considered the transcendental that runs through the other states and forms the basis of the sense of self-identity. Although it is called the fourth level, it is all encompassing. The other three levels are merely relative levels of consciousness. In fact, on close examination from the Vedantic perspective there is little difference between the states of waking and dreaming. They are both classified as maya or illusion. To identify with either state is pointless since they are both unreal. For example, dream food satisfies dream hunger just as waking food satisfies waking hunger. Situations in the dream world last as long to the dreamer as situations in the waking state last for the awakened person.

Another way of understanding these phenomena is to accept all levels as being equally real in the sense that waking, dreaming, and deep sleep are all manifestations of the same pure consciousness. Then all experiences, thoughts, or images can be identified, impartially witnessed and let go of.

From the perspective of dream analysis and philosophies like Vedanta the nature of the world reflects individual fragmentation.

Loss of identity and disunion with the inner whole and the Self is projected externally. People see negativity and despair outside because this is what they feel inside. Internally oriented processes like meditation, contemplation and dream analysis offer potent vehicles to mend the inner splits, guiding both individual and world community towards harmony, completeness, peace and love.

A Personal Life-Changing Dream

When I was living at the Himalayan Institute in the late 1970s, I was undergoing psychotherapy with Arvin Vasaveda, an Indian psychotherapist who had studied with Carl Jung in the 1950s. He had a wealth of knowledge, so I thought this would be a great opportunity to work with a person who not only had so much experience in Jungian dream analysis but also was steeped in the study of Indian philosophy. We met weekly near the campus of the University of Chicago. At that time, I was also having some difficulty communicating with my mother as she couldn't accept my fascination with Eastern thought and that I was trying to integrate this curiosity with my medical practice. I thought working with Arvin could be helpful with improving communication with my mother. At the same time, I was trying to get closer to my father, which caused my mother to be even less pleased because of my parent's nonamicable divorce.

To exemplify how a dream could profoundly affect and influence a person's life, I would like to share a very important and life-altering dream of mine that came during this time. In fact, my sister asked me if she could discuss my dream when she gave the eulogy for our dad after his passing in 2002. Knowing that I was too upset to talk myself during his funeral, I of course said yes.

I discussed this curious dream with Arvin, but I continue to think about it more than forty years later. I dreamed that I was standing in front of a mirror but instead of seeing myself I saw a balding older man who seemed to be looking over my shoulder at the mirror behind me. I felt comforted by this image. I was surprised to see this man looking back at me, especially since I had a bushy crop of wavy hair at the time and I was many years younger than this seeming apparition.

In Jungian dream analysis, one discusses each object, person or feeling and tries to understand what aspect of the dream image or experience represents something about oneself, physically or emotionally. The questions Arvin and I analyzed were: What part of my inner world represents a mirror? Why was I looking at a mirror? What do I associate with this man? Why a bald man? Why do I feel comforted by this image? Who was this man in the mirror since he didn't look like me?

After having spent a whole therapy session on the dream, I discovered much to my amazement that the man standing behind me represented my father, who was quite bald in real life. And although I never realized it consciously, it was my father that had always stood behind me and supported me. Through his continual encouragement to follow my desires and aspirations, he helped me establish a strong sense of self. Like the mirror in the dream, I am indeed a reflection of my dad, especially with respect to what we valued most: integrity, fidelity and love for family. I actually learned that I strongly identified with him, although we were very different with respect to interests and talents. Even though my father was not verbally effusive, he made me feel loved and cared for through his words of support. He was always there for me, although we hadn't lived together since I was ten years old. After the divorce, he continued to visit me and my sister twice weekly, attended my sporting events and accompanied me to college and medical school. He loved my kids and doted on them and consistently gave them little presents.

When I told my dad about the dream and its interpretation, he seemed to be very moved. Sometimes in life it not only is difficult to understand subconscious feelings about love and admiration, but even when realized, it often is difficult to verbalize these feelings. The dream gave me both insight and a psychological tool to tell my dad about how much he meant to me and how grateful I was to him and his wife Jackie, and that they continued to be a strong presence in my life, despite the divorce and my mother's negativity about him. This represented a major turning point in our relationship, as not only did I share some painful memories, but he really began to open up to me about his life and his worries and successes. What a gift!

Gestalt Psychology

Gestalt therapy can also be used in the treatment of psychological and psychosomatic ailments. In this approach, the person learns to experience directly the diverse aspects of their personality. Through experiencing and analyzing the component parts of a situation, the totality and inner meaning of the situation are perceived on a deeper level. The person actively participates in their own life drama by assuming various roles that reflect their inner mental state. For example, in the above-mentioned snake dream, the person would act out the roles of the woman who fears the snake, the snake itself, or perhaps the rocks the snake slides over or the clouds overhead, while watching the whole scene. By assuming the emotions of each character, bits and pieces of underlying or unconscious attitudes, desires and fears emerge. These are experienced directly and provide the patient with first-hand knowledge of their real feelings. The therapist guides, pushes, and prods the patient to go through and feel the Gestalt of each experience.

Humanistic Psychology

Abraham Maslow believed that human beings were continuously evolving, imbued with an inner impulse to "self-actualize," and that they could reach "full humanness." What inhibits this expansion is a "defense against growth," as a person fears not only their lowest attributes but also their highest potentiality. As a result of this inhibition, the person evades their innate abilities and talents and circumscribes their mission in life and their creative destiny. In such a case conflict or ambivalence might set in, where the person could experience their negative side, characterized by passiveness, hostility or greed. In moments of "peak experience," however, they could attain inner fulfillment, expressed as a sense of merging with nature, or with a representation of the divine or God.

On the one hand, Maslow pointed out that a person might admire the world's great leaders, saints and geniuses, as one loves those aspects inherent in oneself. Yet one could also feel in awe, uneasy and inferior because successful people also remind one of their imperfections. Hostility is the predictable and understandable consequence directed at those one admires as well as at oneself. One then sets up defenses to hide this anger or repress these feelings. The result is an evasion of both one's negative qualities and positive attributes.

Maslow also maintained that self-growth or mastery was predicated on having adequate satisfaction of the four primitive urges: food, sex, sleep and self-preservation. When these necessary life-sustaining requirements are adequately met, physical and emotional energy is not dissipated in the perpetual act of trying to attain them and can be rechanneled for self-actualization. Maslow would agree with the yoga concept that emotional problems can stem from unfulfilled desires of the above-mentioned four basic urges and needs.

While Maslow focused on concepts and theory of self-actualization, Roberto Assagioli's system, called Psychosynthesis, another branch of humanistic psychology, uses the yogic methods of meditation and concentration with the aim of enhancing transpersonal and spiritual development. Both systems focus on development beyond the usual range of human capacity.

Meditation and Psychotherapy

Psychotherapy and meditation are two very helpful tools to understand and redirect suppressed emotions. Both act as vehicles for unconscious mental phenomena to be brought into conscious awareness. Once brought into consciousness, hidden desires, memories and fears can be analyzed, and new understanding of inner dynamics can lead to the resolution of these conflicts. In meditation the practitioner can study the mind directly through intense concentration, self-observation and introspection. This is in contrast to Western psychology, which generally studies the mind by observing external behavior.

Change of attitude and habits can take place only if a person first understands the sources of conflicts. Meditation allows a practitioner to carefully observe the contents of the mind and the character of their mental and emotional life, and to trace emotions to their source. On the other hand, psychotherapy depends heavily on verbalization, which can distort the real meaning of the inner world, which is nonverbal. The therapist's interpretation also leaves room for misconceptions and miscommunication because of his or her fallibilities, opinions and countertransference (the therapist's transfer of emotions to the patient in response to the patient's transference of feelings for others onto the therapist).

The growth process of psychotherapy involves making the patient aware of how various unconscious conflicts and defenses have led to personality and emotional imbalances. If a person has feelings that could not be expressed in a safe way, those feelings may be pushed deeper into the unconscious. Generally, unpleasant feelings and thoughts do not simply go away just because one avoids them. Instead they get buried in the unconscious like dust hidden under a rug. When this happens, one loses control over those thoughts, yet the train of associations arising from them continues to affect one's behavior. This can lead to emotions that can be misdirected or expressed in less than healthy ways. If, for example, a young girl who was constantly criticized and demeaned by her father was unable to react or share her feelings of fear and anger, then she might repress these feelings. Later, when she is in an intimate relationship, she may express anger at her male partner as a surrogate figure, not realizing it's really the parent she is upset with. One stagnates and cannot grow without awareness of suppressed thoughts and emotions that create internal conflict. When repressed and suppressed feelings and latent tendencies surface, they can be observed, analyzed and released, leaving the inner psychic world clearer. The distractions and inhibitions of random thought and fantasy are eliminated. In addition, verbal expression of anxieties often allows for release of associated tension.

Meditative techniques work in a somewhat similar way but on a nonverbal level. While one is witnessing the mental flow, repressions surface and aspects of the unconscious and feelings and thoughts that were previously hidden rise into conscious awareness. The objective is to watch those feelings and thoughts arise with a quiet, nonjudging awareness. A person may then acknowledge that identification with persistent fears or obsessions may be preventing them from feeling inner strength. When the mind is quiet, and fears or obsessions diminish, a person may feel less vulnerable to previously challenging circumstances. This strength facilitates a feeling of completeness that allows the person to adapt to changes in the environment without feeling threatened. The completeness leads to a feeling of wholeness within and less dependency on the ever-changing environment for nurturance.

While psychotherapy reveals patterns of thinking and emotions, it often does not lead to any change in the thinking process. Mantra, on the other hand, can change energy patterns within the mind, thereby helping to dissolve problems and eradicate deep-seeded latent impressions (samskaras) stored in the unconscious. Mantra can also neutralize emotional scars and wounds to create new habits and impressions. Memories and thoughts have a vibratory frequency that determines the rhythm of one's consciousness. The silent repetition of a mantra during meditation with focused attention allows one to go deep within the unconscious to change old habits and patterns of the mind.

Another way in which meditation differs from most schools of psychotherapy is that it leads the person beyond problem solving and conflict resolution. The process of meditation sets the stage for self-awareness and expansion as the meditator directs his or her focus of concentration inwards. As the person sits silently, they withdraw from sensory perceptions and objectively view the thoughts, fantasies and images of the mind. By witnessing the internal mental world with neutrality or detachment, they become aware of disturbing thought patterns and how they lead to emotional and physical suffering. This problem identification is similar to that found in psychotherapy and is the first step in catalyzing change in habits and attitude.

After witnessing troublesome thought and emotional patterns, the practitioner of meditation realizes the fleeting, ever-changing nature of the mental field. Acknowledging the impermanence of thought makes one aware that there is an element of unreality associated with the patterns of the mind.

When applied to actual living situations, meditation can enable a person to feel the full range of emotions while maintaining a sense of impartiality and neutrality. Thus, when a stressful event occurs, one's reactions can be viewed with inner objectivity, and emotions can be directed in more constructive ways. By following the path of meditation, one learns to experience the wide range of human feelings in an intense and direct way, including the unpleasant emotions of anger, jealousy, fear and sadness. At the same time, meditation teaches not to overly indulge these feelings and to avoid hanging onto or surrendering to them. Ultimately, meditation leads to liberation from disturbing and distracting emotions, thoughts and desires and replaces these disturbances with a sense of inner quiet, freedom and joy. The meditator comes to know of the quiet, calm center that lies beyond the mind. The meditator considers this state of mind not as an end but as preparation for a stage when the mind becomes an open, receptive field ready to receive true inner knowledge and to experience the deepest, most subtle levels of existence.

The psychotherapeutic benefits of meditation can be more clearly understood by the following analogy: The mind is like the ocean, the surface representing the conscious mind with its innumerable fluctuating waves of thought and emotion. Lying beneath is the great ocean expanse analogous to the unconscious. The turbulence of the surface thought waves obscures the depths of knowledge underneath. The process of meditation calms the tumultuous ebb and flow of the sea's outer layer of wave activity. Bubbles and currents, which represent unconscious repressions and habits, are allowed to rise to the surface to be observed. Since no energy is supplied to suppress them, the bubbles gently burst and dissipate. This averts the creation under the surface of further increased pressure that can produce tidal waves (emotional storms). As the ocean becomes quiet and still, the deeper mysterious layer of the ocean floor (unconscious) can be observed and experienced. In this way the individual wave (separate ego) is again merged with the greater ocean (universal Self). The results are tranquility and true knowledge, and the individual experiences union and peace.

Supervision During Meditation

Meditation is almost always a safe and effective practice on the spiritual path or as treatment for those medical and psychological ailments for which it is indicated. There are a few situations however, where a person should not attempt to meditate unless it is part of a more extensive therapeutic process. The advice of a skilled meditation teacher who has expertise in the field of psychology should be sought to answer specific questions and to guide the person in appropriate practices.

People with psychiatric illness such as schizophrenia, bipolar disorder or those who have had psychotic episodes in which they have experienced paranoid feelings should only practice meditation under close supervision of a meditation teacher and mental health care worker. Medication for these serious mental health disorders is almost always necessary. Sometimes when meditation is practiced for longer periods of time, there can be an exacerbation of the experience of depersonalization and preoccupation with irrational worries. When prescribed for these conditions, meditation and simple breathing exercises should be practiced for very short periods of time. People who are narcissistic might experience an intensification of their self-involvement if they practice meditation for long periods.

Those who have an excessive fear of losing control may be troubled by the idea of meditation. They may have the mistaken idea that meditation is a form of thought or mind control. The goal of merging one's individual consciousness with universal consciousness may be frightening to those who feel insecure and worry about their ability to express their individuality or fear loss of identity. Such individuals will need concomitant psychotherapy support and close guidance from a meditation teacher so they do not become more self-absorbed.

Clinical Applications of Psychotherapy and Meditation

Holistic practitioners are in a unique position to observe how psychological conflicts can lead to physical problems.

Having a theoretical framework that is very broad based and includes several models of psychosomatic integration enables the clinician to evaluate emotional components of illness. The holistic physician also has diagnostic and therapeutic tools that include such diverse aspects as orthodox laboratory evaluation, written psychological testing, homeopathic case taking and more traditional elemental classification found in Ayurveda, Chinese medicine and yoga. To effectively treat psychological problems, especially in association with physical ailments, holistic physicians individualize their therapeutic modalities. For example, a blatantly schizophrenic or suicidal patient might need hospitalization or psychotropic medication. A person with phobias might need to undergo psychotherapy, get regular therapeutic massage or use homeopathic remedies. Someone with anxiety that seems to stem from eating specific foods might need a carefully planned diet along with vitamin and mineral supplementation and an aerobic exercise program. An executive in a highly stressful position might need to learn relaxation techniques, meditation and alternative methods of expressing frustration.

The holistic practitioner who uses psychotherapy needs to decide what approach to use. Jungian analysis might be selected for a client who dreams in symbols or has a spiritual outlook on life. On the other hand, a person whose conflicts seem to stem from early childhood might benefit from a Freudian psychoanalytic approach. A patient who can fantasize and role act might be helped by a Gestalt approach. A phobic person might be advised to use cognitive or behavioral therapy. Nutrition, vitamin supplementation, exercise, relaxation and meditation, along with medicinal therapy including herbs, homeopathic remedies or even allopathic medication could also be utilized concurrently with these psychotherapeutic techniques.

The therapy a holistic doctor decides to prescribe or undertake depends on his or her background, training and expertise. A person trained in formal medicine might not have the necessary skills to personally conduct psychotherapy and might choose to refer a patient to a holistic psychiatrist or psychologist. On the other hand, a psychiatrist may decide to have a holistic internist thoroughly evaluate medical problems before beginning therapy.

A curious thing happens, however, as physicians practice holistic medicine and view things from a multidimensional perspective. The specialty distinctions begin to blur and psychological and medical techniques begin to blend, and the psychiatrist enjoys doing more clinical medicine and the family practitioner practices more psychotherapy. The clinician begins to understand what a rare privilege it is to be allowed to participate in and help treat patients from varying perspectives: how that person exercises, eats, dreams, thinks, acts and feels. As a practitioner learns more about holism and applies that to human problems, their responsibility grows as patients entrust them with ever more subtle aspects of their lives.

As psychology evolves in the humanistic direction, a real understanding of one's mind implies the recognition of the pivotal importance of one's spiritual nature. This concept forms the very core of ancient medical and philosophical systems. A half century ago, Western psychiatrists such as Abraham Maslow and Roberto Assagioli did attempt to explain the underlying nature of psychological health and the experiences that are common to individuals who maximize their creative and intellectual abilities, along with various techniques useful in the quest for inner knowledge, wisdom and self-fulfillment. These conceptualizations are colloquially called the Third Force, or humanistic or transcendental psychology. Unfortunately, especially in recent years, these ideas have been somewhat marginalized by the established psychiatric community, with the very common use of medications, such as anti-depressants, anti-anxiety medicines and mood stabilizers.

Jung, Assagioli and Maslow raised modern psychology to a level where it could begin to administer to all aspects of one's suffering: physical, emotional and spiritual. Forms of psychology such as psychosomatic medicine and humanistic psychology have helped to promote the principle of unity of mind, body and spirit in Western medicine. In addition, humanistic psychology introduces the principle of growth as central to the pursuit of health.

Homeopathy

In 1996, an engineer from Minneapolis, Kurt Swanson, asked me to write the information for a software program on homeopathy. Because I had already co-written one book about homeopathy (Homeopathic Remedies) *and another on holistic medicine, which included a chapter on homeopathy* (Health: A Holistic Approach), *I thought creating a CD ROM on homeopathy would present an interesting new challenge. After one year of hard work, we finished the program and we were pleased to have won an award as the best new software program of 1997.*

Many patients, colleagues and friends, especially those with Apple computers and those who don't especially like using computers, suggested that I write a book based on the same information contained in the CD ROM. Some of the following information is abstracted from my book, The Complete Homeopathic Resource for Common Illnesses. *After many years, the book and accompanying CD ROM are out of print. Because there was much helpful information in that book and as I own the exclusive rights to the original printing, I have taken the liberty to include some of that information in this chapter.*

My Introduction to Homeopathy

My journey into the world of homeopathy opened my eyes to ways of thinking that challenged all of my previous notions of how the world of medicine worked, and it has been an absolutely fascinating ride. It is remarkable to base a prescription of therapeutic medicines, called remedies in homeopathy, on the belief that not only does the body and mind have an innate ability to heal itself, but also that a medicinal substance that can cause symptoms can actually help in the healing process. While I was open to the idea that homeopathy worked by stimulating the vital force, since the vital force is similar to prana in yoga, I did feel I needed to experience the effects of the remedies firsthand to be sure of their efficacy.

After about one month of having moved to the Himalayan Institute and beginning my medical practice at the Center for Holistic Medicine in Glenview, Illinois, Swami Rama and Rudolph

Ballentine, MD took my homeopathic case. I had written down all my symptoms and after discussing at length my concerns, they conferred about what remedy to give me to initiate my treatment. The next morning I took the remedy Sulphur 1M, a one thousand centesimal potency, which is a relatively high potency used for constitutional concerns. While I was curious about what its effects would be, I became busy in the clinic and after about an hour or so I stopped thinking about it. Then in the mid-afternoon, while seeing a patient in the clinic, I got a very heavy feeling in my limbs and felt like I was being gently pressed against the back of my chair. A slight euphoric feeling ensued and I felt quite at peace.

That evening the residents of the ashram were playing volleyball with Swami Rama and I joined in on the fun. To my amazement, I was playing better than I had ever played. While I was always a pretty good leaper, having played basketball competitively in a large high school in Cleveland Heights, Ohio, I had never jumped so high as that evening. Swamiji looked at me and laughed and said the remedy was doing its magic. After a few weeks, a few of my chronic nagging problems disappeared.

Swami Rama continued to prescribe homeopathic remedies for me over the years. Here's a copy of one of his prescriptions in his handwriting.

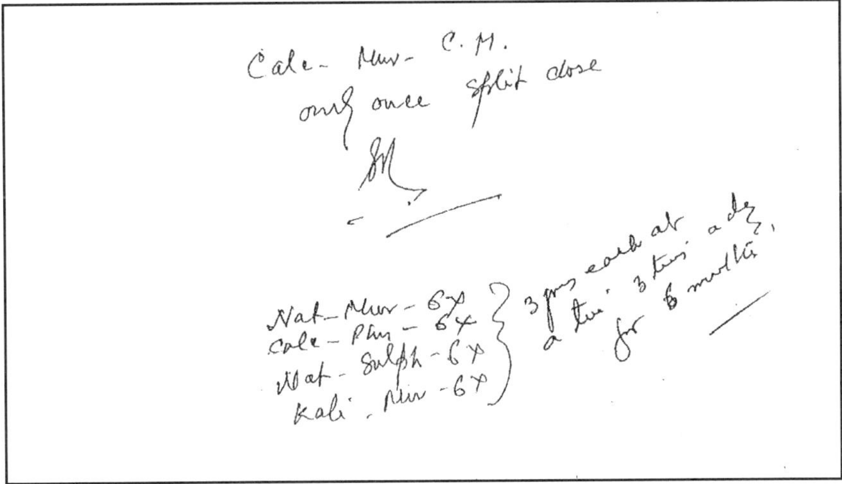

After taking several more remedies over the next few years, I found that some of my other chronic physical and emotional health concerns improved. I was delighted about this and it further enhanced my interest to continue my homeopathic adventure and to help others learn how to use homeopathic remedies. Today, I still remain as excited as ever to prescribe a well-chosen remedy for my patients and always hope to see their conditions improve, as the result of the remedy's capacity to gently stimulate the immune system and to balance the general constitution.

To study and practice homeopathy, a physician has to have all the skills of an allopathic physician, including knowledge of the biological sciences and drug pharmacology of their chosen specialty. Added to this, a homeopath must also become familiar with the wide array of homeopathic remedies that have been made from over 1500 sources. Looking deeply into a person's patterns of illness, matching these symptoms with the essence of the remedy and watching them improve in predictable ways is both exhilarating and intellectually stimulating. It helps one realize that the kingdoms of plants, animals and minerals/metals and humans are all one and the same and that this similarity can be used in the healing process.

Homeopathy is an interesting system of medicine that acts directly through the pranic sheath to restore balance as needed on all levels. It is not only a system that uses medicinal substances to heal and prevent disease but is also a philosophical system that has an underlying spiritual basis. Like yoga and meditation theory, homeopathy maintains there is an underlying energy that animates the human being. And like Ayurveda, homeopathy treats mind and body simultaneously. For this reason, I am describing homeopathy as an example of a therapeutic modality that has its primary actions on the pranic sheath, though it goes much deeper and extends to all levels, even to the subtlest spiritual level.

Origins of Homeopathy

The great German physician, Samuel Hahnemann (1755-1843) rediscovered homeopathy in the early 1800s and it has been practiced throughout the world for almost 200 years. Today homeopathy is widely practiced in North America, India, Mexico, South America, Germany, France, Great Britain, Russia and other European countries. Homeopathy was first introduced in the United States in 1825, and the American Institute of Homeopathy, the first national medical association, was founded in 1844. The second major medical association was the American Medical Association, which was founded three years later in 1847. In the late 1800s and early 1900s, many homeopathic hospitals and twenty-two homeopathic medical schools existed in the United States, including the University of Michigan in Ann Arbor and four medical schools in Chicago.

Samuel Hahnemann, the codifier of homeopathy, was a practicing physician in the early nineteenth century. He had become disillusioned by the dangers of existing therapies at that time, such as the use of toxic doses of mercury for many ailments and the practices of bloodletting and blood leeching. As a result, he turned to the study of the pharmacology and healing principles of ancient and indigenous medical systems. In his studies, Hahnemann became interested in the curative effect that quinine had in the treatment of malaria. He experimented with quinine by ingesting very dilute and activated amounts over a period of time and eventually developed many of the symptoms of malaria. His conclusion was that quinine could cure malaria because it could create the typical symptoms of this particular disease when given to a healthy person. Thus, Hahnemann rediscovered the law of similars.

Law of Similars

The roots of the law of similars are ancient, having been described in the treatises of Hippocrates in Greece and by the Ayurvedic physicians in ancient India. Paracelsus, a fifteenth century European physician, referred to the principle underlying the law of similars in his discussion of the Doctrine of Signatures. He stated, "You bring together the same anatomy of the herbs and the same anatomy of the illness into one order. This simile gives you understanding of the way in which you shall heal.49

Thus, homeopathy is a system for prescribing medicinal substances according to the "law of similars." This law states that the appropriate medicine for a sick individual is a substance that would create a similar set of symptoms if administered to a healthy person. In other words, substances that could produce symptoms when given to a healthy person can, after proper preparation, be used to treat sick people with those same symptoms. The word *homeopathy* is derived from the Greek root *homoios* that means "similar or like treatment" and the word *pathos* that means "of disease." Thus, the word *homeopathy* means "like treatment of disease."

In homeopathy the energy qualities of the remedy (as revealed by the proving of the remedy) are matched with the unhealthy person's energy qualities (as revealed by physical, mental and emotional symptoms). Through the law of similars, unhealthy people can be cured. Perhaps the similar vibratory qualities of the remedy and the sick person produce a harmonic resonance that helps to balance the person's vital force.50

Law of Proving

In light of this discovery, Hahnemann began a systematic study of many commonly known medicinal substances. He and a number of other physicians who were under his tutelage administered very small amounts of these substances to themselves and other healthy volunteers over an extended period of time. Then they carefully noted the symptoms that developed. Through this meticulous work, they were able to collect a vast amount of knowledge regarding the symptoms that these medicinal substances could produce in healthy people. Later they compiled this collection of symptoms to create the *Homeopathic Materia Medica*, the basic reference work of homeopathy still used by all homeopaths today. This process of verifying the medicinal properties of these various substances is called "proving the medicine" and is derived from the German word *prüfung* meaning "test."

According to the law of similars, one of these medicines could thus be administered and result in a curative effect in a sick person with a similar set of symptoms. The law of proving is the systematic verification of the law of similars. During the proving of a substance, healthy people take a remedy over a certain period of time and report any symptoms or sensations that represent a change from their normal state of health. When the symptoms are found to be common to a specified proportion of experimenters (eighty percent), those symptoms are considered the "proving" of that remedy. Hahnemann stated, "There is . . . no other possible way in which the peculiar effects of medicines on the health of individuals can be accurately ascertained. There is no sure, no more natural way of accomplishing this object, than to administer the ... medicine experimentally, in moderate doses, to healthy persons, in order to ascertain which changes, symptoms, and signs of their influence each individually produces on the health of the body and of the mind."51

Approximately 1500 different remedies have been proven over the years. Plants, minerals, acids and extracts from animals, such as snake or bee venom, are among the many agents used in the preparation of homeopathic remedies.

Law of Potentization

When Hahnemann first began treating people according to the law of similars, many of the medicines in use at the time were potentially toxic substances such as mercury, arsenic and snake venoms. To prevent the toxic reaction that usually occurred after taking these substances, he sequentially diluted the substance before it was administered. However, he recognized that though toxicity was reduced by dilution, there was also a decrease in therapeutic effect. As a result of his extensive knowledge of ancient medicinal systems and practices, Hahnemann was aware of a method of increasing the activity of a medicinal solution by vigorously shaking it in its container. Therefore, after each dilution, he methodically vigourously shook the medicines he had prepared. What he disvoered was that as the toxic properties were steadily reduced with each dilution, the therapeutic efficacy increased with the shaking, a seemingly paradoxical effect. This method of increasing therapeutic effect with each sequential dilution by shaking is known as potentization or attenuation. Because of the process of dilution and vigorous shaking, the remedies are prepared and refined in such a way that they work on the energy level. The remedy is then offered to the patient when it matches the energy qualities of the illness. This has the effect of catalyzing a healing response of the body and mind.

The resulting product of potentization is referred to as a micro dilution or potency. The concept of the potency of small amounts of medicinal substances is not novel, as is demonstrated in the case of thyroid hormone. Free thyroid hormone in the human is one part per 10,000 million parts of blood plasma. Potentization also provides a means for releasing medicinal qualities from supposedly inert substances such as common table salt, or as it is known in homeopathy, Natrum muriaticum.

Potentization is controversial because, according to the laws of chemistry, by the time the 12C or 24X potency is reached, there are few if any molecules of the original substance left in the solution. Here C means "centesimal" (diluted 1/100 times) and X means "decimal" (diluted 1/10 times). This is why critics of homeopathy suggest that homeopathic medicines could only exert a placebo effect. However, documented provings of homeopathic medicines using dilutions greater than 12C or 24X provide a strong argument against this. It is unlikely that many different people would experience the same set of symptoms from a given medicine if the medicine were simply a placebo.52

High potencies such as 200X, 200C, or 1000M are effective over a longer period of time, and are used for more chronic diseases and, thus require fewer doses than the lower potency 3X, 6X or 6C preparations that are often used for acute or less chronic illnesses. The higher potency remedies are prescribed for deeper and long-lasting or chronic illnesses. This is called prescribing for a constitutional case.

Homeopaths speculate that the process of potentization liberates the energetic essence of the substance and that the solvent (alcohol and water solution or lactose) acts as a template or vehicle in which the energy of the medicine is imprinted and preserved. This concept of a template can be better understood in light of the effects that pressure has on ice crystallization of freezing water. The late Harvard Physics Department Chairman, P. W. Bridgman, reported different crystallization patterns for water freezing at higher altitudes than for water freezing at lower altitudes. When the ice from the higher altitude was melted and refrozen at lower altitudes, the crystallization pattern of the higher altitude was maintained.53 The effect of pressure on crystallization was demonstrable and indelible. Perhaps the homeopathic remedy exerts a similar effect on its solute.

Vital Force

Homeopathy calls the energy that animates the organism the vital force, which is equivalent to prana, shakti or kundalini in yoga philosophy. The concept of the vital force is fascinating and integral to understanding homeopathic medicine. This concept helps to explain the dynamics of how the potentized remedy interacts with the sick person to affect a cure.

The vital force is not a biochemical entity. Rather, it is more of a bioelectrical or electromagnetic energy that affects a person's mental and physical functioning. It is this energy that animates living organisms and constantly seeks the return to homeostasis and health in an inherently intelligent way. All aspects of nature, whether mineral, vegetable or animal, also have underlying energy patterns. Homeopathic remedies are derived from these three kingdoms. The energy pattern of these remedies is enhanced by the process of potentization and when matched with the energy pattern of the vital force of a person, promotes a healing response.

Homeopathy maintains that the vital force permeates all levels of human existence, body, mind and spirit, and is similar to the energy stimulated by acupuncture needles. The vital force is also similar to the yogic idea of prana and how this subtle energy affects mind and body. People are viewed as a dynamic whole, with the vital force acting as the integrating factor. Healthy people have a particular quality or pattern to their vital force, but when they become sick it indicates this subtle energy has become distorted, blocked, deficient, excessive or simply imbalanced. Even during illness this healing force reacts in the most self-preserving manner and its plan is clearly articulated through the symptom complex. The homeopathic remedy balances and brings the vital force back to a state of harmony, as is reflected in the response of the whole organism to the remedy.

The vital force of homeopathy underlies the physiologic energy of the body. Without this subtle energy, biochemical reactions could not occur. However, technology has not been developed to a sufficient degree to analyze this vital energy. It cannot be assumed from that, however, that the energy is not real. Two hundred years ago people would have scoffed at the idea of electrical energy, and not long ago the concept of nuclear energy or the internet might have seemed preposterous. As technology has advanced, these energies have been isolated, channeled and reproduced with amazing rapidity and skill. Ancient Eastern medical traditions, such as yoga, Ayurveda and Chinese medicine, and even a few branches of Western medicine, have discovered that not only is this underlying subtle energy real but it is fundamental to health and disease. Chinese medicine and Ayurveda, due in part to the technical limitations of the time when they were developed, may have placed less emphasis on trying to understand the specific details of physical anatomy, physiology and biochemistry that modern medicine has extensively explored. However, these older traditions have provided explanations of the subtle forces that animate humans and coordinate their complex functioning. Hopefully, in time it may be recognized in traditional allopathic medicine. Perhaps the modern technologies of nuclear magnetic resonance (MRI), PET scanners, or electron spectrometry will someday be sensitive enough to detect the energy described by homeopathy and ancient systems.

The Chinese call this force *chi,* meaning "life energy." Chi is made up of various components and is simply that quality, which when extracted from food, air and water, animates life forms. Yin (female) and yang (male) are polarities of chi. As the chi energy enters the lungs directly with inhaled air and indirectly from food and water via the stomach and spleen, it is distributed throughout the body in an orderly fashion through the acupuncture meridians. The meridians are pathways for the uniform conduction of chi to all the different hollow (yang) and solid (yin) organs. These are hard to correlate with any anatomical structure and many practitioners feel they are not physical but rather energy channels. This is similar to the yogic idea of prana and the nadis, which carry the energies of prana. In the therapeutic system of acupuncture, needles or finger pressure are applied on the meridians that transmit energy flow. These meridians have no real correlation with nerve pathways. By stimulating certain points, a balancing of energy flow is facilitated in distant organs. Pain reduction or anesthesia is also possible through acupuncture therapy.

Chi represents the power of enduring and continuing, or literally the vitality of the organism. Similar to the prana of yoga and the vital force of homeopathy, chi underlies mental, emotional and physical health. Strengthening and redirecting this vitality is a fundamental goal in holistic healing systems.

Homeopathic View of Health and Disease

Homeopathic philosophy views health as a dynamic ongoing process in which a person constantly faces challenges in a positive way. This way of thinking is similar to the role that meditation plays in a person's life. Health is not simply the absence of disease but represents the person's constant adaptation to internal and external stresses. From this perspective, a person who has a chronic illness such as arthritis but continually strives to have a positive attitude and takes responsibility for doing appropriate joint loosening exercises may be healthier than a person who is pain free but is stubborn, constantly angry or hypercritical. In a similar way, meditation teaches that healing begins on the deepest level of consciousness and the more subtle koshas. As these inner levels heal, the more outer koshas will heal in turn.

Emotional health is characterized by a person who feels and experiences the full gamut of human feelings, including love, anger, jealousy, compassion and sadness. The individual who is emotionally healthy does not become overwhelmed by these feelings, does not feel enslaved by emotions and does not dwell or brood on negative thoughts. Mental health is characterized by calmness, courage, patience, clarity of thinking and creativity. Even after disappointment or loss of a loved one, emotionally healthy people are able to adjust to new life circumstances with reserves of strength.

An understanding of the concepts of health and disease from a homeopathic perspective is fundamental to comprehending the three laws of homeopathy discussed above. The relationship of health versus disease can best be understood by examining the interaction of people and their inner and outer environments. The nervous system, endocrine system and immune system initiate and control the body's response to environmental pressures. These pressures may include internal or external factors such as inherited genetic weakness, emotional stress, mental or physical strain, injuries, environmental pollutants, bacteria and viruses or nutritional deficiencies. If a person's adaptive powers are strong enough to withstand the disruptive effect of these influences, health prevails. On the other hand, disease results if pressures stress the individual's adaptive powers beyond his or her ability to cope.

Homeopathic philosophy contends that from birth until death the individual is reacting with his or her environment in the most intelligent way possible. A vital healing force moves in the direction of greater overall balance for the whole person, and this healing force is clearly expressed in every mental, emotional and physical symptom. The symptoms of an illness are a clear expression of this intelligence at work attempting to reestablish a state of health. In this context, a fever or nasal discharge represents the body's attempt to fight infection, and so a medicinal substance that encourages the immune reaction is needed. This is precisely what the homeopathic remedy does. It works to stimulate the pranic sheath and the different functions of prana in a similar way and in the same direction as the person's own response to illness.

A homeopathic prescriber obtains information about the cause of disease by studying the body's reaction to the disease. This reaction is depicted by symptoms such as fever, cough, diarrhea, swelling or pain. Based on the law of similars, a remedy is chosen that reinforces the symptoms that are representative of the immune system's attempts to heal the organism.

Not only are homeopathic remedies effective in treating disease, they can also prevent it. Even if there is no specific diagnosis of the group of presenting symptoms and all diagnostic studies are within the normal range, homeopathic treatment can precisely be prescribed. This is because the symptom complex is an accurate expression of the subtle and invisible forces underlying the disease process. There are many signals or sensations that may appear long before actual tissue damage takes place. By administering the appropriate homeopathic remedy, a disease process may be halted before it progresses to pathological changes. In this respect, homeopathy is a preventive medical system.

Individualized Treatment

Homeopathic remedies are like packets of subtle energy that can affect very subtle and deeply rooted patterns of physical, emotional and mental concerns. Homeopathic treatment is individualized, just as in yoga and meditation mantras and specific yoga postures are prescribed according to individual needs. Homeopaths closely observe and follow their patients just as yoga teachers do. Homeopaths believe one can heal oneself by activating the vital force and internal defenses. Yoga also teaches one can heal oneself by maintaining a good diet, a regular regimen of exercise, regulation of the breath, correct thinking and a regular practice of meditation.

Susceptibility to Disease

Homeopathic philosophy has long understood the importance of susceptibility to disease. Even though people are continuously exposed to bacteria and viruses, not everyone gets sick. There are even potentially deadly bacteria growing in everyone's body. This includes meningococcus in the nasal-pharynx, which can cause severe meningitis, pneumococcus that grows in the bronchial tubes and can cause pneumonia and the trillions of bacteria in the intestines (microbiome) that can contribute to various forms of colitis but also function as a whole to promote healthy digestion and immune functioning. An individual's underlying susceptibility and the ability of the immune system to maintain health determines if one will get these diseases. This susceptibility or predisposition to illnesses can also help explain why certain people respond to loss of a loved one or job with anger or extreme depression, while others may feel sad yet continue to lead productive lives.

Homeopathic practitioners recognize that the underlying susceptibility to disease is based on such complex factors as hereditary predisposition, childhood experiences, emotional traumas, accidents, life habits and psychological attitudes. All of these factors affect and interact with a person's immune and nervous systems to lower or increase susceptibility to disease. Homeopaths believe this interaction is coordinated in an intelligent, coherent way by the vital force. The homeopathic remedy acts on the vital force when it has become imbalanced, as evidenced by subjective and objective symptomatology. The remedy activates the vital force when the immune system and other psychological and physiologic factors need stimulation, such as in the case of colds, influenza, injuries or depression. The homeopathic remedy also acts to reduce the activity of the immune and nervous system when they are over stimulated, such as in allergies, rheumatoid arthritis or anxiety.

Internal Cause of Disease and the Chronic Miasms

Miasms are inherited and acquired tendencies to disease. They are the manifestation of physical genetics, unconscious belief systems, samskaras and archetypical psychological structures transmitted from generation to generation. Miasms furnish the underpinnings of thoughts, ideas and eventually action. Hahnemann has described three basic miasms: *psora, sycosis* and *syphilis.*

Psora

Psora is the basic miasm as it is considered to be the root cause of disease, and thus underlies susceptibility to disease. Psora can be likened to the roots of a tree. If the roots of a tree are diseased, then the trunk, branches and leaves will also be diseased. Homeopathic philosophy echoes what yoga and Vedanta advocate: harmonious interaction between body, mind and spirit is critical for good health. This is maintained by careful self-observation and a healthy lifestyle. Humankind, in the play of consciousness, has been given the gift of free will to act and express oneself as desired. However, the desire for self-expression without the deep internal recognition of the underlying unity of consciousness, can lead to physical, emotional, energetic and spiritual imbalance, referred to as psora in homeopathy.

Psora is first described as being a mental and emotional irritation. Thus, it is characterized by irritation and hypersensitivity on the mental level and inflammation and itching on the physical level. Psora brings tumult to the mind, affecting thinking and feeling processes as well as leading to the loss of personal will power. This in turn can lead to actions that are not in harmony with the health of body and mind. Psora is characterized by increased sensitivity and lack of structural integration along with restlessness in thoughts and feelings, diminished will power, anxiety and fearfulness. Ayurveda would call this state rajasic.

On a psychological and spiritual level, psora represents negative thinking, attachment to the results of one's actions and the desire to possess too many unnecessary objects. When a person is not satisfied or peaceful, increased cravings for food and unhealthy activities can lead to misguided actions. As one acts on excessive desires and, as a result, overeats, has unhealthy sexual relationships, sleeps too much or is overly attached to possessions, homeopathic remedies are needed to help readjust these tendencies. This is the basis and rationale for constitutional treatment in homeopathy. In order to cure psora, the homeopath uses highly diluted, energized medicinal substances that initiate healing from the deepest parts of one's being.

Yoga and Vedantic philosophy emphasize that the quality of viveka is essential to help discriminate between what is real and permanent and what is not real and impermanent. This enables a person to practice vairagya, to show dispassion and learn nonattachment to objects of the world and, at the same time, to explore the knowledge of the inner Self. Since the deepest spiritual level is imbalanced in psora, spiritual practices can be prescribed to enhance the curative effect of the homeopathic remedy. Yoga practices such as pranayama and meditation can help to control and direct the mind and senses, thus helping to eliminate subtle desires (vasanas) that act as obstacles to the freedom of emotions and mind. These can then be replaced with devotion to the spiritual path, ultimately leading to the experience of universal consciousness.

Psora is considered by homeopaths to be a disruption or disturbance in the vital force. Psora can manifest in the body as an external expression of this irritation, like rashes or eczema, especially if thoughts or feelings are suppressed or unacknowledged. This can also occur if body rashes are consistently suppressed by steroid creams or salves, which have the effect of driving the disease process inwards. If mental irritation is suppressed or emotions not channeled well, more serious types of illnesses can occur and other deeper, more problematic miasms can result. Two other miasms are the sycotic and syphilitic miasms. Homeopathic philosophy reasons that miasms result when negative thinking leads to negative actions. Thus, psora is the result of negative thinking and attachment to desires and the temptations of the world. The sycotic and syphlitic miasms result if a person acts on such negative thoughts.

Without psora there can be no disease. Psora begins in the center of one's being and moves out towards the body, causing illness that is treatable and reversible. On the other hand, when the expression of disease by the vital force is suppressed and driven inwards, the sycotic and/or syphilitic miasms appear. They not only deepen the physical problem but also lead to more serious emotional and mental illness.

Sycosis

On the physical level, sycosis is the miasm that results in infiltrations, overgrowth of tissues and induration, and it is common to develop different types of growths, tumors and warts, which homeopaths believe reflect the tendency to become suspicious and brooding. On the mental level sycosis is associated with secretiveness and manifests as more serious types of generalized anxiety disorders and obsessive thought patterns. Ever anxious that one's weaknesses or anxieties will be found out and suspicious that others will discover their fears and weaknesses and then hurt them, the person under the influence of the sycotic miasm has the tendency to brood. As one's conscience fails, they become mischievous, selfish and sometimes mean and irritable.

Syphilitic Miasm

The syphilitic miasm tends to result in ulceration and degeneration of body organs and on the mental side leads to mental dullness and unrelenting depression as well as more degenerative emotional disorders such as serious problems with substance abuse and deviant behavioral problems.

Summary of the Miasms

To summarize the homeopathic miasms, psora makes the mind overactive, the sycosis miasm makes the mind mal-active and the syphilitic miasm makes it underactive. Psora is quick, sycosis is malevolent, and syphilis is slow. Psora represents a loss of wisdom and intelligent decision-making, sycosis leads to mischievous behavior and the syphilitic miasm represents dullness and sluggishness. Thus, from a homeopathic perspective, the disease process that goes from psora to the sycotic and syphilitic miasms represents a de-evolutionary process.

With respect to the homeopathic miasm concept of disease causation, yoga and meditation philosophy present a similar idea. Homeopathic notions of psora (negative thinking, attachment to results of actions, the overwhelming desire to possess what is not necessary and the overriding need to express oneself that is not in harmony with other people or the world around them) is similar to the yogic idea of attachment to objects and the suffering that this causes, whether the objects are things of the world or one's thoughts or feelings. Both yoga philosophy and homeopathy agree that when one is not on the path of love, harmony and non-attachment to one's egocentric desires, suffering and illness occur. Similarly, not following the principles of the yamas and niyamas eventually leads to disharmony, chaos and unhappiness and ultimately results in illness and disease.

External Cause of Disease

Besides the internal causes of disease that have to do with mind, emotions and habits, in Ayurvedic and Chinese medicine there are external environmental factors that are the cause of disease. Extremes of weather can be injurious to the various elements and the internal organs associated with the elements. In a traditional medical practice, it is very easy to see seasonal patterns with arthritis, strep throat, skin problems and allergies. Even viruses that cause human disease have a seasonal pattern. This includes polio and summer, influenza and late fall and winter, and chickenpox and spring. (And as I edit this book, we are hoping that as springtime turns to summer, the current Covid-19 pandemic may diminish its activity, as other corona viruses tend to become less active in the warmer weather). In a similar way, homeopathy pays exquisite attention to detail in its survey of the sick person's vitality, and every experienced homeopath is aware of how weather and temperature can precipitate many different diseases in people who are sensitive to climate changes.

Aggravation

The homeopathic remedy may cause an initial aggravation of symptoms. The premise of homeopathy is: a medicinal substance that causes symptoms when given to a healthy person can also cure a sick person who has similar symptoms. Homeopathic treatment works by amplifying the immune system and metabolic functioning to help the person become stronger, to eliminate biological susceptibility and enervating emotional patterns, and to combat disease to become healthier. Because of this activation of the healing processes, sometimes the symptoms get worse before they get better.

Hahnemann wrote in his treatise, *The Organon of the Healing Art,* "In the healthy human state, the spirit-like life force (autocracy) that enlivens the material organism as dynamis, governs without restriction and keeps all parts of the organism in admirable, harmonious vital operation as regards both feelings and functions, so that our indwelling, rational spirit can freely avail itself of this living, healthy instrument for the highest purposes of our existence."54

In a similar way, during the practice of meditation, a person may experience unconscious feelings that rise into the conscious mind while they are sitting still and observing their thoughts. Sometimes emotions that may have been buried or suppressed can be unsettling and can create agitation or anxiety. In this sense, the person feels worse. However, as the person allows the feelings to surface where they can explore their roots, it is an opportunity to let those feelings go and move beyond the unconscious hold of the repressed feelings. Then the person can feel even better than before.

Suppression

If medicinal treatments are given for ailments without a thorough understanding of their origin and without an understanding of the whole person and the predictable patterns of disease progression or regression, the natural defense mechanism may be suppressed, and a poorer state of health may result. For example, a typical problem often seen by homeopathic prescribers is infantile eczema. Allopathic doctors usually treat skin eruptions with cortisone creams but neglect the underlying process and individual symptom pattern. Topical treatment of eczema is often suppressive and forces the disease process inwards. If the suppression is chronic, the skin symptoms may improve while the destructive force shifts to the internal organs. Classically, the lungs are affected and bronchial infections and possibly asthma result. In fact, homeopaths believe that most cases of asthma and eczema are the same disease. The eruptions and skin appearance so characteristic of eczema can be pushed even further inwards to affect the mental state of the child.

More on Homeopathy and Yoga Philosophy

Homeopathy and yoga are evolutionary systems that have faith in man's inherent and essential goodness. Both systems observe that, by not following healthy habits and/or being overly selfish in attitudes and activities, symptoms of disease and distress can result.

Both homeopathy and yoga work towards the transformation of the individual on physical, energy, emotional, mental and spiritual levels. From psychological and spiritual perspectives, both systems have the ability to take one from illness to health as well as from ignorance of the true Self to the knowledge of pure consciousness.

Homeopathy, being a European derived medicinal system, shares similar philosophies with yoga as well as with the spiritually inclined alchemists of the middle ages. The alchemical process is not really a quest to transform common metal into the element gold, as is commonly thought, but is a metaphor that represents the transformation of the physical nature of human beings (metal) into the spiritual qualities of the light and brilliance of enlightenment (gold).

Externally, homeopathy is a medicinal system to help the sick return to a state of balance and health. But on a philosophical level, alchemists and homeopaths, like yogis, have consistently worked to extract from our dark and restricted emotional and mental lives, the free and autonomous inherent spirit that is every human's birth right.

Yoga philosophy and meditation, like homeopathic philosophy, maintain that by eliminating distracting fluctuations of the mind, the individual soul has the opportunity to experience universal oneness, often described as a wave of individuality merging into the larger ocean of universal consciousness. From early childhood, people add multitudinous layers of sensory and mental perceptions that hide the truth of their true natures from their awareness. Yogis, mystics and sages have developed various methods and techniques to help lift these veils of ignorance that keep humans in bondage, emotionally, psychologically and spiritually. From a Tantric and yogic perspective, this evolutionary transformation begins as a person moves their spiritual awareness from the chakras at the base of the spine upwards towards the higher chakras.

Homeopathy and Kosha Association

Hering's laws of cure in homeopathy describe how during the process of healing a person improves in a specific pattern: from the most important organ or function to the least important, from above down, from inside out, from the mind and emotions to the physical and in the reverse order of the appearance of the symptoms. Meditation also teaches that one needs to heal the mind, thought processes and emotions first by following such disciplines as the yamas and niyamas, and then slowly progressing through the other steps of raja yoga. The homeopathic remedies are likewise associated with symptoms, patterns, archetypes and constructs that extend from the physical to the spiritual as do the chakras and koshas.

Homeopathy and Chakra Associations

With respect to the chakras, differing remedy characteristics and the illnesses they can treat can be understood as a reflection of the imbalances and disharmony of a particular chakra. Below are specific remedies and the associated chakras they act upon. For those readers who have not explored homeopathy in much detail, these remedies will be unfamiliar to them, but I've included them here as they do illustrate the connection between yoga philosophy and homeopathy. One can learn more about these remedies by reading one of several available books on homeopathic materia medica.

For example, the first chakra is associated with the issues of feeling grounded and secure as well as bowel function irregularities such as constipation, and also problems such as low back and sciatic nerve pain. A remedy such as Calcarea carbonicum, which helps people with issues of bowel functioning as well as emotional concerns of insecurity, can be considered a remedy whose action is that which organizes itself around first chakra functioning. Other examples of remedies associated with specific chakras are:

- *first chakra:* Graphites
- *second chakra:* Sepia, Pulsatilla, Lillium tigrum, Staphysagria, Cantharis
- *third chakra:* Nux vomica, Gratiola, Sulphur, Carbo veg, Arsenicum album
- *fourth chakra:* Natrum mur, Phosphoric acid
- *fifth chakra:* Phosphorus, Lachesis,
- *sixth chakra:* Agaricus, Stramonium, Hyoscamus

Homeopathy and Ayurveda

There are similarities between the Ayurvedic tridosha qualities of pitta, kapha, vata and the homeopathic portraits of Sulphur, Calcarea carb and Lycopodium. It is beyond the scope of this book to explain this connection, but the subtle characteristics of these three homeopathic remedies and of the tridosha energies are remarkably alike.

Homeopathic Case Histories and Anecdotes

A few medical cases will help the reader better understand how homeopathy works. I estimate I have seen over 70,000 patients throughout my forty-four years of medical practice, so it would be impossible to describe all the remarkable results I've seen.

Several years ago, two siblings, a boy and a girl who were two years apart in age came to see me. Each had a sore throat, fever and mildly swollen tonsils and lymph nodes around the neck. An allopathic physician would treat them with an anti-pyretic like acetaminophen or ibuprofen and an antibiotic if a bacterial infection were suspected and proven through culture. A homeopath on the other hand would see these two cases as two different illnesses. After determining this was not a streptococcus infection through a negative strep test and therefore most likely a viral infection, I went to work and asked about their symptoms. The boy's symptoms were as follows: red flushed face, irritable, thirsty, 101F temperature, felt very hot internally and skin felt dry and hot. In homeopathy, these are typical Belladonna symptoms.

His older sister's symptoms were: weepy, wanted sympathy, was chilly but liked the window open as she liked the cool outside air to blow on her skin, and she had no thirst. This case matched the homeopathic picture of Pulsatilla. These represent two cases of an upper respiratory illness, probably caused by the same virus, but having two very different expressions of the illness and thus needing two very different remedies to initiate healing.

In another example, two children who were suffering with middle ear infection (otitis media) provided a similar instance of specificity in homeopathic prescribing. One child appeared extremely irritable and oversensitive and was sweaty, thirsty and susceptible to drafts, wishing to be well covered with blankets. The pain in the ear was worse with cold applications and better from warmth. Homeopathically prepared Hepar sulph (calcium sulphide) produces these symptoms in a healthy person and acted curatively in this particular case.

The other child displayed a mild and weepy disposition, wanting to be held and comforted. Lack of perspiration, thirstlessness and wanting to be uncovered and outside in the open air were apparent. The ear pain improved with cold packs and became worse from the application of heat. Pulsatilla was needed to cure this child and Hepar sulph would probably not have helped at all. The reaction of the mind and body as expressed through perspiration patterns, thirst and reaction to weather and temperature were totally opposite in these two children. The selection of the remedy, which is most similar to the symptoms, will lead to a rapid and lasting cure of the illness.

These were two cases of similar syndromes, but because each of these children's vital force and immune responses produced a very different picture, I treated them with completely different remedies. The homeopath sees this as two very different cases and thus uses different medicinal substances to initiate a healing response from the underlying vital force.

It's important to remember that these two remedies were chosen because of the provings of these plant substances. Originally, when healthy people took both Belladonna and Pulsatilla in controlled settings, they developed symptoms that characterized these botanicals. When a sick person has these symptoms, the homeopath gives them the matching remedy. This represents the first law of homeopathy. A remedy given to an ailing person will cure the case if that remedy would cause similar symptoms when given to healthy persons.

In a more chronic case, I was astounded when early in my career a woman came to see me and my colleague with a huge horny-shaped wart that had been on her left heel for a decade. All allopathic treatments had failed. After examination of the wart, I gave her a few doses of the remedy Thuja. Shortly thereafter, one morning she awoke to find that not only was the wart gone, but it was lying next to her on the bed. Thuja is very well known as a great wart remedy in homeopathy, so much so that in the nineteenth century people often referred to homeopaths as the wart doctors. Even my father, a highly respected podiatrist, asked me late in his career if I would show him how to use Thuja as he had heard of its great therapeutic benefit in treating stubborn warts. I told him of course I would help him, but that homeopathy was complex. For example, a wart that is on the right side of the body, is crusty, deeply imbedded in the cuticle of the nail or is calloused, may need a very different remedy, such as Causticum. Skill and careful case taking is very important when prescribing remedies as the symptoms need to match the picture of the remedy as demonstrated by its original proving.

The Chakras as a Holistic Medical Model

At this point I will give a description of the chakras. I have described the koshas, the other major paradigm I use as a model for understanding and treating people, in Part II. I will present case histories based on the chakras and koshas at the end of the book.

The chakras are energetic formations that exist on a very subtle level, animating the human bodymind complex. Each chakra has its characteristic vibratory patterns and frequencies. In deep meditation humans can experience these as color, form, yantra and sound frequencies as described in this section.

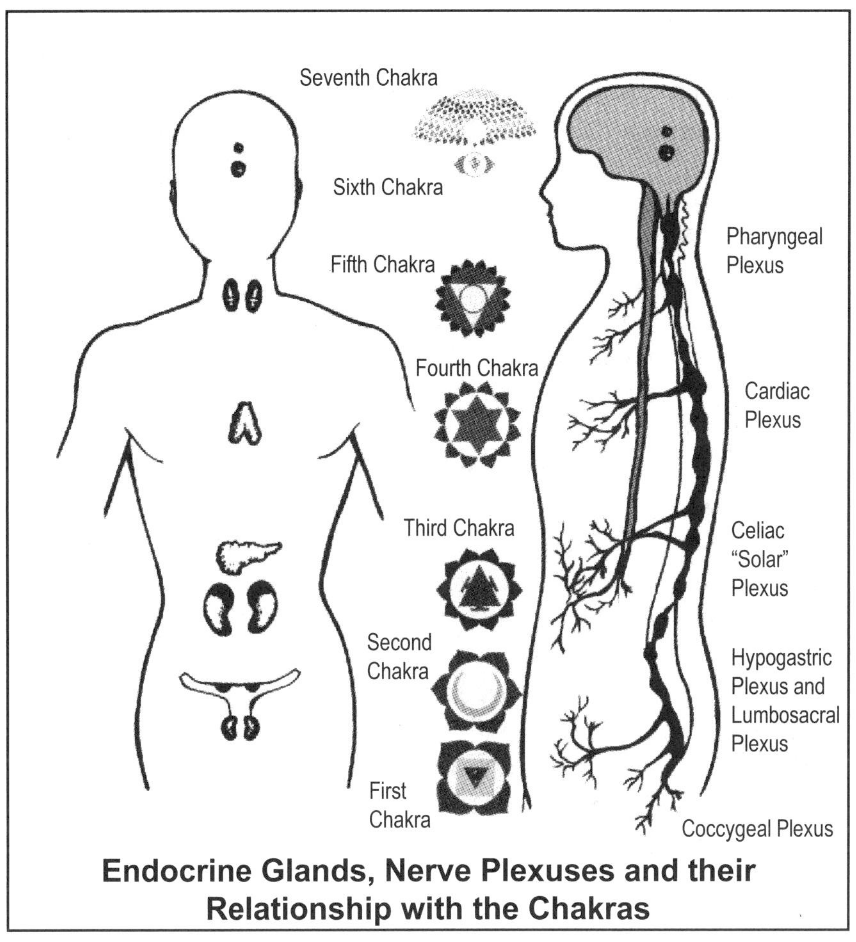

Endocrine Glands, Nerve Plexuses and their Relationship with the Chakras

Swami Rama, who was not only a yogi but also a homeopathic doctor, taught me that the system of the chakras could be used as a healing model. In this medical paradigm, it is easy to understand how disease is associated with body, breath and mind. An understanding of the chakras can help a healer or physician perceive the connection between deeply rooted health issues and patterns of behavior that manifest in a person's life.

The chakras are arranged in an evolutionary hierarchy like seven floors connected by a spiral staircase (ida and pingala nadis). They represent highly complex energy patterns that have many psychological correlations that are expressed through emotions, behavioral attitudes and desires. These patterns represent archetypes or symbols of highly complex psychospiritual qualities. Depending on a person's focus, body issue or state of mind, he or she can be dominated by the psychospiritual qualities of a particular chakra center.

The stories in each chakra are unique with variations found in the fables, myths, and fairy tales that have been narrated through many cultures. Within the experiences of each chakra, there are specific psychological and emotional dramas with main and supporting actors such as family, friends, colleagues and enemies. When one gets stuck in the drama of a specific chakra, they become bogged down in the old habits that characterize that chakra and are lost in the endless recreation of past wounds and memories.

If the flow and movement in an individual chakra become imbalanced, resulting in an excess or deficiency of energy, characteristic emotional, mental and physical ailments result. For example, esophageal and stomach pain due to acid reflux in someone who also harbors unexpressed anger, helps me organize my understanding of the case as a third chakra problem associated with digestion and assimilation issues and repressed feelings of inadequacy. The holistic physician can offer not only medicines but also homeopathic remedies, herbs, yoga postures, nutritional advice, breathing techniques, mantras and other spiritual practices to help balance, activate or pacify the problems associated with the chakras. These are all tools to help bring about healing so everyone can become free of the specific physical and emotional problems associated with the chakras. Through hard work, therapy, healthy life habits and the practice of meditation a person can raise their consciousness to the next emotional, mental or spiritual level.

The goal of the practice of meditation on the seven major chakras is to activate the chakra centers through intense concentration and to heal imbalances as well as to raise the latent energies from the lower more physical chakras to the higher more spiritual ones. In most people, the chakras function at a minimum level and are not in harmony with each other and can be compared to closed lotus flowers. Through intense concentration and meditative practices, the chakras become increasingly harmonized with each other until they vibrate in unison, like lotus flowers opening to the sun in full bloom. When this occurs, the body, emotions and mind are balanced and one experiences higher states of awareness.

First chakra

Muladhara, the first chakra, means "foundation." It is located at the base of the spine and is associated with the earth element and the power of gravity, the electromagnetic energy that holds things down. Thus, muladhara is related to the cellular and molecular level that also holds things together and gives life structure and form. In addition, the first chakra is the foundation that allows us to form connections and relationships with fellow humans and our culture. In association with the earth element, the first chakra connects a person to land, culture, tribe or social group. The sense associated with the first chakra is smell, a vital element that can attract people to each other or repel them away from each other.

Not only do the chakras govern and vitalize the physical functioning of certain areas of the body, there are also mental and emotional qualities associated with each chakra. Physically, muladhara chakra is associated with the lower bowel and excretion and chronic bowel disorders such as constipation, colitis or loose stools. Sacral spine problems, sciatic nerve pain, hip disorders, osteoporosis and arthritis are also associated with the first chakra. In addition, the legs and lower parts of the body as well as solid tissues such as the teeth and bones all come under the influence of the first chakra.

Psychological issues related to the first chakra are concerned with trust, being nurtured, emotional security, being grounded and financial security. Thus, psychological problems of the first chakra can manifest as distrustfulness and viewing the world as hostile, fear of being abandoned and difficulty setting limits and bonding with others. Other emotional problems associated with the first chakra include feeling disconnected from one's body, restlessness, being disorganized, having financial difficulties and feeling unfulfilled with one's profession. First chakra imbalance is also at the root of dietary disturbances such as obesity and eating disorders (anorexia or bulimia as the extreme examples). Problems with being overweight in turn can lead to diseases such as hypertension and diabetes. Other psychological problems include laziness, chronic tiredness, addictive behavior, and rigidity in thought, speech and action.

Healthy first chakra characteristics are good vitality and health, the ability to relax, balanced emotional stability, trust in relationships and in the world and a sense of prosperity.

My personal experiences with first chakra issues are as follows. Since childhood, I have had scoliosis and associated chronic pain in the lumbar and sacral area of my back and more recently unrelenting right leg pain while walking and standing. Since the lower back and legs are connected to first chakra functioning, I have used meditation and visualization on the first chakra to help bring healing energy to this area. I have also practiced tai chi and have done yoga postures that stretch and strengthen the first chakra area. I believe these practices helped mitigate and control my back/leg problems for many years. Finally, in my late sixties I realized I had to have surgery to release the pressure on two of the sciatic nerve roots as I was feeling more and more pain. As my leg and back pain have improved considerably since surgery, I continue to do the practices described above for continued healing and strength.

As the first chakra is also connected to issues of family, culture and our relationships with others, focus and concentration on this center can be quite helpful for emotional stability. Personally, during certain life events, I have spent considerable time in meditation focusing on the first chakra and moving energy from this center up through the higher chakras. This was especially true during conflict with my mother over my life choices, after my son Nathaniel's death and during my separation and subsequent divorce. This practice has had the effect of grounding me emotionally and helping me to integrate change and grow as a person.

And now as I am writing and editing this book, we in the US are going through some very tough times. There are demonstrations in the cities about police killings of African Americans and calls for social justice. There is some rioting in the streets, confrontation with police and fires burning. Sadly, my daughter's Barre Code studio in downtown Chicago has been damaged as a result of the chaos. We are also in the midst of the Covid 19 pandemic and there are worries that diminished social distancing during these demonstrations may lead to another upsurge of infectivity and subsequent increasing disease.

Global warming due to fossil fuel consumption has been steadily worsening. This has resulted in rising levels of our lakes and oceans, and we are experiencing more intense hurricanes and increasing frequency of devastating forest fires. To me, these are also first chakra issues that manifest not only as instability and illness on an individual basis, but also on a collective level, the latter characterized by the breaking down of social norms and increased stress on the earth's environment. If our very foundations are weakened, we as a nation (and world) face more social disorder, prejudice, political polarization and unemployment. While I realize I can't change the world by myself, I do feel I can make a bit of difference by sending out messages of peace, inner strength and emotional balance through my meditation practic in which I have been focusing on the first chakra to stabilize myself and my emotions and to take this energy up to the fourth chakra. From this heart-based center of consciousness, I send out love and compassion to citizens of this country and to the world at large.

More importantly, the first chakra is the resting place of the latent kundalini shakti. Visually, the first chakra is described as four red lotus petals surrounding a circle that contains a yellow square within an inverted red triangle. Within the triangle is the coiled kundalini energy. This resembles a serpent wrapped around itself three and one-half times with its head facing upwards into the central canal (sushumna). The deity associated with the first chakra is Ganesh, who helps remove obstacles on the path to liberation and helps open up the first chakra for the ascent of the kundalini shakti. Kali, the deity associated with kundalini shakti is also associated with the first chakra.

Kundalini shakti is the primal force of the seen and unseen universe and is manifested and expressed in humans through the chakras. When this energy is activated by yogic practices, the kundalini force is directed upwards to the higher centers. As a result, the individual experiences the world through the particular frame of reference of the chakras, according to which level the kundalini has ascended. For example, if one's mind and energy are primarily expressed through an imbalanced first chakra, they may experience the world as threatening and may feel insecure. If one is overly focused on third chakra issues, one might experience the world and other people in terms of power and control. When the mind and kundalini are expressed through the fifth chakra, one becomes creative and communicates more effectively.

To help heal issues and problems with first chakra functioning, the following yoga postures can be helpful: standing poses, bridge, boat, tortoise, lotus, tree, sitting meditation postures as well as the anal lock and ashwini mudra. Tai chi standing postures like the horse stance or bow and arrow stance are also very helpful. Repetition of the bija mantra *Lam*, while focusing on the symbol (yantra) of a red downward pointing triangle, is used for meditating on the first chakra.

Second Chakra

The second chakra, located slightly above the genital area, is called *svadisthana*, which means "one's own abode." Physically it is related with the nerve plexus and glands associated with the sexual organs. The element of the second chakra is water. It symbolizes the ability to change, like the transformation of ice to water and liquid water to steam. Just as hydrogen and oxygen come together to create water, sexual union can create a new life. Like water itself, a healthy second chakra enables change, flow and the ability to yield. Thus, it allows for the movement of inner physical and psychological forces. If one considers the first chakra to be like a riverbank, the second chakra is the water flowing within the boundaries and walls of the river. The sense associated with the second chakra is taste. Fluids such as saliva allow the different tastes to be appreciated.

On a physical level, the second chakra is in the area of the reproductive organs (ovaries, uterus, testes and prostate), the urinary tract, the lower abdomen in general and the lumbar area of the lower back. Diseases of the urinary system and reproductive organs including chronic bladder infections, prostate issues, menstrual problems, uterine fibroids, infertility and sterility represent second chakra issues. In addition, knee pain is also associated with the second chakra.

Second chakra functioning also encompasses sexual relationships, sexual desire and the sexual act. Sexually healthy people care deeply about their partners, often see the divine in them and love them fully, without feeling overly needy or possessive. An example of this is the passionate love and physical relationship between Shiva and Parvati.

Overexpression of the energy of the second chakra leads to problems such as being manipulative, infidelity, sexual addiction, obsession with pornography, being overly emotional (e.g hysteria), being sexually abusive and becoming overly attached to a person as a sexual object. When one is overly involved with seeking sensual pleasures, he or she will often find such experiences fleeting and insufficient, and the sexual partner may be experienced as being simultaneously alluring and fearful.

It follows that a low level of second chakra energy could be associated with emotional coldness, withdrawal from relationships, depression, a deadening of the senses, sexual rigidity, impotence, lack of interest in sex, fear of sexual contact, guilt and a general denial of sensory pleasure.

Psychological issues of the second chakra manifest as psychological movement away from the culture, tribe or social group to experience separateness and individuality. In general, deep feelings and emotional expression are associated with the second chakra. In the yogic tradition, emotions are a reflection of the four main human needs: food, sleep, sex and self-preservation. Emotions are often instinctual responses, arising from the unconscious mind. Like water, emotions flow and have a life of their own, often in contradiction to the rational, conscious mind.

Humans have often struggled with expression of sexual intimacy and have had to make difficult decisions and have had challenges to their inner moral standards along the way, both as adolescents and adults. Sexual expression, being a second chakra characteristic, has always represented a powerful urge, at times leading us to ecstatic moments of intimacy and at other times to manipulative behaviors or to frustration and loneliness. Generally, the challenge has been to love fully, with faithfulness and fidelity. Sometimes attaining this goal is successful and fulfilling but sometimes one can lose their way. Using the many modalities inherent in the yoga and holistic medical systems, the issues that reflect second chakra functioning can be helpful on the inner journey.

To help heal second chakra issues the following asanas can be helpful: cobra, locust, bow, all twists, forward bends and sitting meditation postures. Other yogic practices such as the anal lock and ashwini mudra can also be useful. Tai chi standing postures like the horse stance or bow and arrow stance can also be used therapeutically, similar to their effect on the first chakra.

Ruma and I have been walking three to five miles daily past a winding river and into a nearby forest during the current Covid 19 sequestration. Each day the woods have been very different as late winter birthed into early and late springtime, and now mid-autumn. New green undergrowth, majestic leafing oaks, emerging delicate wildflowers and perfuming honeysuckles and lilac bushes are there to delight our senses. The lush summer leaves have given way to beautiful orange, red and yellow colors. We have enjoyed touching the innumerable deciduous and shapely arbor leaves as we try to identify each tree species, aided by our newly downloaded plant identification app. The exquisite olfactory sensations and luminescent visions of the rapidly growing plant life are punctuated by happily chirping birds seeking their mates. Returning from our walks, we generally drink lemon-flavored sparkling water and share a light and healthy snack, thereby completing the journey through our five senses. This is the essence of the second chakra sensual experience.

There are times, however, when experiencing the fullness of the senses is blocked by physical illness, such as bladder problems, female menstrual cycle issues or sexual organ disorders. Emotional difficulties, problematic living situations and relationship issues can also interfere with the fullness of one's sensory experiences. I have certainly had moments when life's vicissitudes have prevented me from fully enjoying all the sensory gifts that have been given to us. Having experienced much loss through the death of my entire birth nuclear family has caused life to lose some of its luster. On the other hand, I have also experienced the amazing births of my children and grandchildren, bringing unlimited joy to my innermost being. I have loved, lost love and found it again. Health issues have depleted me at times, but fortunately have never knocked me out and I feel I have always learned valuable tools from these tough experiences.

The yantra for the second chakra is a circle surrounded by six dark vermilion lotus petals. Inside the circle is the color white with a silver crescent moon resting near the bottom. The sound (bija mantra) associated with this chakra is *Vam*. It is helpful to repeat the bija mantra *Vam* while meditating on a silver crescent moon at the second chakra.

Third Chakra

The third chakra is called *manipura,* which means "filled with jewels," and is located behind the navel near the spinal cord. It is associated with the celiac plexus of nerves, the adrenal glands and the pancreas. This area is often referred to as the solar plexus. Because of its ability to signal hunger or fear, it is also called the second brain. The third chakra is associated with the physical organs and tissues within the middle and upper abdomen. This includes the liver, gall bladder, spleen, stomach, lower part of the esophagus, the small intestine, adrenals and the linings of the abdominal cavity including the mesentery and peritoneum.

The element of the third chakra is fire, so it is the center of transformation where one thing becomes something else, such as the transformation of food into energy by the fires of digestion, metabolism and assimilation. The pancreas and adrenals are responsible for the secretion of insulin, glucose, adrenaline and cortisone, which also play important roles in transforming food into energy. Light, color, form and sight, all of which are involved with the phenomenon of fire, are the qualities and senses of the third chakra.

Physical health problems that reflect third chakra imbalance are gastric and duodenal ulcers, acid reflux, diabetes, hypoglycemia, gall stones, liver disease, pancreatitis, hypertension, chronic fatigue syndrome and adrenal fatigue.

This is the center where energy from the two lower chakras is transformed and stored. Asian martial arts describe this center as the middle dantian, the storehouse of power. It is at the core of one's physical strength, whether it involves striking a blow in the martial arts, the twisting motion of a golfer or a baseball batter trying to generate power. Yoga and other exercise forms like pilates often focus on exercises and techniques that strengthen this core. Anyone who has ever been punched in the center of the abdomen can testify how it knocked the energy and breath out of them.

On the psychological level, the third chakra represents the transition from identification with the group and family of the first chakra and the association with another person on an intimate manner of the second chakra to the sense of independence and individuality in the external world in general. This is the center of ego and competitiveness. And so there are issues of power over other people, of dominance and submissiveness and of a need to expand one's sphere of influence. The need to prove oneself and gain financial wealth and power are predominant. Anorexia and bulimia are two emotional disorders associated with problems of the third chakra (as well as the first chakra). And so it follows that people who experience life through the third chakra often have fiery and powerful personalities and tend to be motivated by the desire for external recognition, fame, power and material wealth. Physical strength and beauty are important to them and they may be arrogant and ambitious. They tend to demand attention from others and may even try to control others' actions and beliefs.

Overexpression of third chakra functioning can lead to aggressive behavior, pushiness, obstinacy and being controlling and dominating with friends, children or co-workers. They can be arrogant, overly prideful, manipulative, always having to be correct in arguments, headstrong and have a bad temper and fly off the handle easily. They are often rigid in their desires and behavior. Such persons can overwork, over drink, over study, be compulsive, be demanding at work or with children and generally have type A personalities.

With healthy expression of third chakra activity, one explores ways to assert themself in the world and begins to individuate as a separate person. One finds the inner strength and will power to assert oneself in the world when necessary and recognizes when it is more appropriate to step back and be more pliable and receptive. It also helps transform the emotions of attachment for others that are characteristic of the first and second chakras to the powers of individuality and expression of self or ego. One learns to develop good ego strength and autonomy and comes to understand who one is as an individual, rather than just in connection with family, friends and loved ones. At the level of the third chakra a person develops a personal sense of power and control. Persons with a healthy and balanced third chakra have a good image of themself, a good sense of humor and are spontaneous in their words and actions.

Healthy integration associated with this chakra allows for striking a balance between being active and assertive when necessary and being receptive or passive as required. There is a desire for success as well as an acceptance of failure. As one continues to move on the spiritual path, a balanced third chakra instills confidence and self-discipline. Healthy living involving the third chakra allows one to become nonattached to the fruits of their labor, and they work hard for the good and safety of others without looking for personal gain or power. Even when they are assertive to get things done, they do it in a pleasant and nonaggressive manner. This is typical of someone who practices karma yoga.

On the other hand, people with a weak energy field associated with the third chakra may have poor self-esteem, experience low energy levels, feel like they are victims and feel sorry for themselves, blame others for their problems, have feelings of shame, are undisciplined and can be quite passive when they need to assert themselves.

Swami Rama would say the ego is like a good shoe. It is important to have shoes that will help one walk comfortably and safely during their lives. In an analogous way, it is important to have a strong ego to navigate the vicissitudes of life. But when the shoe has worn out, one should not be attached to it but instead should toss it away rather than continue to wear it, as it will only cause discomfort. In a similar way, the ego can only take us so far before it interferes with ideas of living humbly in the moment.

To help heal issues with third chakra functioning, the following yoga practices and postures can be helpful: sun salutation, bow, upward bow, forward bend, bridge, locust and all sitting meditation postures. The whole tai chi form is also helpful. The breathing techniques of diaphragmatic breathing, kapalabhati and bhastrika help energize the third chakra. Other yogic practices such as the stomach lift, agni sara and nauli can also be useful.

When I was a young boy, I was extremely competitive, athletically and academically. I didn't like to lose at anything. Making the little league all-star game was a must, and making the Cleveland Dream Team for baseball and scoring a bunch of points for my high school basketball team were essential for my happiness. Also, being academically successful in my class was critical to my self-esteem. Occasionally, I even cheated at poker with my friends to win and of course to not lose money.

As I got older this super competitive drive morphed into my need to date the prettiest and smartest women. I even got in a fight with a friend when I probably mistakenly thought he was flirting with my college girlfriend. Well, after yelling at him and then getting sucker punched in my mouth in retaliation, knocking my front two teeth lose, I realized something needed to change. My third chakra was completely out of whack. It was then and there that I embarked on a journey to get my ego under control and quiet my supercharged nervous system. I found yoga and meditation.

Repetition of the bija mantra *Ram* while focusing on the yantra configuration of an upward facing equilateral triangle are useful for third chakra balancing. The third chakra is visualized as a circle surrounded by ten dark blue lotus petals. Inside the circle is a red triangle that is pointed downwards but which inverts to point upwards during meditation. The female deity, Durga, can be meditated upon at the third chakra, as she represents the slayer of the ego, which often obstructs the aspirant on the spiritual path

Fourth Chakra

The fourth chakra, located in the area of the heart near the spine, is called *anahata,* which means "unheard sound." The fourth chakra is the center of the expansive force, that of air. In air, there are forces that push molecules apart, creating energy like that of two magnets pushing each other apart. The sense is touch, which is associated with the pressure force of air on the human body. On the emotional and mental level one "touches" the soul of another when giving nurturance, love, compassion or forgiveness.

Physiologically, the fourth chakra is associated with the cardiac plexus of nerves as well as the breath and the air-filled chest cavity that includes the lungs, heart, thymus gland, breasts and middle back area. On a physical level, the heart nourishes the cells and tissues with blood, the lungs nourish the body with air, the breasts nourish the baby with milk and the thymus gland produces immune cells that nourish the body for self-defense and immunity. Problems on a physical level include illnesses such as heart disease, arrhythmias, chronic bronchitis, asthma, emphysema, breast disorders, nursing problems, immunity issues and mid-back pain.

The fourth chakra, being the central chakra of the seven major chakras, provides the necessary support for the individual to progress to the three highest chakras. It represents the transition from the more biological and instinctual urges of the three lower chakras to the more highly evolved spiritual qualities of the higher chakras. Now the person can move beyond the issues of survival and self-preservation of the first chakra, the issues of the senses and sexuality of the second chakra and the issues of expression of the individual ego of the third chakra.

Once a person is firmly established with pride, dignity and a strong self-identity, they can experience loving feelings for themselves and for others. Positive fourth chakra qualities include loving kindness, compassion, empathy, the ability to forgive and generosity of spirit both for others and for oneself. When the heart chakra is open, one realizes the divine is present in everyone. Loving all sentient beings regardless of race, gender, degree of handicap, age, sexual orientation, gender identification or religion is a sign of a fully developed and open fourth chakra. However, when the heart chakra is underdeveloped, many emotional problems can occur, such as being unable to be intimate, to love others or to be emotionally vulnerable. The person can be consumed in self-absorption and remains isolated and withdrawn. A person with a cold heart can be demanding and overcritical.

On the other hand, when an excess of energy exists within the fourth chakra, a person may have poor boundaries in relationships, be possessive and demanding and have difficulty establishing meaningful relationships.

Those who are able to experience life through balanced energy of the fourth chakra practice loving kindness and develop a deeper capacity for expressing love, generosity, forgiveness and compassion. Such persons are a source of inspiration to others who feel at peace in their presence. The capacity for empathy and deep feelings for other people represents an evolutionary step towards higher consciousness.

While my physical heart has always been strong during my lifetime, my emotional heart has taken some blows. The fourth chakra, the pranic heart center, has needed some healing over the years. Below, I discuss the methods to heal the heart chakra area and I'm very thankful for having tapped into good nutrition and homeopathy as well as yoga, pranayama and meditation techniques. To heal issues and problems with fourth chakra functioning, the following yoga practices and postures can be helpful: back bends, fish, camel, cobra, upward dog, cat stretch and all sitting meditation postures. The whole tai chi form also is helpful. The breathing and pranayama techniques of diaphragmatic breathing, kapalabhati, bhastrika and breath retention help energize the fourth chakra.

I have always tried to avoid being rude or haughty with other people and have felt and tried to express empathy for other's pain. This aspect of my personality was certainly compatible with my training to be a physician. The birth of my eldest son Abe also opened me up as the love for him just exploded out of my heart. Then Nathaniel's death took the breath out of me and I learned about the pain and suffering of losing a child. I directly experienced loss at the deepest level, but it also taught me about compassion and love and to truly experience other people's suffering. Ethan and Ari's birth further opened my heart to love and I feel so grateful for all of it.

The fourth chakra is visually described as twelve deep red lotus petals surrounding a circle. Inside the circle are two blue-green triangles that intersect, one pointed down and the other pointed up. In the Jewish religion this shape is referred to as the Star of David. Inside the six-pointed star is a dark area, often described as a black cave. Inside the cave is a lit candle with a flame that doesn't flicker. This flame is often referred to as the reflection of the soul. The soul is the eternal and nonchanging center of consciousness, which channels the energy and creative forces of the universe through the individual. The bija mantra associated with this chakra is *Yam.*

From the yogic perspective, the great love between Rama and Sita can be contemplated when concentrating on the fourth chakra. Radha can also be invoked when meditating on the fourth chakra as she is the devoted partner of Krishna. The union of these two couples is a metaphor for the power of attraction, love and commitment in relationships.

Hrit is a lesser-known chakra closely associated with, connected to and located slightly below the anahata chakra. Great depths of emotion and feelings of devotion are associated with this center. Some consider hrit to be the seat of the soul. It is described as being surrounded by eight gold lotus petals resting on a circle. Inside the circle is another circle red in color and inside this is an orange circle.

There are several mantras that connect the individual to the heart and hrit chakras. The bija mantra for the fourth chakra is *Yam.* The *Maha Mantra,* which is *Hare Krishna, Hare Krishna, Krishna Krishna, Hare Hare* is a powerful invocation to the opening of the fourth chakra. *OM Hrim Shrim Klim* is a powerful feminine mantra associated with the fourth chakra. Another Sanskrit heart-centered mantra is *OM Hrim Hamsa Ha So Ham Swaha.*

The *Shema,* which is the most important Jewish prayer that is said upon waking, falling asleep, at synagogue services and upon dying, can be recited with focus on the fourth chakra. The words to this prayer are: *Shema Yisroel Adonai Eloheinu Adonai Echad.* This means: "Hear O Israel (all sentient beings) the Lord is our God the Lord is One." It goes on to say, "And you shall love the Lord our God with all your soul and with all your might." The spiritual significance to this prayer is that all sentient beings are connected and at one with God. It is interesting that the symbol for the Jewish faith, the Star of David, is like the symbol for the fourth chakra in the yogic and Tibetan Buddhist systems of chakras. The mystical interpretation is that all people and their individual souls are one with God.

The meaning of the great Buddhist mantra, *OM Mani Padme Hum,* is: "I give reverence to consciousness itself experienced as the jewel in the lotus." The jewel and the lotus refer to the soul and the heart. This is often chanted with attention on the fourth chakra.

Fifth Chakra

The fifth chakra is *vishuddha,* which means "purified." It is the center of electromagnetic forces and fields. The element associated with this chakra is ether, or space, which contains the other elements of earth, water, fire and air. Ether encompasses all the quantum frequencies of energy, including heat, light and sound. Thus the sense associated with the fifth chakra is sound, inclusive of speech, music and hearing. When the fifth chakra is strong, one may have a nice singing voice and be able to use mantras with ease in meditation.

Visuddha is located between the throat and the cervical portion of the spinal cord and is associated with the cervical nerve plexus as well as the nerves of the larynx and the thyroid gland. The thyroid gland is involved with the rate of metabolism, energy production, the rate of cell activity and the control of body temperature, all of which are connected to the energy of body functioning. The fifth chakra is also associated with the throat area, the Eustachian tubes, hearing, and the carotid body within the carotid artery, which detects changes in the composition of arterial blood, mainly oxygen and carbon dioxide. The larynx, the lower jaw and the neck are also part of this chakra area. Illnesses on a physical level could be hypothyroidism, Grave's disease, thyroiditis, chronic sore throats or laryngitis, stiff neck, recurrent ear infections, hearing problems or deafness.

The fifth chakra is the chakra of communication. It also is associated with the inner voice of creativity. In a sense, the universe is the broadcaster, the brain is the radio, energy waves are the means of communication, and the fifth chakra decides what station the person attunes to. Those who experience life through the fifth chakra may develop a melodious voice, be musically inclined, have a good command of speech and the ability to write well, or have the capacity to understand spiritual writings and to interpret the deeper significance of dreams.

The other important aspect of healthy fifth center functioning involves the receiving side. Being able to listen well not only means to listen to others who are speaking to you but also reflects being receptive to one's inner voice of reason and creativity. I feel I am a good listener in general, especially with my patients, but also with family and friends. But it wasn't until I decided to meditate and quiet my mind that I was able to tap into and take advice from my inner spontaneous creative guide.

Emotionally this chakra is associated with being supported and taken care of and nurtured. The fifth chakra has to do with communication between people as well as to the world of ideas and the surrounding environment. One with balanced energy at the fifth chakra is truly receptive and responsive and able to listen carefully and thoughtfully. While it may seem that the capacity to be nurturing (fourth chakra) is a higher spiritual attribute than receptivity (fifth chakra), from a yogic perspective the capacity to be truly open and receptive is higher. The receptivity associated with the fifth chakra not only has to do with listening to others but more importantly to the higher Self, from where creative urges and insights originate. The level of the fifth chakra is also where one can experience the grace of divine inspiration or grace from the teacher who is a representative of higher knowledge. Grace is said to descend, to be received and focused within the fifth chakra. As trust develops, the spiritual aspirant becomes more open to the highest levels of more complete states of awareness.

Deficient functioning in the fifth chakra area can result in difficulty in communicating thoughts or feelings. One may have problems finding the correct words to express an idea. People with low functioning associated with this level of consciousness may be reticent to speak and generally are on the shy side. Their voice may be weak, or they may be tone deaf.

Excessive functioning of the fifth chakra can lead to problems being truthful, giving people mixed messages, being overly critical of oneself or others, being bossy, loud and dominating, being a poor listener, talking excessively and having conditions like attention deficit hyperactivity syndrome.

I never felt I was particularly artistic, musically inclined or talented at creative writing. As I reached young adulthood, I saw myself as an athlete, a future physician and a person devoted to family, hoping to marry one day and have children. One of my first experiences with creative writing occurred when I wrote my master's thesis on vegetarianism. My mentor at the time said she really liked what I wrote and suggested that I continue on to get a PhD and continue my research into the health benefits and history of plant-based diets. I respectfully declined her offer to be my doctorate mentor as I needed to get back to my medical practice and caring for my growing family.

When I began to study with Swami Rama, he asked me and two colleagues to write a book on homeopathy, called *Homeopathic Remedies for Physicians, Laymen and Therapists*. There were very few modern books on homeopathy at the time and I was happy to be a young co-author. Since then, I have written three other books as well as this one.

In yogic philosophy, the center of creativity is a fifth chakra function. From this perspective I would say that my writing reflects some activity in this chakra. Fifth chakra issues of creativity for the individual bring together inspired thinking and synthesis of ideas that come forth from the deep subconscious and unconscious. Generally, for myself, I get inspired to write, paint or even sing when my mind finally ceases its chatter. If I over think, what comes out is less spontaneous and more infused with what I think I should do.

I don't really call myself a musician but I have worked hard to refine my voice and learn to play harmonium so I could lead kirtan in my group, Ann Arbor Kirtan, which I started fifteen years ago. I have taken voice lessons from four different voice teachers. I've enjoyed this activity and I feel I have adequately challenged myself to constantly improve my musicality. Before my foray into kirtan, I had co-created a CD, called *Kundalini Rhapsody*, with my colleague and friend, Muruga Booker, a prominent percussionist. We led groups at various musical venues, where he would drum and I would chant bija mantras through the chakras. We humorously advertised our musical events as: *A Yogi Physician and a Yogi Musician Provide Entertainment for Inner Attainment.* It was a lot of fun.

Another creative endeavor I have most recently engaged in is art—painting and drawing. I have always been unbelievably deficient at any form of art. Anyone who has seen my doodles and rudimentary stick figures would attest to this fact. But through trial and error and quite a bit of humility, humor and practice, I have found a small niche in abstract and colorful, fauvist type acrylic paintings.

I share all these attempts at creative endeavor as an example of my taking risks to do things that don't come easy for me as examples of the importance of making effort to open up the fifth chakra. Meditation, yoga postures and the practice of tai chi have also been important in my fifth chakra expression.

To help heal issues and problems with fifth chakra functioning, the following yoga practices and postures can be helpful: neck exercises, plow, fish, shoulderstand, lion, back bends, fish, camel, cobra, upward dog and all sitting meditation postures. The breathing techniques of diaphragmatic breathing, ujjayi, bhramari, sitali, sitari and breath retention in general help energize the fifth chakra.

Kirtan or yoga chanting may be a spiritual practice that one might enjoy because kirtan is part bhakti yoga (yoga of the heart, fourth chakra) and mantra and nada yoga (yoga of sound and vibratory frequency, fifth chakra). Authors, artists, musicians, research scientists, poets and other people who need to tap into their inner creative abilities often have highly functioning fifth chakras. When these people have blocks in being able to access their creative reservoirs, meditation with specific mantras on the fifth chakra can be very helpful to tap back into the creative self.

Vishuddha is described as sixteen dark purple lotus petals surrounding a circle. The space inside the circle is dark blue in color and in the center is a white circle resting within a white triangle. This is described as the full moon seen against a blue sky. Repetition of *Ham,* the bija mantra for the fifth chakra, is useful for fifth chakra balancing.

Another mantra associated with the fifth chakra is *Aim,* although it is not the bija mantra for this center. It represents the mantra for Saraswati, the goddess of wisdom, art, knowledge, learning and communication. Focusing on the deity Saraswati along with the mantra *Aim* at the fifth chakra, helps one to better express oneself creatively and to experience higher truths.

Sixth Chakra

The name of the sixth chakra, *ajna,* means "command." It is located behind the area between and slightly above the two eyebrows in the center of the forehead. The sixth chakra is beyond any sense association or element. It can be described as clear illumination or pure mind.

The sixth chakra, also referred to as the third eye, is associated with the higher functions of the mind such as intuition, wisdom, good decision-making and clarity of vision. Being able to analyze dreams to help bring unconscious thoughts and concerns into conscious awareness as well as having the ability to creatively visualize are also functions of the sixth chakra, along with having a good imagination and being able to think symbolically.

The sixth chakra, unlike the other chakras that are influenced by the five senses, is the integrating center where all the senses come together to formulate one's view of the world and reality. It is called the third eye or the eye of insight because it sees inwards into the conscious and unconscious mind. Experiences of paranormal activity and phenomena are localized in the area of the sixth chakra.

This includes clairvoyance, telekinesis, clairaudience, synesthesia and telepathic communication.

Wisdom and intuition are the qualities that are associated with the sixth chakra. They come from having experienced the world and life's vicissitudes over time and having come to understand how important thoughtful decision-making is. Wisdom facilitates clear decision-making. Especially when applied to the spiritual world, wisdom not only reflects having good judgment and knowledge of a situation, but also involves being gentle with others and having the ability to discriminate right from wrong, and whether action needs to be taken in response to an event or whether it can be let go of. How best to handle a delicate and potentially reactive event requiress skill, patience and wisdom.

Intuition reflects the ability to understand something immediately without the interference of conscious reasoning, and often involves instinctive feelings rather than critical thinking. Intuition and insight develop when deep understanding is immediate and accurate, leading to clarity in judgement and decision-making. My own experience with intuition often plays out when seeing patients. I sometimes sense a person's underlying physical and emotional health issues almost immediately, even with a new patient. I believe that having this ability stems from having seen over 70,000 patients over many years and observing how they walk, how they fold their hands, how they smell, the tone of their voice and the expression on their face. I also make it a point to observe how each person breathes. Do they tend to hold their breath, is their breathing rapid, irregular or shallow? This always helps to better understand the patient's health concerns.

Because my practice of meditation has helped me quieten my mind, I can better see, hear and understand a patient's concerns without any of my own thoughts and preconceptions getting in the way. I believe that habitually resting my concentration on the sixth chakra, the third eye, helps to build the quality of insight. The third eye sees inwards, unlike the two physical eyes that look outwards. On a spiritual level, insight is a deeply felt experience with an associated perception and awareness of life's many mysteries. In yogic philosophy, this means an experience of union with the

Chakra Associations with Physical, Emotional, and Spiritual Qualities

Chakra	Nerve Association	Gland Association	Physical Quality	Physical Illness
Muladhara	Sacral and pelvic nerves, Coccygeal plexus		Bowel function	Irritable bowel syndrome
Svadisthana	Hypogastric plexus, Lumbar-sacral plexus	Sexual organs, Testes Ovaries	Reproduc-tion, Sexuality	STDs Urinary tract infec-tions
Manipura	Celiac plexus	Adrenal, Pancreas	Digestion	Ulcers, Indigestion, Diabetes
Hrit	Cardiac plexus			
Anahata	Cardiac plexus	Thymus	Breath, Circulation	Asthma, Heart disease
Vishuddha	Pharyngeal plexus	Thyroid, Parathyroid	Metabolism, Speech	Low thyroid function, URIs
Ajna	Midbrain	Pineal, Pituitary		
Indu	Brain			
Guru	Brain			
Sahasrara	Cerebral cortex of the brain			

Chakra Associations with Physical, Emotional, and Spiritual Qualities

Psychological & Spiritual Quality	Psychological & Spiritual Problem	Color & Shape of Yantra	Color & No. of Lotus Petals	Sense & Element	Mantra
Strong foundation, Security, Kundalini	Survival, Fear, Paranoia, Insecurity	Yellow square, red triangle	Red, Four	Smell, Earth	LAM
Healthy sexual expression	Sexual concerns	Silver crescent moon	Red, Six	Taste, Water	VAM
Sense of self, Power Ego, Dominance & submissiveness	Inferiority complex, Anorexia	Red triangle	Blue, Ten	Sight, Fire	RAM
Love, Devotion		Red circle, Orange circle	Gold, Eight		
Compassion, Loving Kindness	Apathy, Grief, Hatred	Blue-green, Star of David	Red, Twelve	Touch, Air	YAM
Receptivity, Communication, Creativity	Inhibition of speech and creativity	White moon on blue sky	Purple, Sixteen	Hearing, Space	HAM
Intuition, Wisdom, Insight		White circle with OM symbol	Blue, Two	Pure Mind	OM
Bliss, Taste of Nectar		Silver crescent moon	Blue, Sixteen		
Sublime Mantras & Vibrations		Red triangle	Red, Twelve		
Enlightenment, Highest Consciousness		Pure light, Rainbow lotus petals	Pure light, 1,000		

higher Self. When one meditates on the sixth chakra, one can see inwards into the different levels of the mind, and observe thoughts, worries and fears float by.

Sixth chakra imbalances are associated with poor memory, being unable to concentrate or visualize, lacking common sense and not being perceptive. To help heal issues and problems with sixth chakra functioning, the following yoga practices and postures can be helpful: all yoga postures that involve focusing of mind and body, headstand, all sitting meditation postures and the tai chi form where body, breath and mind are in coordination. The breathing and pranayama techniques of diaphragmatic breathing and alternative nostril breathing, with or without breath retention, help to focus energy at the sixth chakra.

Ajna is described as a white circle with a light blue lotus petal on each side, giving it the appearance of an eye. Inside the circle is a small white triangle pointed down. The sound associated with this center is the universal mantra *OM*. The deity is Brahma as he is associated with the consciousness out of which the manifestation of the universe occurs.

Many meditative traditions focus on this center to enhance mental clarity and the ability to concentrate. When the kundalini energy rises to this level, a person experiences expanded states of consciousness.

Indu is a minor chakra located above ajna chakra. This chakra is visually described as a circle surrounded by sixteen light blue lotus petals. Within the circle is a silver-white crescent moon. Indu is said to be the source of soma, the sweet nectar that drips down with the cerebral spinal fluid from the third ventricle of the brain into the spinal cord. When a person experiences higher states of consciousness, this nectar can be tasted in the throat.

Guru chakra is another lesser known but very important chakra located above the ajna and indu chakras and below the seventh sahasrara chakra near the back of the cerebral cortex of the brain. This chakra is visually described as a circle surrounded by twelve red lotus petal. Within the circle is a red inverted triangle, which in deep meditation turns upwards and represents the fire of knowledge. It is associated with very subtle mantras and sublime images of great luminosity. One who meditates on this chakra and establishes consciousness here attains great spiritual knowledge and feelings of bliss.

Seventh Chakra

Sahasrara, which means "a thousand petals," is the seventh and highest chakra. The seventh chakra is associated with higher brain functioning and the cerebral cortex. All sounds, elements, and senses are absorbed and integrated into the seventh chakra. Shiva is the deity associated with the crown chakra as he is closely associated with pure consciousness. When kundalini reaches this level, the individual self merges with and is absorbed into universal consciousness. Here there is no distinction between the knower and the known; there is only perfect knowing. The experience of the oneness of consciousness at this level is said to be nameless and indescribable, though the qualities of existence, consciousness and bliss are close approximations of this state. Names used to identify this experience are: universal consciousness, absorption in the absolute, Brahman, God consciousness, nirvana, samadhi or the void. A very advanced practice at the seventh chakra is to focus on the Shri Yantra.

Sahasrara is described as appearing like one thousand lotus petals of pure light emanating like an umbrella or crown from the top of the head. At times, during meditation the crown chakra can be visualized as though it is arranged in the variegated colors of the rainbow.

The Centers of the Tree of Life

As in the chakras of the yoga model of consciousness, meditation on the ten sefirot in Judaism can balance and awaken latent forces and qualities inherent in each of the centers, including factors and influences that create physical, emotional and mental problems or illnesses. In both systems, the ultimate goal is liberation from suffering and merging with the divine, or God.

First Sefirah

Located at the base of the spine, the first sefirah is called *malkhut* (kingship). As the just and righteous king and queen rule to make the people who live in their kingdom feel secure and taken care of, malkhut provides security and support. Shekinah energy is stored here, as is kundalini stored in the first chakra in the yogic model. Malkhut is associated with feminine earth energy, often referred to as mother earth. By having a well-integrated first sefirah, one feels connected to other human beings and is grounded and secure. Malkhut is associated with the feet.

Second Sefirah

Similar to the second chakra in yoga, the second sefirah, called *yesod* (foundation), is associated with the sacral area and genitals. Yesod is connected to the powerful forces that connect spirit and matter to bring human life to incarnate. However, the psychological aspects of yesod represent not only the creation of a new life but also the higher, more evolved aspects of love and compassion. Yesod represents the creative aspect of one's nature, where two opposites attract and create something new.

Male and female principles commune here and it is the center of sexual energy. When the sexual act between a man and woman is connected to and blessed with love, the Shekinah energy is guided to the fourth sefirah, allowing this center to expand.

Also, as the second sefirah blossoms, the creative power is manifested intellectually and into the higher aspects of art, music, writing and scientific exploration associated with the sixth sefirah. Therefore, a healthy and balanced second sefirah is connected to both the fifth and sixth sefirot, allowing for the evolutionary progress of pure love and creativity. In Jewish thought the higher aspect of God's creative urge and love for manifestation can come to full fruition when the fifth sefirah is balanced and open.

Third and Fourth Sefirot

The two names associated with the third and fourth sefirot are *netzach* (eternity and victory) and *hod* (splendor). Netzach is associated with the right leg, hod with the left leg and both are associated with the abdominal organs and the solar (celiac) plexus.

As in the third chakra in the yoga system, these two sefirot are located around the solar plexus. In the tree of life system, they are connected to the emotional side of one's nature, representing one's emotional needs and sense of self. The feelings that make a person fully human are aspects of netzach and hod. Energy from the lower two sefirot, malkhut and yesod, is also stored in this center.

Netzach, which means victory, represents the pacification and victorious redirection of emotions seen in the two lower sefirot. The eternity aspect of netzach means that as one learns how to control one's inner emotions and redirects these to more spiritual domains, that person reaches the heavens and their true eternal nature. This is the experience of the splendor (hod) of God and the divine nature of one's being, characteristic of the fourth sefirah.

When one is established in these centers, altruistic goals replace the need for fame, conquest and glory. A righteous teacher or *rebbe* can help a person remain humble and balanced when on the path of self-awareness and ascension on the tree of life.

Fifth Sefirah

The name for the fifth sefirah is *tiferet* (beauty). Tiferet is associated with the heart and general torso. As in the fourth chakra in the yogic system, love and compassion are qualities that personify this heart center. Religious pursuits and spiritual truths are associated with tiferet. The beauty referred to in this sefirah has to do with the inner beauty that ensues when one's consciousness is infused with selfless love and the beauty of the soul.

The love associated with the fifth sefirah is of a divine nature, enabling one to love God and all sentient beings as being one and the same as God. The ability to see and experience the godliness of all creation exemplifies an evolved fifth sefirot. Other important aspects of a highly developed tiferet include the desire to serve humankind and eliminate social inequity, hunger and poverty. The Hebrew idea of bringing the Kingdom of Heaven into the everyday world is similar to the fourth chakra attribute of love and compassion.

Sixth and Seventh Sefirot

The sixth and seventh sefirot names are *chesed* (mercy) and *gevurah* (power). Chesed is associated with the right arm and gevurah with the left arm. Mercy refers to the grace from the divine that gives the ability to create, such as in artistic talent or musical expression. Gevurah represents the power of speech, communication and of healing others, much like the attributes associated with the fifth chakra in yoga. It also represents the powerful expression of words for the good of humanity. As discussed earlier, there is a direct connection between the second sefirah and the sixth in that the aspects of sexuality that result in the creation of a new human being are now also used to create other forms of self-expression, such as the ability to verbally communicate well and succeed in such areas as art, music and science. Here in the sixth and seventh sefirot, love from the fifth sefirah merges with the mercy and power of these two higher sefirot to help guide the spiritual aspirant to continue the journey towards merging with the divine and God awareness. The power to heal, which is considered to be a state where there is receptivity to universal forces of unity, is said by Kabbalists to reflect open sixth and seven sefirot.

Eighth and Ninth Sefirot

The eighth and ninth sefirot names are *chokhmah* (wisdom) and *binah* (understanding). These centers represent the bridge that connects the physical body and the spiritual body through the activity of the mind. Transmutation of mundane thought into more spiritual awareness and creative endeavor begins in these siferot. One begins to perceive and experience higher planes of existence. This area, like the sixth chakra in yoga, is said to be located in the center of the forehead. Intuition and decisiveness represent the wisdom aspect of these siferot. At this level one comes to understand more of the great mysteries of the universe and the spiritual nature of one's birthright and begins not only to ascend to the Kingdom of Heaven but also to truly and deeply experience themselves as divine beings. When this center is highly developed, one is able to receive inner spiritual insights and to communicate thoughts and creative energies to other receptive people.

The female energy, Shekinah, ascends through the left and right channels and it is here, in chokhmah and binah sefirot, they merge into a single path to ascend further to the highest sefirah, the crown center, keter. It is when one merges and becomes absorbed with these three highest sefirot that one merges with God.

Tenth Sefirah

Keter, the tenth sefirah, is the center where the energy of Shekinah that has risen from below unites with the energy that descends from the Heavens *(ein sof)*. One is filled with the light of pure, divine awareness as universal consciousness and the individual merge to become one. This is similar to what happens in the seventh crown chakra in yoga in the experience of samadhi.

Eleventh Sefirah

Another sefirah, not classically considered part of the ten sefirot, is called *daat* (knowledge). This is a hidden center and represents the experience of the highest knowledge of the seen and unseen cosmos (God). It forms when the sefirot of chokhmah, binah and keter fuse into one center. It is often represented by a triangle with keter at the apex.

Chakra Case Histories

In my medical practice as well as in my meditation classes, I teach how and when to focus on different chakras for specific therapeutic purposes. We work on strengthening and balancing specific physical, behavioral and spiritual characteristics associated with individual chakras. Now I will discuss several case histories to illustrate this work.

Case History Focused on the First Chakra

A fifty-five-year-old woman, DB, described herself as an empath because she could deeply feel other people's pain and suffering. She was quite intuitive and often felt she could sense what other people were thinking. She enjoyed communication with others and was a good listener. She came to see me because, while she could help others, she felt insecure and off center in her own life. A particularly troublesome worry was that her husband would leave her for another woman, despite his continual reassurance this wasn't true and there were no real grounds for this concern.

Chakra Perspective

DB appeared to have more highly developed fourth and sixth chakras as she was sensitive and loving towards others as well as being quite intuitive. On the other hand, her chakra system was not really well integrated since she exhibited first chakra weakness as she felt ungrounded and insecure, particularly about her husband's fidelity. Her third chakra functioning was also underdeveloped as she felt a sense of powerlessness and inability to manage anxiety.

Her physical complaints primarily centered around first chakra deficiency as follows: irritable bowel syndrome, where she had alternating diarrhea and constipation and a lot of gas; she was slightly obese with a BMI of 32; balance was a problem for her and she often fell and injured herself.

Treatment

I taught her diaphragmatic breathing and progressive relaxation to help her relax and have better regulation of the three lower chakras. The rhythmical movement of the abdomen during breathing stimulates all the digestive organs as well as the reproductive system. To help strengthen the first chakra, we worked on the standing yoga postures such as the triangle and warrior poses. I also taught the horse stance of tai chi in which one stands with the knees bent and back straight while visualizing the feet gripping the ground and penetrating nine feet into the earth. We also worked on shaking qi gong, where she gently bounced with arms, legs and neck loose and with the whole body vibrating and shaking. I also recommended walking thirty minutes four times weekly as part of her regime. Leg presses were recommended for greater hamstring and quadriceps strength, all of which are oriented to help balance the first chakra. These practices were complemented with dietary changes to help her lose weight and a homeopathic remedy (Calcarea carbonica) to further manage her weight and to help heal the large bowel issues.

To increase self-confidence and a stronger sense of herself (ego strength), we worked on a special concentration technique where she visualized the third chakra having a red upward pointed triangle, breathing energy and light from this point up through the spine to the crown chakra with inhalation and back down the spine with exhalation to the third chakra. To help integrate all of this, I asked her to meditate on the fourth chakra to continue to explore and strengthen her already heart-centered and devotional approach to life. She used the mantra *Yam.*

Outcome

From a chakra perspective, this woman resembles a tree that has beautiful branches full of flowering blossoms (represented by a more developed fourth, fifth and sixth chakra) but whose root structure is not strong (weak first, second and third chakra) and thus could be easily toppled in a strong wind. Another image is that of a big beautiful house full of expensive art work, wood paneling and luxurious items but with a weak foundation that could not withstand storms or floods. Over time, she experienced improvement in balance, bowel functioning and a better sense of self-confidence and self-esteem.

Case History Focused on the Second Chakra

JB was a thirty-two-year-old psychotherapist who was having difficulty conceiving. She was very tearful when talking to me about her troubles. She and her husband had been trying for over two years to have a baby but didn't want to go through an infertility clinic or have to take medication to stimulate ovulation. With more in-depth counseling, she revealed to me that she and her husband argued quite often, after which he would annoy her with his passive aggressive words and hostile glances. Having sex at specified times to enable conception was a burden and created anxiety and tension in the relationship. She wasn't even sure her marriage was going to survive the ordeal.

Chakra Perspective

JB exhibited difficulties in second chakra expression. She was somewhat stubborn and lacked the ability to be flexible and emotionally available in her relationship with her husband. She was rather withdrawn and distant and denied herself the simple pleasures of life, such as enjoying a good meal or going to a movie. Sex had become a burden for her and she could not express feelings of tenderness.

Treatment

Initially we did some work on anger management, which involved not losing her temper while openly telling her husband what made her upset. She also encouraged her husband to directly disclose his frustrations, rather than simply retreating to his abundant tools in his basement workshop where he would simmer in silence for long periods of time. She was a paradoxical breather as her abdomen moved in as she inhaled and moved out as she exhaled. Not only is this an inefficient way to breathe but it also creates a feeling of energy depletion as well as anxiety. Specific therapeutics included simple diaphragmatic breathing and alternate nostril breathing to balance the active and passive sides of her nervous system. I also taught her how to use second chakra visualization focusing on its symbol of a white crescent moon enclosed in a circle with six scarlet lotus petals surrounding the circle. I introduced the second chakra bija mantra, *Vam,* to activate the energy associated with this center of consciousness. I had her move energy up the spine during meditation so as to move her restricted procreative energy and her frustrations up towards her heart center where the qualities of caring, compassion and forgiveness towards her husband were centered. Yoga postures that helped activate her second chakra issues included the spinal twist, which stimulates the pelvic organs and the knee to chest pose, which also gives a nice stretch to the second chakra area.

I prescribed the homeopathic remedy Pulsatilla as it matched her early symptoms of crying easily and tendency to change moods quickly and unexpectedly. I later prescribed Natrum muriaticum because not only did she constantly crave salty foods, she revealed she had experienced verbal and some physical abuse earlier in her life, which led her to dwell on the past.

Outcome

Happily she did finally become pregnant and delivered a healthy baby. The marriage, however, only lasted a few more years, but because of both her and her ex-husband's hard work, they separated with respect and are now good co-parents.

Case History Focused on the Third Chakra

MB is a thirty-five-year-old man who works in a rapidly growing startup tech company. His group is working on a very interesting app for cell phones and also does data analytics for several major businesses. With the newness of the company and with stock options as compensation, he is very motivated to work many hours. To do this, he drinks five cups of strong dark coffee daily and his diet is full of refined sugar and greasy fast foods.

He is hoping for a Google or Facebook-like success where the original founders and workers became millionaires or even billionaires. As a consequence, he sometimes sleeps at the office because he allows himself only a few hours of sleep so he can get going early in the morning.

His wife has become really annoyed by his absence and feels quite alone in caretaking their three-year-old daughter. He is super crabby and irritable when at home, staying busy on his cell phone and avoiding eye contact with his wife. Their sexual relationship has greatly suffered as her growing anger and his continual distraction have led to physical and emotional distancing.

Physically he is suffering from upper abdominal burning pain, relieved by constant chewing of antacids, which I diagnosed as GERD (gastroesophageal reflux disease). He also has irritable bowel syndrome, as his symptoms are explosive diarrhea alternating with constipation.

Chakra Perspective

MB's picture is classic for third chakra imbalance. His is driven to succeed at all costs, he is distracted and irritable and his digestion and metabolism are completely unhealthy. His first chakra is also affected as he is ungrounded and has lost his sense of family and community in his quest for money and success. His second chakra imbalance is evident in that while he had a healthy and active sexual relationship with his wife and was very attracted to her, his desire had considerably lessened due to his preoccupation with work. When he does initiate lovemaking with his wife, she rejects him as she feels alone and unloved. This in turn causes him to feel uncared for and frustrated.

Treatment

It was his wife who had initially come to see me and who told me the story, both because of her concern for her husband's obsessive preoccupation with work and making a lot of money, but also because she had been thinking of separation, despite loving her husband. I asked that she tell him directly of her deep frustrations and that their marriage was at risk. A couple of weeks passed and finally we got a call from MB to say he wanted to come in for an appointment. We talked for a long time about what was happening in his work and private life and about his wife's feelings about his attitude and behavior. Though he was open to change he couldn't see a path forward.

We began the analysis by ordering blood tests, stool tests for blood and parasites (he had traveled to Southeast Asia), abdominal ultrasound and upper endoscopy to rule out a duodenal or gastric ulcer. All his testing was normal, except for elevated blood pressure and LDL cholesterol. As he realized that his life was out of balance, we first delved into his past and his family of origin. His parents had been working class and somewhat economically disadvantaged. He had a strong need to succeed and show his parents and his community that he could be very successful financially. From a chakra perspective, this symbolizes an imbalance in the first three chakras as he feels insecure about his ability to support himself. I taught him aswini mudra and showed him how to do yoga postures that stimulate the lower chakra centers such as a modified spinal twist. To help stabilize his lower chakras I taught him the triangle, the warrior pose and the tai chi warm-up postures, the horse stance and the bow and arrow.

I also taught him a short meditation practice where we focused on raising energy through the chakras through breath awareness to help cool his third chakra area. I recommended that he visualize a red triangle pointed upwards in his third chakra area with cooling energy moving up the spine to the crown.

As his condition was rajasic in nature, dietary suggestions included cooling foods such as cooked grains, vegetables and lean fish to help calm down the GERD. I asked him to decrease his coffee intake as that was exacerbating his reflux and making him feel agitated. A healthy alternative is a light green tea, which would give him some caffeine but also create some relaxation as green tea has l-theanine. Green tea is also very healthy in that it contains polyphenols, which have anti-inflammatory and antioxidant effects.

We mutually agreed that he should make an effort to always be home for dinner and to help put his daughter to bed. Then he would spend time with his wife after this for at least one hour just talking and sharing tidbits about the day before returning to work for a few more hours.

The homeopathic remedy that most closely matched his symptoms was Nux vomica, as this remedy is most useful for someone who overdoes things to the point that their life becomes out of control and they suffer illnesses. Any kind of overindulgence can be helped by Nux vomica such as too much work, food, alcohol, study, exercise, talking or TV watching.

Outcome

MB joined my meditation class to further enhance his practice and he worked on some moderate weight loss. His blood pressure came down to high normal (without allopathic medicine), his lipid profile improved and his home life was considerably more harmonious. They decided to have a babysitter once weekly and resumed making love by creating a time each weekend to relax and just have time for themselves. Although he was still driven to become successful and very wealthy, he realized there were other things in life that were meaningful, most importantly his health and family. From a yogic chakra perspective, balance of the various energy centers was a key to bringing more joy and happiness into his life and overall body and emotional health.

Case History Focused on the Fourth Chakra

SK is a sisty-six--year-old man who was in semi-retirement following a long career as a mechanical engineer. He had been a practitioner of meditation for many years, delving into both Buddhist and yogic philosophy. Three years previously while he was away from home at a conference in California, his fifteen-year-old son was killed in a tragic motor vehicle accident. When he first heard what had happened, he immediately felt pain in the center of his chest. The shock of the terrible news took his breath away, exacerbating long standing asthma, and he felt he was going to die from oxygen deprivation. He couldn't cry, not only because of the shock but also because he had always been a rather stoic person, having been taught by his parents that men don't cry.

Although it was never articulated, he felt his wife blamed him for not being at home in New York at the time of their son's death. She became emotionally distant, refusing any physical intimacy and withholding conversation except when absolutely necessary. This added to his loss, loneliness and grief.

His chest discomfort continued for six months and after a stress echocardiogram and angiography, it was determined that he had coronary artery disease and was in heart failure. Subsequently, he had a stent placed in his left anterior descending artery (widow maker artery). While his chest pain became less, he continued to remain in heart failure. Several medications were prescribed but nothing seemed to help his failing heart. The physicians caring for him were at a loss to understand why he wasn't getting better.

Chakra Perspective

In my opinion, he clearly was suffering from a broken heart. No matter the appropriate medicine, he continued to have cardiac problems. From a yogic perspective, the mental body is intimately connected to the physical body, mediated through the energy body. In this case, SK's heart problems were partly the manifestation of the loss and sadness of his child's death. His wife's self-isolation contributed to his aloneness and sadness. In addition he had no outlet to express his feelings of sadness and guilt for not being at home when his son died. Not being able to talk about his feelings exacerbated his frustration. From a chakra perspective, his imbalance was in the fourth chakra, the heart center.

Treatment

I recommended individual psychotherapy as I believed this could help him tap into inner suppressed feelings associated with childhood and very controlling and critical parents, which resulted in expression of repressed anger and sadness. Therapy could also be an outlet for his current grief and loss, all in the safe environment of a therapist. I suggested marital therapy as well.

We worked on improving his diet and moved more towards a mostly vegetarian heart healthy diet to help lower his cholesterol. For example, I recommended less red meat and larger amounts of a combination of legumes and whole grains, which are associated with lower cholesterol levels and less atherosclerotic heart disease. Since vegetarians have lower amounts of gut microbe-derived metabolites like trimethylamine N-oxide (TMSO) that are biologically active and associated with atherogenesis and thrombosis, I also suggested a high potency probiotic to enhance intestinal microbiome health.

We worked on yoga postures to open up the chest, such as the camel, bridge, cobra and fish. I also taught him alternate nostril breathing to balance the right and left energy channels and to calm him. After learning how to slow and regulate his breath, we worked on lung and heart stimulating breathing techniques such as kapalabhati and bhastrika. Vigorous walking was recommended to improve cardiovascular health as well as to help lower his lipid levels.

Since he regularly meditated and was familiar with the chakra system, I recommended using the fourth chakra, the center of love, compassion, loving kindness and self-forgiveness, as the focus of his concentration. I suggested he use the fourth chakra bija mantra, *Yam,* while focusing on the fourth chakra for his morning meditation, and to quietly sing the mantra *Om Hrim Shrim Klim Ham Sa Ha So Ham Swaha* as a walking meditation. I taught him the melody to the latter chant. Since he was also Jewish, we discussed his repeating the *Shema* prayer upon waking and going to sleep. This would help lessen his feelings of aloneness and enhance a connection to something larger than his own self-suffering.

I prescribed the homeopathic remedy Natrum muriaticum in high potency (10M), which is the classic grieving remedy where people isolate themselves rather than reach out to others for consolation and comfort. Later I added the remedy Cactus grand 30C and Calcium fluoride 6X to help improve heart muscle strength and contractility.

Outcome

About six months after initiating most of my suggestions, the ejection fraction of his heart went from twenty-six to forty-six, which reflected greater heart strength and meant he was out of heart failure. He lost seven pounds and his muscular strength improved considerably. He was better able to communicate his grief and loss to his wife and they were enjoying time spent together. While he has made some progress, he realized that to continue to heal in body, mind and spirit he needed to continue to incorporate holistic and yogic approaches to health. From a yogic perspective, his fourth chakra strengthened.

Case History Focused on the Fifth Chakra

RB is a well-known artist who has been quite successful as he has sold many wonderful paintings, and his work is prominently displayed in several art galleries. But over the last two years he had been unable to create new and original art. He has become very frustrated and has begun to isolate himself from friends and family. He also stopped communicating with long-time art dealers and agents. He clearly had a bad case of creativity block, resulting in depression and anxiety.

Chakra Perspective

RB showed fifth chakra issues of not being able to communicate and express himself effectively. The fifth chakra is the center of creativity and communication. He exemplified a situation that is common with artists, writers and scientists who become stuck in their work and have difficulty tapping back into their creative tendencies. He also felt he couldn't communicate his inner frustrations with colleagues, friends and family because he felt they weren't really listening to him.

Treatment

We revised his diet to include more fluids, especially warm drinks that would soothe the throat area. I encouraged him to practice yoga postures that stimulate the throat area, including the shoulderstand, bridge, wheel and fish pose. Breathing techniques that help open and stimulate the fifth chakra include bhramari with its wonderful stimulating effects on the vocal cords and ujjayi, which gently stimulates the upper throat and larynx.

I instructed him to follow the above-mentioned yoga postures and breathing exercises by meditation on the fifth chakra using the mantra *Ham*, the seed mantra for the fifth chakra. Homeopathically, I prescribed Staphysagria, as his withdrawal was the result of repressed anger, frustration and resentment, all characteristics of this remedy.

Outcome

RB soon began painting again and interacting with colleagues and family, which brought him great joy.

The Holistic Approach: Case Histories Using Koshas and Chakras as Models

The yoga concepts of the koshas, chakras and raja yoga are integrating approaches to therapy that are flexible and adaptable to each person's unique needs. By presenting the following case histories it is my intent to illustrate the direct correlations between mental and emotional conflict and imbalances in physical health. Using the yogic systems of raja yoga, the chakras and the koshas as my basic model, I will analyze a particular ailment from an integrated approach to illustrate that a disease can be understood and treated simultaneously from the perspective of ancient holistic models (Ayurveda, meditation and yoga) and modern holistic models (nutrition, exercise, breathing techniques, stress theory, psychotherapy and homeopathy). It is also my intent to show that all these therapies have similar underlying principles and can be used synergistically to analyze and treat an ailing person.

The common diseases I have chosen to discuss using these paradigms are: asthma, gastric ulcers, thyroid diseases, lower bowel disorders and skin disorders. As an underlying psychological paradigm, I use psychosomatic medicine, which is an offshoot of the psychoanalytic perspective. This does not mean that other diseases that are not classified as psychosomatic will not respond to a holistic approach. In fact, almost any ailment, even infections and back problems that manifest primarily on a physical level with less obvious mental and emotional involvement, can be treated holistically. I am grateful to my teachers, Swami Rama, Rudolph Ballentine and Swami Ajaya for having introduced me to this overall approach and to their fascinating book, *Yoga and Psychotherapy: The Evolution of Consciousness*

A Holistic Approach to Asthma

I will now look at asthma from the various levels of consciousness, incorporating the yogic concepts of the koshas and the chakras along with the various ancient and modern therapies that have been presented in this book.

Physiologically, asthma is characterized by a constriction of the muscles that surround the bronchi, with resultant narrowing of the bronchial tubes, making it difficult to breathe, especially on exhalation. The friction produced by air passing through the narrowed passageways creates the characteristic asthmatic wheeze, which is usually worse on exhalation. Excess mucus accompanies the bronchial constriction because the tiny mucus-producing goblet cells become overactive due to irritation. The parasympathetic hormone acetylcholine and histamine in allergic cases, are the biochemical substances that mediate the bronchial constriction and excess mucus secretion.

Causes of Asthma

Psychosomatic Medicine Theory

Psychosomatic medicine offers an interesting explanation of how emotional conflicts can lead to an asthmatic condition. According to this theory, the asthmatic individual is often excessively dependent upon his or her mother or another adult who has assumed an overly demanding parental role and unconsciously desires to "merge" or "reunite" with this person. There are two major ways in which a person deals with uncomfortable emotional impositions such as an overbearing and demanding parent. One response is to actively rebel and fight. If this rebelliousness is stifled by a punitive parent, the sympathetic nervous system, which stimulates active internal functions like raising blood pressure, may become activated. The other mechanism for dealing with an overbearing parent is to passively withdraw to avoid the influence. If this is prevented by the parent (or society) who respond by making more demands, activation of the parasympathetic nervous system can be triggered, which stimulates passive internal functions, including constriction of the muscles that surround the bronchi as occurs in the case of asthma.

According to psychosomatic theory, the asthmatic's unconscious wish for bonding and deep connection with a parent to confer protection and eternal love is often symbolically expressed in recurring dreams of water (amniotic fluid). Some people feel very uncomfortable with these dependent feelings and fantasies, and consequently they create defenses. The asthmatic defense against maternal dependency is to try to escape these obsessive and confusing feelings. This withdrawal response, which is a passive restrictive reaction, can be blocked by actual or threatened separation from the mother figure. This may be internalized through overactivation of the parasympathetic nervous system, which correlates with the passive psychological state, resulting in the release of acetylcholine and bronchial muscle constriction. This is in keeping with the fact that the passive or expiratory phase of respiration is the most markedly affected in asthma. The difficulty with exhalation may also be symbolic of the asthmatic's inability to "let go" of the deep maternal or paternal attachments.

From this perspective, asthma revolves around the need to be protected and encompassed. Asthma can thus be called a "suppressed cry for the parent's help." Insecurity often underlies this unconscious dependency and, as a result, overcompensation might occur, perhaps assuming the form of competitiveness or excessive striving. This can be seen in children who try to win their mother's approval by outdoing their siblings. Anxiety often accompanies this behavior, which can be explained in part by the decreased supply of oxygen to the brain that occurs in an asthmatic attack and also by the hyperreactive sympathetic system. The sympathetic nervous system and the adrenal glands, which are actually enlarged sympathetic nerve endings, can become exhausted because they attempt to counterbalance the overactive parasympathetic system, which is responsible for producing the acetylcholine that causes the bronchial constriction of asthma. Adrenalin, which is secreted by the adrenals, acts to dilate (open up) the bronchial tubes and at the same time can cause palpitations, sweating, flushing and racing thoughts, all of which characterize the anxious state. On the physical level, asthma can be exacerbated by imbalances in nutrition, irregular breathing habits, improper posture and lack of exercise.

Ayurveda

According to Ayurvedic medicine, asthma is considered to be a state of decreased pitta or fire, and similarly, in Chinese medicine it is thought to involve a lack of the yang fire element. Ayurveda further describes asthma as a combination of excess kapha and vata. This is consistent with modern physiology: a kaphic condition is characterized by excess production of mucus, and vata refers to imbalance of the element air. These are the two principle disturbances in asthma. However, Ayurveda goes further to state that vata potentiates the detrimental effects of excess kapha when the two are combined. Ayurveda further categorizes kapha (mucus) by describing its consistency, odor, color and taste. These concepts have great therapeutic significance, not only because herbs are prescribed according to the type of kapha, but also because specific foods can be given to counteract and rebalance the effects of vata and kapha.

Both Chinese and Ayurvedic medicine maintain that liver dysfunction is a major contributing factor in allergies and asthma, and homeopathy also recognizes the association between liver problems and asthma. The liver is the second largest organ in the body after the lungs and has many very important functions, including metabolism of fats, proteins and carbohydrates, production of bile, enzymes and hormones and detoxification from the blood of drugs, chemicals and other waste products. Liver problems are very common today, and symptoms vary according to the degree of pathology. If the ailing liver cannot get rid of metabolic waste and toxic materials, these substances may be excreted through other routes such as the mucus membranes of the nose, throat and bronchi. Also, if the digestive tract is not functioning properly, excess and unhealthy mucus can accumulate and aggravate the allergic or asthmatic tendencies. From an Ayurvedic perspective, a sluggish congested liver results from overeating, not chewing food properly, chemical additives, environmental pollutants, a lack of physical activity and stress. Symptoms of constipation, bad taste in the mouth, fatigue, nausea and headaches are characteristic of liver distress.

Chakra Analysis

The yogic concept of the chakras also provides a paradigm in which to integrate various physical and psychological aspects of the asthmatic condition. Asthma can be understood to involve the third, fourth and fifth chakras.

The third chakra, located in the proximity of the solar plexus at the level of the navel, is associated with emotional issues of dominance and submissiveness. Symbolically, it is represented by fire, which is in keeping with its control of the physiological processes of digestion and metabolism and also its function as a center of somatic and psychic energy. Asthmatics have a disturbance in this chakra as they are overly passive and dependent, or else they overcompensate for their dependent feelings by being dominant and aggressive. As discussed earlier, the adrenal glands are often affected in chronic asthma.

The fourth chakra is an obvious center for asthma. The fourth chakra is in the proximity of the area that contains the heart and lungs and is symbolized as a six-pointed star (chakra system), a cross (Christianity) or as the Star of David (Judaism). It is psychologically associated with love, devotion and nurturance, all positive attributes of motherhood. It can be inferred that the typical overbearing nurturing figure can create tension, constriction and oppression in the asthmatic child's fourth chakra. This can lead to tightness of the bronchial tubes and shortness of breath. Apathy, or the inability to give love and affection, may also occur if the child fears rejection and withdraws into their own inner, "constricted" world. This withdrawal can be unconsciously expressed through activation of the parasympathetic nervous system, which constricts the bronchial tubes. Fourth chakra weakness is also potentiated by third chakra weakness as it is difficult for the higher center to be balanced if the center below it cannot transfer energy upwards.

The fifth chakra also is occasionally involved in asthma. This chakra is associated with communication and growth. The asthmatic often cannot express their real feelings, which can lead to tension and constriction in the throat area, thereby inhibiting the smooth flow of breath. Asthma, in such a case, might be focused in the upper part of the respiratory conducting system, the upper bronchi, trachea or larynx. The normally smooth laminar flow of air is impeded by narrowed passageways.

Holistic Treatment

Many of the therapies already discussed are useful in treating these imbalances at the chakra level.

Nutrition

Because the third chakra is responsible for "fire" production, treatment oriented towards stimulating the gastric or abdominal fire is appropriate. This is accomplished by eating pitta foods, as these are substances that produce fire that can "burn up" the excess mucus and use up the excess air. For example, bajra flour (black millet) and buckwheat flour are especially potent in decreasing mucus and increasing pitta. In general, the fire element is increased by eating cooked foods. Peppercorns fried in clarified butter (ghee) in a fixed daily ratio also increases pitta, while adding honey to yogurt tends to cut down on the mucus-producing quality of yogurt.

Nutritional observances to decrease the production of mucus from the lungs and bronchial tubes are important. Asthma can be minimized by avoidance of mucus-producing foods such as dairy products, glutenous grains (wheat, rye, oats, and barley), refined sugars and flour, starchy fruits like bananas and red meats. Other foods to avoid are those that contain sulfites (a preservative) as these substances can worsen asthma. Sulfites are found in wine, dried fruits, pickled food, maraschino cherries, shrimp and bottled lemon or lime juice. Foods preferred are the other whole grains (corn, quinoa, millet, buckwheat, and brown rice), fresh vegetables, fruits, legumes and peas, nuts, seeds and low-fat meat or fish such as salmon.

Vitamins considered beneficial in asthma are B, C, E, pantothenic acid, and the mineral manganese. Vitamin C helps to protect the respiratory mucous membrane lining, minimizes allergic tendencies, decreases infection and counteracts the stress associated with asthma. Vitamin E helps increase oxygenation to cells and Vitamin B complex helps to stabilize the nervous system. Pantothenic acid (one of the B complex) has been reported to stimulate depleted adrenal glands. Manganese has also been reported to decrease the incidence of allergic asthma in patients deficient in that mineral. Herbs that decrease mucus, and are sometimes useful in asthma, are goldenseal root, lobelia, slippery elm and wild cherry bark. Ayurveda uses herbs prepared according to Ayurvedic principles to help the liver function more effectively.

Besides asthma being a disease of smooth muscle constriction and excess mucus production in the bronchial tubes, it is also an inflammatory disorder. It is often advised to eat foods and take supplements that are anti-inflammatory. This includes foods high in resveratrol (red grapes), turmeric and mushrooms such as maitake, shitake and reishi. A good way to take turmeric is to make golden milk. This includes two cups of almond milk, one teaspoon of ground turmeric, one teaspoon of ground ginger and ¼ teaspoon of black pepper. This is brought to a simmer for ten minutes, strained, and it's ready to drink.

Antioxidants that decrease oxidative stress and damage also support the immune system, so ample supplementation and healthy foods are important. This includes taking alpha-lipoic acid, rosemarinic acid (found in rosemary and oregano) and ginseng. Cysteine and glycine are precursors that make the all-important antioxidants glutathione and can be readily found in carrots, asparagus, cooked spinach, broccoli, edamame, split peas and lentils. The supplement N-acetylcysteine can also be taken to increase glutathione leverls. Prebiotics that enhance the microbiome are very important in immunity since close to seventy percent of the body's immune system resides in the GI system. Beta-glucans, whole grains and seaweed are good prebiotics. Also, probiotics such as sauerkraut, fermented foods and low-fat yogurt can be helpful. Green tea, astragalus, olive leaf extract and melatonin all have a lot of polyphenols and antioxidants that enhance the healthy functioning of the immune system. These recommendations can apply to any illness that is inflammatory in nature.

Overeating causes accumulation of intestinal gas and puts pressure on the diaphragm, especially if one has acid reflux. This may cause tightness in the chest and trigger asthmatic flares. Gas-producing foods can include legumes, cabbage, carbonated drinks, onions, garlic and fried foods. Although it's rare, some people with asthma are sensitive to the salicylates found in coffee, tea and some herbs and spices. Chemical preservatives, flavorings and colorings are almost always found in processed and fast foods. Some people with asthma may be sensitive or allergic to these artificial ingredients. People with food allergies may also have asthma. Dairy products, shellfish, wheat and tree nuts are among the most common allergens.

Posture and Exercise

The asthmatic individual usually exhibits characteristic problems in body posture. Not uncommon are shoulders hunched forward, accentuated cervical (neck) curves and tightened chest and back muscles. The physical posturing of the asthmatic must first be improved by correcting the forward position of the shoulders and the thoracic spinal kyphosis (hunchback), which serves as body armor to "protect" the asthmatic. Specific yoga postures can be used to realign, relax, strengthen and straighten muscles, bones, joints and ligaments. Examples of hatha yoga practices that are helpful to stimulate the third chakra are: the abdominal lift, spinal twist, cobra and peacock. In addition, many yogic practices can be directed towards opening and balancing the heart chakra. Asanas such as the cobra, camel and bow are helpful to relax tension in the chest.

An active exercise program is also advisable to help asthmatics increase aeration in the lungs where stagnant trapped air accumulates, expand their lung reserves and to increase oxygenation to the brain, heart and other vital centers. Caution should be taken not to overextend and cause further injury to the areas of tissue damage. Studies suggest that swimming may be particularly beneficial in helping to reduce the frequency and severity of attacks in some asthmatics.55

Cleansing Techniques

Yoga cleansing techniques can be helpful in eliminating excess mucus. In the upper wash two quarts of warm saltwater are quickly swallowed and then vomited. The upper wash is not recommended for persons with cardiovascular or kidney problems. This practice is done in the morning and helps eliminate mucus from the lungs (mucus is swallowed during the night while one is lying down). The upper wash helps to develop greater control over the vagus nerve, which is in part responsible for the vomiting reflex, and which also mediates the parasympathetic bronchial constriction.

Breathing Exercises

Asthma is associated with prolonged and difficult breathing, especially exhalation. This can lead to increased accumulation of carbon dioxide and an acidic body condition, each of which can cause mental and sensory dullness, low energy and depression. Breathing exercises are helpful because they can create a state of heightened awareness by regulating abnormal respiratory patterns and thus improving oxygenation. They can also help to modify and quiet the parasympathetic nervous system, which in turn will reduce the asthmatic symptomatology. As diaphragmatic breathing is the key to all other breathing exercises, it should be learned before doing any other breathing exercises or pranayama. Awareness and regulation of the diaphragm and abdominal muscles are essential for control of the autonomic nervous system. Breathing exercises such as diaphragmatic breathing, the complete yogic breath, kapalabhati, bhastrika and nadi shodanam (alternate nostril breathing) help expand lung capacity, regulate pranic flow and can help the asthmatic develop control of respiratory movements.

Complete Yogic Breath: Three different movements can occur during the process of breathing: the movement of the diaphragm, the movement of the intercostal muscles, and the upward and downward movement of the clavicles (collarbones). This complete, orderly, sequential manner of breathing is not practiced in a normal relaxed state, but it can be used to bring maximum oxygenation to the system, as is needed in active exercise. All areas of the lung are aerated, and stagnant carbon dioxide is removed, thus helping to improve the symptoms of respiratory problems like asthma. The complete yogic breath involves using all three respiratory phases to completely flush and aerate the lungs. The great amount of oxygen inspired during this exercise increases the energy available to the brain, muscles and organs of the body. A person often spontaneously does the complete breath, especially after a stressful situation, when he takes a slow, full deep breath. If practiced regularly, this exercise helps the bronchial tubes and respiratory conducting system remain free of spasm. It is possible to palliate an acute asthmatic attack by doing the complete breath in a relaxed manner.

Kapalabhati is both a breathing exercise and a hatha yoga cleansing technique that flushes out the respiratory passages, including the sinuses, nose and bronchi. The expiratory phase consists of a rapid contraction of the abdominal muscles, followed immediately by a passive slow inhalation, while the abdominal muscles relax and move outwards in preparation for the next active exhalation. Kapalabhati helps to eliminate excess carbon dioxide, drains the sinuses, eliminates mucus and improves concentration. In asthma it should not be done too vigorously as forcing the breath in and out can exacerbate bronchial spasms.

If you add breath retention (should not be done by a beginner) after the pumping movement in kapalabhati, the transfer of oxygen into the blood will be enhanced. As retention continues oxygen levels decrease and carbon dioxide levels increase. This, if not done too vigorously, can help to calm the anxiety and fear as oxygen hunger intensifies in an asthmatic attack.

The restricted breathing of asthmatics can be relieved by kapalabhati, especially at the beginning of an attack or during a mild attack. On a daily basis, kapalabhati relaxes the bronchial tubes and lungs and may help prevent further episodes or infections.

Nadi shodanam cleanses the respiratory tract, balances the left and right lungs and sides of the brain, and allows more stale air to be eliminated when exhalation is twice as long as inhalation.

In a sense, breathing is the ultimate form of being fed, as every individual receives nurturance through the breath in the form of prana from the universe. The infinite cosmos acts symbolically as the greatest of all mothers as it supports, stores and gives prana to all life forms. By learning to breathe rhythmically and effortlessly, a person with asthma can tune into the universal source of life and subsequently move closer towards satisfaction of dependency needs at the deepest level.

Psychotherapy and Meditation

Understanding how the psyche and emotions affect the body helps in both the prevention and treatment of asthma. Guilt can often result from conflicting feelings of dependency and frustration or anger towards an overbearing parent. This can be lessened by learning to express these feelings verbally. The psychotherapist helps reduce the strength of emotions by allowing the patient to transfer dependence onto him and then helping the patient understand the conflict. Understanding can lead to acceptance of one's feelings and then the therapist can initiate active attempts to change behavioral patterns. Analysis of dreams helps the individual to comprehend the inner symbols that reflect unconscious motives and desires.

Techniques of concentration and meditation on the solar plexus can also be prescribed to balance third chakra activity and focus awareness and energy. Certain concentration exercises and meditative techniques on the heart center also facilitate greater awareness of this center. Yoga meditation based upon chakra concentration and awakening of the primal energy (kundalini) are among the most comprehensive and sophisticated of all meditation teachings. The goal is to create a state of peace, harmony, deep understanding, love and pure joy.

Homeopathy

Homeopathy can be very effective therapy for asthma. It is interesting to note that many homeopathic remedies that are helpful in asthma are also prominent liver remedies. These include Natrum sulphuricum, Nux vomica and Arsenicum album.

With respect to the koshas, when analyzing a disease like asthma and a remedy associated with treating it, we can describe how the remedy helps people get healthier on the different levels of consciousness (koshas). For example, on the physical level the remedy Arsenicum album helps people to have less bronchial spasms, less stomach pain, less burning; on the energy level to breath more deeply, to be less restless and do less night pacing; on the mental level to be less aggressive and hostile; on the emotional level to be less controlling; and, spiritually to be less rigid and compulsive with themselves, other people and their environment.

The vital force follows particular patterns in asthma, as reflected by the total symptom picture, so that different remedies are prescribed to match the different patterns. Specific examples are as follows: Nux vomica for asthma coming on after overeating; Ipecac for asthmatics who must vomit to get relief; Carbo vegetabilis for elderly asthmatics who turn blue (cyanosis) and like to be fanned; Kali carbonicum for asthma attacks awakening the person punctually at 3:00 a.m.; and, Pulsatilla for asthmatics who are weepy, thirstless, chilly and have thick, yellow mucous phlegm associated with a loose cough.

At this time, I would like to make an important point of clarification. When discussing remedies, the homeopathic physician often describes a remedy as either being representative of the symptom picture that emerges from the medicine's proving or the symptoms of the patient being treated. Because both situations reflect similar symptom pictures, these descriptions are used interchangeably. Two remedies, however, are most eminent in the treatment of asthma. These have interesting associations with both unconscious symbolization and psychosomatic medicine theory. Arsenicum album is a remedy that results in extreme anxiety and restlessness, burning pains relieved by warmth and asthma becoming worse around midnight, often awakening the person from sleep. Because of the extreme agitation and increased heat production (burning secretions), the remedy corresponds more with the chronic compensatory sympathetic nervous system response pattern in asthma. In other words, the sympathetic system tries to balance the initial parasympathetic response that is characteristic of asthma.

Natrum sulphuricum is suitable for asthma made worse by dampness or wet weather, in which the tongue and phlegm may be yellow or green in color and the liver is often dysfunctional. Depressed moods are also very apparent. Natrum sulphuricum is said to be one of the deepest acting of all asthma remedies and is often the first remedy given to children with asthma. It is associated with the more intense parasympathetic response, which mediates bronchial constriction and is affiliated with depression, withdrawal and general sluggishness. In this case, the compensatory sympathetic response does not occur. Because Natrum sulphuricum is aggravated by water or dampness in any form, such as being in the rain or near lakes or other bodies of water, it may be associated symbolically with the mother principle. The mother figure also is characterized by water, the life-giving sea, and it is within the womb's amniotic fluid that the embryo grows. In essence, Natrum sulphuricum symbolically corresponds to the deepest of all places, the vast ocean of the unconscious mind.

As a holistic physician, I must add that I recognize that sometimes allopathic medicine is needed. Being holistic means that I have many tools in my medical toolbox and that I observe, analyze and treat the whole person. When using drugs, I always try to use the least amount of medicine with the least side effects and which is the most efficacious. I have found Symbicort to be a good medicine for ongoing mild to moderate asthma. This medicine has a mild inhaled steroid to decrease the inflammatory part of asthma and is very minimally absorbed systemically. In addition, a short-term and long-term bronchodilator to open up the bronchial tubes and allow for expulsion of excess mucus is also helpful.

A Case History of Asthma

Mr. D is a thirty-one-year-old man who first developed asthma in 2011. His medical history included eczema as a child and nasal allergies in his early teens. He described himself as "a person who doesn't like being out of control" and said he is generally passive, fearful of responsibility and worries about being taken for granted. He has recurring feelings of guilt and is in general depressed, discontented and withdrawn. He tends to withdraw from conflict and, while often feeling angry inside, has great difficulty in expressing this emotion. He has specific problems communicating with his parents and has found it impossible to argue with his mother. In fact, anger coming from his mother would precipitate an asthmatic attack because he interpreted her anger as rejection.

He found that lying in the fetal position and the child's pose (balasana) helped relieve his shortness of breath. This is a common characteristic of an asthma patient.

Specific Treatment Plan

Mr. D was treated in a multilevel way. The yogic model of the koshas and the chakras provided a framework for an approach that included the many aspects of his disease.

Nutrition

He was taken off all dairy products and after allergy testing for foods indicated he was allergic to most gluten-containing grains, he was advised to limit wheat, barley, rye and oat intake. Vitamins A, C, B-6, pantothenic acid and zinc were also prescribed. In addition, he was advised to take an herbal tea combination of ephedra, mullein, calendula, comfrey root, ginger root, licorice root and pleurisy root three times daily.

Breath

He was instructed to do breathing exercises that included the complete yoga breath, kapalabhati and diaphragmatic breathing twice daily, along with progressive relaxation, where the person systematically relaxes each part of the body from the head down to the toes. He was taught to do visualization in which he imagined his bronchial tubes to be greatly expanded hollow tubes that allowed large volumes of air to enter and exit. Yoga postures included the fish, bridge, modified wheel and the sun salutation, all of which open up the chest.

Psychotherapy

Concurrent psychotherapy was begun with special emphasis on working out anger and on dream analysis. The patient slowly began to recognize his repressed frustration and that he needed to assert himself more with his parents. He was able to redefine important familial boundaries and to separate psychologically from his family. Recurrent dreams of doing poorly on school exams and of losing important possessions, which reflected an inner fear of rejection and failure, began to be replaced by dreams of success. His attitude and self-confidence also improved. He explored meditation, focusing on the heart center with the mantra *Yam*. This helped him relax and allowed him to get in touch with anxieties of loss and fear.

Homeopathy

Slowly, the intensity of his asthma attacks diminished, and subsequent minor bouts of wheezing were easily handled by the appropriate homeopathic remedy and an occasional puff of albuterol. Gradually, he was able to avoid medications (albuterol and a steroid inhaler) and put on low potency homeopathic remedies that included Natrum sulphuricum for asthma coming on at 4:00 to 5:00 a.m. or during damp weather, Arsenicum album for asthma occurring between 12:00 to 2:00 a.m. with associated extreme anxiety, and Ipecac for asthma associated with vomiting (for relief of symptoms). The constitutional remedies that were given included Sulphur, Thuja, Staphysagria and high potency Natrum sulphuricum.

A Holistic Approach to Gastric and Duodenal Ulcers

Now I will examine the various aspects of ulcerative disease as they involve physical, emotional, mental and spiritual factors, and also present some alternative ways of treatment.

Causes of Ulcers

Physiology

The acids present in the stomach are powerful enough to dissolve metal. To prevent the acid from eating through the walls of the stomach, thick tenacious mucus is produced to line the walls and protect the delicate cells from the noxious acid. This mechanism breaks down when too much acid or not enough mucus is produced. As a result, the acid comes in contact with the stomach lining and begins eating its way through. If the process is minimal, it may not be noticed at all or may simply appear as common "heartburn." If allowed to continue unabated, a large crater (ulcer) or even a hole may be produced in the stomach. Before the drugs to inhibit acid secretion came on the market, this problem was one of the more common manifestations of disease in the gastrointestinal system.

Gastric ulcers occur in the stomach and duodenal ulcers in the duodenum, the first section of the small intestine. Initially, the only symptom may be a sensation of burning in the stomach, which can be relieved by eating, especially more bland foods or milk products, as such food neutralizes the stomach acid. If the condition progresses, the ulcer may erode through a blood vessel and bleeding occurs. This may show itself either by the vomiting of blood or more commonly by black bowel movements, indicative of digested blood in the stool. Finally, the ulcer can erode through the stomach wall. When this occurs, the stomach secretions pass into the abdominal cavity, leading to peritonitis, a potentially fatal condition where the abdominal cavity becomes inflamed and infected.

It is important to understand that an ulcer does not develop overnight. It usually takes weeks, months or years of gastric malfunction to induce ulcer formation. Certain conditions are known to favor ulcer development, such as the use of coffee, alcohol and cigarettes. Drugs like aspirin, ibuprofen and cortisone can also predispose a person to ulcer development.

The stomach is in direct communication with the brain via the autonomic nervous system. Specifically, the vagus nerve (the parasympathetic mediator) as well as the sympathetic nerves, innervates individual gastric cells. Activation of the vagus nerve signals the stomach to secrete digestive juices and to increase blood circulation to the stomach. For example, when a person sees a freshly baked loaf of bread and smells its rich aroma, nerve impulses are sent through a series of neural pathways from the eyes and nose to the hypothalamus, which then relays messages to the vagus nerve and eventually to the stomach to get ready for work.

An opposite response might occur if a person walks down a dark street and sees someone coming in the other direction looking menacing. Immediately the sympathetic nervous system becomes activated. In this case, the blood vessels of the stomach contract to inhibit blood flow to the stomach so that blood can be redirected to the heart, brain and skeletal musculature in order to react to the potentially dangerous situation. This is perceived as a knot in the stomach, and if something is eaten at this time, it will not "sit" very well. Thus, the parasympathetic nervous system stimulates digestion and the sympathetic inhibits digestion.

Oversecretion of stomach acid is the result of chronic stimulation by the parasympathetic vagus nerve. Before the advent of medications such as omeprazole (Prilosec), one of the more common allopathic approaches to an ulcer that did not respond to restrictive dietary treatment, was to perform a vagotomy, a surgical procedure in which the vagus nerve is cut so that the stomach's normal means of being stimulated by the brain was severed. It should be remembered that the vagus nerve has its origin in the deep recesses of the brain. There are many factors that influence the response of the vagus. Besides normal physiologic reflexes that mediate functioning of this nerve, the emotional center or limbic system as well as the higher or cortical centers of the brain also has an effect. It is through this mechanism that emotional reactions such as anger or fear can influence the functioning of the gastrointestinal system.

Psychosomatic Theory

According to psychosomatic medical theory, the basic unresolved psychological issue in some patients with ulcers is a conflict between the ego's desire to assert itself and demonstrate its strength and independence and more infantile needs to be nurtured and loved. In such a conflict, if the ego is weak and the infantile needs are strong, the person may choose to deal with the conflict in a passive way by withdrawing from it. However, societal values may view overt withdrawal from conflict as a sign of weakness. Therefore, the person compensates by withdrawing symbolically through activation of the parasympathetic nervous system, which leads to gastric acid overstimulation.

Psychological factors and stressful situations have long been known to strongly influence stomach function and are a major consideration in the development of ulcer disease. The unfulfilled need to gratify feelings of dependency is consistent with the eventual formation of an ulcer. Being fed is the earliest way the infant or young child is able to resolve anxiety. The child identifies nourishment with a decrease in stress and with security. For some, this craving for oral gratification persists throughout life, and lighting a cigarette, biting the fingernails or constantly munching on a piece of candy serve as the prime method for dealing with anxiety. This is how the need and desire to be loved becomes converted into the need to be fed.

In this way the ulcer patient's anxiety is compensated for internally by the unconscious activation of the neurogastric pathways rather than by more conscious and external healthy ways. The increase in acid production is the body's way of preparing itself for the nurturing it desires but is unable to obtain. "In such a situation, the stomach responds continuously as if food were being taken in or about to be taken in . . . the greater the rejection of every receptive gratification, the greater will be this unconscious 'hunger' for love and help. The patient desires food as a symbol of love and help rather than as satiation of a physiological need."56

Chakra Association

In the yogic model, the first chakra is associated physiologically with the act of intestinal elimination, and some practitioners link it psychologically with security and possession. Security and the desire for survival are the most primitive of all needs. All organisms, from the simple ameba to the complexities of a human being, have this instinct. It is so inbred into one's being that it need not interfere with conscious processes. A healthy balance of energy at the first chakra is very important because it can establish a secure and protected feeling in the individual, which provides the foundation and strength upon which to build a healthy body and mind. Although egotism is eventually overcome, a strong intact ego and sense of self are mandatory for the balanced functioning of the higher chakras. If the first chakra energy is dissipated, then a person's psychophysiological matrix will be weakened and may manifest as chronic constipation or diarrhea on the physical level, and/or anxiety and paranoia on the mental level.

In yoga psychology an ulcer also represents an imbalance in the third chakra (solar plexus). This chakra, situated near the center of the digestive tract, is associated with metabolism of food and is related to oral psychological attitudes as well. Imbalances manifest here as digestive or metabolic difficulties such as ulcers or diabetes mellitus. The yoga model implies that power conflicts are most likely to develop problems around the third chakra area, such as gastric illnesses. Individuals with difficulties at this area present themselves in one of two ways. Either they are overly self-assertive, characterized by the go-getting, hard-driving, nobody-is-going-to-get-in-my-way businessman, or the opposite passive, disgruntled individual who is silently disenchanted and feels like "the whole world is picking on me." In either case, the common denominator is the "me against them" attitude. Both types are often classified as characteristic ulcer personalities.

Holistic Treatment of Ulcers

Nutrition and Ayurvedic Medicine

According to Ayurveda, the stomach and duodenal area correspond to the primary seat of the dosha pitta, or the digestive fire. It is here that the food is metabolized, and prana is liberated to provide the energy needed to sustain life. If a person experiences burning abdominal pain, the Ayurvedic physician will explain that there is too much pitta and will treat the patient to reduce it. This therapeutic approach includes several different treatments. First, the patient is advised to eliminate foods that create excessive quantities of pitta, like hot or spicy foods and stimulants such as coffee, tobacco and alcohol. Raw foods such as nuts and salads would also be eliminated because these foods are very complex structurally and require more pitta or digestive fire to be broken down. A diet is prescribed based on foods with a cooling or kaphic effect such as milk and yogurt or well-cooked vegetables and grains. Cooked foods are more digestible and stimulate less pitta to insure their assimilation.

These dietary recommendations are very similar to the standard ulcer diet. While the Western physician recommends a diet based on the principle of reducing or neutralizing the effects of the surplus acid, the Ayurvedic physician is simply trying to eliminate excess pitta. One point of interest here is that drinking milk has classically been known to reduce ulcer pain, yet the exact reason for this has escaped Western physiologists. Claims that milk effectively neutralizes acid or "coats the stomach" have not been substantiated. However, in Ayurvedic terms the reasoning is simple. Milk is a kaphic food and therefore stimulates mucus production. This excess mucus provides an increased protective barrier against the acid and therefore reduces inflammation and pain.

Ayurveda also considers the psychological factors that increase pitta, such as anger. To be "red with rage" may not only represent a psychological attitude, but also will manifest in the body as increased anger or pitta. People with fiery temperaments have too much pitta and therefore may have too much fire stored in the "pitta center" or solar plexus.

Exercise

The establishment of a consistent, progressive program of physical activity such as a regimen of brisk walking or jogging can be helpful in ulcer disease. Jogging or other aerobic exercise can be an outlet for the release of anxiety that has taken the form of muscular tension. In view of the proposed psychosomatic model and the role of anxiety in the genesis of ulcers, the relaxation of muscle tension and the sense of well-being associated with vigorous exercise are very important.

Hatha yoga's role in ulcer disease relates to the understanding that the student develops concerning the relationship between mental and physical tension. General muscular tension reflects mental unrest, and this tension becomes "stored" in the muscles that line the digestive tract. A regular all-rounded hatha practice results in release of skeletal muscular tension that also facilitates relaxation of the muscles that line internal organs. A person who has an active ulcer should be careful not to put undue pressure on the abdomen and should avoid the spinal twist, peacock and bow.

Breathing Exercises

Because of the close relationship between the breath and the emotions, breathing exercises help to decrease the anxiety associated with the conflict of ego strength. The chronic activation of the parasympathetic nervous system associated with ulcers can be relaxed by breathing exercises, especially the practice of diaphragmatic breathing. Since the breath provides a bridge between the voluntary and autonomic nervous systems, it can be a tool for consciously regulating autonomic nervous system activity.

Psychotherapy and Meditation

The use of meditation and relaxation to treat ulcers has been used traditionally in the East, but is a relatively new approach in the West. For example, to decrease the quantity of pitta and reduce the excess fire, the Ayurvedic physician may not only prescribe a diet, but will often give the patient a therapeutic herb or perhaps a mantra or meditative practice.

Meditation and/or psychotherapy are of paramount importance in holistic medicine therapeutics to help prevent or heal GERD or ulcers. The suffering individual needs to understand the psychological disturbances that underlie his gastric problems. By becoming aware of emotional conflicts that are associated with ulcer disease, a person can actually transform his discomfort into a learning experience. And so, awareness is the first step, followed by learning to integrate the knowledge gained through self-awareness into practical methods to eliminate the digestive problems.

Both psychotherapy and meditation can lead to enhanced awareness of how physical habits, personality traits and emotional conflicts lead to disorders of the digestive system. Through slow, methodical psychological insight, energy can be redirected from creating abnormal physiologic conditions like ulcers and lower bowel disorders to help better integrate body, mind and spirit.

Homeopathy

Arsenicum album and Nux vomica are two of many homeopathic remedies that are very effective in treating ulcers. The reader will notice that the remedy Arsenicum album is mentioned under two disease discussions: asthma and ulcers. It is one of several remedies called polychrests that are useful in a broad spectrum of ailments and so are frequently used in clinical practice. Arsenicum album is a remedy that affects almost all organ systems, and it is a good example of a remedy that can be used to treat many diverse problems. I have indicated that a certain emotional and psychological type needs Arsenicum album irrespective of the category of disease. This illustrates that it is the person that is being treated and not just the illness. Arsenicum album is characteristically prescribed for an individual who is subject to states of fearfulness, restlessness and insecurity. There is a "morbid dread of friends and family deserting them," of being left alone, perhaps to die.

Physically, there can be diarrhea, usually with burning in the rectum. There are burning discharges from most of the body orifices including the eyes, ears, nose, bladder, lungs, vagina, uterus and skin. The excessive burning pains, which are characteristic symptoms of the Arsenicum picture, indicate that the third chakra or solar plexus area is overactive. The inner heat increases in intensity, creating burning discharges and ulcerations of the mucous membranes, especially along the upper respiratory passages and in the solar plexus areas itself. Yoga philosophy would say that samana, the prana responsible for digestion and metabolism, is hyperfunctional. Because the inner fires are exaggerated, the fuel is quickly consumed and the system is left devoid of its heating element. The feet and hands become frigid and blue, the blood vessels feel "as though ice water runs through them" and the perspiration becomes cold. These latter symptoms are definitive hallmarks of Arsenicum album.

From a yogic standpoint, the first and the third chakras are involved in the Arsenicum album state as seen in the ulcer patient. Characteristic of the Arsenicum album pattern of pathology, this insecurity and anxiety can be compensated for by the need to control everyone and everything that may affect one's security.

This resultant struggle for control or power may become evident as imbalances in the third chakra.

Nux vomica is another remedy that is frequently indicated in the treatment of ulcers. The patient for whom Nux vomica is suitable is often the overly ambitious person who is interested primarily in self-fulfillment. He can be selfish, caring mostly for his own needs and often overlooking the emotions and requirements of others. The strong need of the Nux vomica personality to be nurtured and satisfied can be inferred from his marked predilection for overindulgence in food, drink and stimulants. The Nux vomica patient is often a typical ulcer patient, whose conflict leads to difficulties in digestion (nausea, vomiting, belching) and ulcer formation, all third chakra symptoms. As in the Arsenicum album type, the conflicts at the third chakra cause the system to create an overabundance of heat. This helps explain the Nux vomica symptoms of the "skin feeling hot, especially during fevers, despite an inner feeling of coldness" and "a great need to be covered up."

Case History of Duodenal Ulcer

When the typical hardworking executive finds himself in a particularly precarious or stressful situation, the pressure to assert independence and strength may clash with more childlike or infantile desires to be nurtured, passive and dependent. One practical solution, at least as far as his or her unconscious mind is concerned, is to develop an ulcer. This kind of conflict can occur in people from all walks of life. An ulcer creates a situation which permits one to rest, withdraw and accept comfort and support.

A forty-year-old man, RF, developed a duodenal ulcer after years of having tolerated excessive belching and heartburn. He is a busy executive who spends long hours at work, worries about corporate finances and spends little time with his family. He relates having a difficult time showing affection outwardly and often avoids emotional expression by overworking. His parents always had a difficult time showing or telling him that they loved him. Despite a cool exterior, inwardly he felt insecure and vulnerable. He wished he could be more open, but whenever he felt the urge to express himself emotionally, he quickly closed off to try to appear calm.

His current illness came on when his business developed financial problems. He felt as though he were a failure, had anxiety attacks and developed severe ulcerative pains in the abdomen. His facade of authority and power was eroded, and he had a strong desire to run away and be nurtured by his mother and father (who unfortunately responded by being cold and critical). This conflict of trying to appear outwardly strong while feeling weak inwardly and wanting to withdraw seemed to result in the activation of the parasympathetic type response and subsequent development of ulcer symptomatology.

Specific Treatment Plan

Diet

Nutritional management was integral in controlling his ulcer disease. Alcohol, tobacco, coffee and spicy foods were eliminated because of their irritating qualities. The patient was placed on a diet of lean meat including fish and poultry. He was instructed to eat frequent small meals and to avoid raw food because it could irritate the ulcer. Cooked vegetables and cooked whole grains, yogurt and probiotics were to be included in his daily diet. Slowly chewing crushed almonds was helpful to absorb acid. I also recommended apple cider vinegar, ginger, aloe vera juice, bananas, DGL licorice and turmeric, all of which can be helpful to absorb acid or to decrease gastric acid irritation.

Homeopathy

Medically, he had tried the proton pump inhibitor, Omeprazole, which was helpful to decrease stomach acid secretion while he was taking it, but each time he stopped it the symptoms would return. I then decided to give him the homeopathic remedy Sulphur, as it helps clear the energy body that has been negatively affected from years of suppressant medication. Also, Sulphur is a good remedy to start a chronic case. Sulphur is also helpful for those who have habitually abused stimulants, which he had done. Nux vomica given at night helped to quiet the digestive symptoms and calm his overactive mind and anxiety.

Meditation

In addition, we worked on incorporating two short meditations during the day, each type using simple awareness of the breath as the object of his concentration. I taught him how to visualize the third chakra symbol of an upward facing red triangle and to imagine that cooling energy was moving up to the crown of the head and back down again. I also taught him how to use the mantra *Ram* in coordination with moving this energy upwards through the chakras.

Within three months after making these changes, he was virtually without digestive system symptoms for the first time in years. During this three-month period, he began psychotherapy, which helped him substantially to identify feelings of fear and sadness and how to express these feelings more directly with his family and friends. Thus, coping with his illness started this patient on a path towards self-knowledge and a fuller, more rewarding life.

A Holistic Approach to Thyroid Disorders

Physiology

The thyroid gland is an endocrine organ that is divided into three major parts: right lobe, left lobe and the isthmus, which interconnects the lobes. It is located alongside and slightly below the laryngeal protrusion (Adam's apple). The major function of the thyroid gland is to produce an iodine-containing hormone called thyroxin, which is responsible for controlling the rate of body metabolism and is needed for normal physical and mental growth.

Hypothyroidism

Deficiencies in this hormone lead to premature cessation of bone growth and mental retardation in children and hypotension, depression and poor metabolic functioning in adults. Underactivity of the thyroid leads to weight gain, dry skin, decreased sex drive and miscarriages. Overproduction can lead to anxiety, weight loss, racing heart and palpitations. Thyroxin's role in reproduction, development and maturation is well established. Levels of thyroxin rise in pregnancy, and this hormone is responsible for stimulating genital duct formation in the male.

On the emotional and mental levels, thyroxin exerts important influences, as the qualities of alertness, sensitivity and clarity of thought are dependent upon adequate supplies. Deficiency causes mental sluggishness and depression, while excess thyroxin causes hypersensitivity where the person can become anxious and suffers from insomnia.

The anterior pituitary gland in the brain secretes a hormone called thyroid stimulating hormone (TSH) that causes the thyroid to produce more thyroxin. TSH in turn is controlled by a substance made in the hypothalamus called thyroid releasing factor (TRF). TRF may be affected by higher brain centers such as the cerebral cortex and limbic system. This may provide the explanation of how thoughts and emotions can affect the production of thyroxin. Thyroxin itself has a negative feedback on both TSH and TRF, which means that when blood levels of thyroxin are high enough, thyroxin will signal directly to the pituitary and hypothalamus to stop secretion of their hormones and vice versa.

Hyperthyroidism

Hyperthyroidism, also called thyrotoxicosis or Graves Disease, is characterized by overproduction of thyroid hormone. Symptoms associated with this illness reflect an exaggeration of all the normal functions controlled by thyroid hormone. Among these are anxiety, extreme restlessness, weight loss despite increased appetite, sweating, hair loss, palpitations of the heart and bulging of the eyes (exophthalmos). These symptoms are quite similar to those found in the anxiety-stress syndrome of the sympathetic nervous system.

Causes of Hyperthyroidism

There are several common causes for hyperthyroidism: (1) overactive nodules of thyroid tissue or tumors of the thyroid; and (2) generally enlarged and overactive thyroid gland due to inflammation or viral infection. The thyroid gland can also be enlarged when it is underactive. Iodine is important in the synthesis of thyroxin, and iodine deficiency occurs in certain locales where iodine levels in the soil are low, such as in the Great Lake areas where the glaciers leached the iodine out as they retreated upwards towards the Arctic. In such cases, the gland works harder and enlarges in an attempt to produce enough functional thyroxin to provide for the body's needs. Here the thyroid gland is hypofunctional because of missing iodine.

Thyroid hormone functioning increases when there are longstanding stresses on the body or mind. It acts in a similar way to the sympathetic nervous system hormone adrenalin, although the latter hormone is generally released during acute sudden stress, while thyroxin is secreted during chronic stress states. The association between thyroxin and adrenalin is also seen in people with hyperactive thyroid glands who overreact to small amounts of adrenaline.

Psychosomatic Theory

According to psychoanalytic theory, the most frequent conflict that sometimes typifies the hyperthyroid patient is difficulty in exchanging the roles of being nurtured and nurturing others. At the root of this conflict is an intense insecurity characterized by a fear of death or loss of maternal support, accompanied by a concurrent worry about taking over the burden of motherhood. It is not surprising that the great majority of hyperthyroid patients are female. These people psychologically struggle against this insecurity by trying to control the expression of emotions externally or by increasing their sense of responsibility. The first psychological defense of not expressing emotions leads to tension and rigidity in the throat and larynx area and results in a chronic inability to communicate. The second defense is curious. In an effort to overcome the anxiety or fear of the loss of maternal support, the person may compulsively try to master that which is feared. And so "pseudo-maturity" develops, resulting in an attempt to assume a parental role in order to decrease the discomforting feelings of insecurity. This self-reliance, however, is hollow because such a person is not internally ready for this role.

A common way to combat the fear of maternal loss is by becoming pregnant or by becoming a mother figure to siblings. Becoming pregnant combats the fear of death through the act of bringing another life into the world and it also counteracts the fear of losing the mother by "becoming a mother." Being motherly to siblings can bring about vicarious gratifications of dependency needs.

Feelings of insecurity often originate in early childhood, especially when there is parental death or divorce, parental indifference or from actually witnessing the death of someone close. A long-term facade of maturity may then be assumed to disguise or conceal the feelings of insecurity or nurturance needs. As long as the defense (hyperactivity, pregnancy, etc.) remains intact, the individual may continue to live normally within the pseudo-mature role. However, when stressful situations such as illness or miscarriage threaten these defenses, or when a child leaves home, the underlying anxiety surfaces. This creates more stress on the part of the maturation system associated with the thyroid gland, already under chronic activation since childhood because of the constant demands for accelerated maturity. When the vicissitudes of life overwhelm the struggle to control anxiety and dependency needs through premature self-reliance roles, hyperthyroidism can result.

Chakra Association

According to the yogic model, physical, mental and spiritual issues relating to the fifth chakra predominate when the thyroid becomes diseased. This chakra is said to be associated with the capacity to be nurtured, feelings of trust, communicative functions and the creative potential. Being nurtured involves the ability to be receptive, open and trusting towards the provider. Nurturance can be in the form of food, material goods or emotional support. The child receives sustenance from the mother, while the adult obtains nurturance from the external environment, interpersonal relationships and the inner Self. Guidance from one's conscience or inner feelings is also a form of nurturance.

According to this theory, the giving of nurturance is a concern of the fourth chakra, which involves feeling love for others. Receiving nurturance is, in a sense, a higher capacity than giving it, and the ability to accept love and guidance from within and without is a function of an integrated, balanced, well-focused fifth chakra. Trust is also a quality of the fifth chakra. When a person fears rejection, as can happen in hyperthyroidism, there is a tendency to mistrust others and fear of being hurt or abandoned. This is in accordance with the psychosomatic model, where the most prominent emotional conflicts associated with hyperthyroidism are the fear of maternal loss or rejection and feelings of insecurity. There is an overpowering fear that one will not be taken care of or nurtured.

The ability to communicate with clarity is also an important aspect of the fifth chakra, since the larynx and voice box, essential for speech and verbal expression, are located in the throat area. The physical counterparts of emotional shock or anxiety that manifest in the throat area are the feeling of "a lump in the throat" and a tight or constricted sensation in the throat. People who have tension in this area often "lose their voice" or "can't find the right words to express themselves." Hyperthyroid people often have similar blocks, either because of a severe emotional shock that precipitated the hyperthyroidism or because of chronic repression of fears and anxieties.

Creativity, which is said to be characteristic of a focused and well-balanced fifth chakra, involves the ability to tap into one's inner potential. Deep within the unconscious are hidden abilities, knowledge and sources of great inspiration. Insights gained from this vast reservoir allow individuals to express themselves creatively. The results can be seen in great achievements in art, music or literature and also in skill and productiveness in any endeavor that involves precision or ingenuity. This creative urge is often blocked in persons with thyroid problems. The characteristic defenses of the hyperthyroid individual are psychological barriers that inhibit the inner flow of creative thought and understanding. A person who utilizes various defenses in their relationships is employing conscious effort, which requires great amounts of energy. The unconscious potential is kept in abeyance by the hyperactivity of conscious preoccupation. To experience truly creative inspiration, the conscious mind and egoistic tendencies must not be allowed to interfere with the fresh, pure aspects of the unconscious mind. The individual must be open to receive nurturance from within and to be a channel and receptacle for the finer secrets of life that emerge from deep inside the creative centers.

Creativity leads to evolution and growth of consciousness. As a person integrates more and more of the unknown with the known, the universe becomes more understandable and controllable. The fifth chakra is the steppingstone to the two highest chakras, and it is at the highest centers of consciousness that integration leads to true intuitive knowledge and expanded awareness.

Holistic Treatment

Nutrition

Since hyperthyroidism is an illness of hyperactivity and oversecretion of thyroid hormone, it would be considered a pitta condition. Therefore hot, stimulating foods need to be avoided. This would include spicy foods in particular. More sattvic foods like beans and whole grains and dairy products are encouraged.

Hatha Yoga and Cleansings

In hypothyroidism treatment oriented towards the fifth chakra includes yoga postures that stimulate the throat area: the lion, shoulderstand, fish, bridge and general stretching exercises for the neck and shoulders. The lion's pose is also helpful if practiced twice a day. On the other hand, these yoga postures should be avoided in hyperthyroidism until proper treatment has been initiated.

The upper wash, in which a large amount of warm salty water is swallowed and then regurgitated, not only helps rid the system of excess mucus but is also beneficial in several other ways. This should only be practiced under the supervision of a medical provider well versed in hyperthyroid disorders. Tension in the throat is often associated with the fear of letting go of emotions. Vomiting, an act of letting go or releasing, can relieve these physical and emotional tensions. Individuals with problems in the throat area often fear vomiting, and the upper wash can help to gradually eliminate this fear.

Breathing Exercises

Breathing exercises are very valuable in thyroid disease, especially bhramari and ujjayi, which directly stimulate the thyroid area. Diaphragmatic breathing accompanied by relaxation techniques helps to reestablish a smooth air flow through tightened throat areas where the thyroid gland is situated. Kapalabhati, through its more vigorous vibrational stimulation, can positively affect the thyroid gland's deficient functioning.

Psychotherapy and Meditation

Learning to verbalize internal problems through psychotherapy often helps to release throat tension. Free verbal expression of locked-in feelings and thoughts can help open up the throat chakra. Similarly, crying, laughing and singing may provide an outlet for tension, making possible relaxation of the throat. Techniques of concentration and meditation on the throat help to focus awareness and energy. They help to decrease the tendency towards dissipation of energy and to control and direct it for more creative purposes.

Homeopathy

There are several homeopathic remedies that can help to treat hyperthyroidism. By acting on the vital force, which in this case is in a state of chronic overstimulation, the similar remedy helps to reestablish physiologic balance and to catalyze psychological growth. After taking the homeopathic remedy, the patient carefully notes changing symptoms and emotional attitudes that affect the entire system. In working with the physician, the patient learns to recognize personality patterns and underlying conflicts that may predispose him to the thyrotoxic condition. Recognition of these conflicts is a most important step in changing habits and psychological attitudes. More mature methods of handling problems can be substituted for immature coping and defense mechanisms.

Natrum muriaticum (sodium chloride) is the primary homeopathic remedy to consider in the hyperthyroid condition. This substance is interesting, both from a physiologic viewpoint and from a psychological-symbolic perspective. On the physical level, sodium chloride helps to maintain normal blood volume and blood pressure. Most molecular particles depend on a normal concentration of sodium in water to facilitate their free movement through the body's tissues. In the Eastern tradition of Ayurvedic medicine, salt is considered a very powerful stimulant, and one is cautioned to use it with discrimination. Chinese medicine views salt as a yang substance which if taken in excess can lead to yang symptoms such as aggression and heat production.

In the West, sodium chloride (table salt) is overused because artificial foods are devoid of taste, and salt brings out added flavor. Also, because salt is a stimulant, it is used to provide a physical and mental lift. In the United States salt is not only added in the preparation of foods but is also used as a preservative in most prepackaged foods. The result is an intake of as much as fifty to one hundred times the daily requirement. Because of this, symptoms can occur that mimic those of thyrotoxicosis, such as anxiety, palpitations and sweating.

From a psychological standpoint, Natrum muriaticum is symbolic of the ocean, since salt is the main substance found within the sea. Because the earliest plant and animal life began in the ocean, it represents the primordial pool from which all life stems. It is symbolically equivalent to the mother archetype. The ocean, like the mother, is the giver of life. The water sac (amniotic fluid) that bathes the growing embryo in the womb is comprised of saltwater and is another instance of the relationship between the ocean, the origin of life and the mother. Emotional problems centered on the mother figure are typical of thyroid hyperactivity.

The other remedy that is often used, and which typifies the overactive state of thyrotoxicosis is Iodine. Iodine is important in the synthesis of thyroxin and imbalances in its metabolism greatly affect the functioning of the thyroid gland. When indicated, iodine used homeopathically helps to balance the overactive thyroid gland. It is interesting to note that iodine is commonly added to table salt to be sold in locales that are iodine deficient.

Hypothyroidism, or low thyroxin production, is characterized by sluggish metabolism, slow heart rate and slower mental activity. The remedy most closely associated with these symptoms is Calcarea carbonica, which is calcium carbonate derived from the oyster shell. Symbology applies here, too. The oyster lives in the salty sea and is surrounded by a firm, rigid shell that protects the animal but also restricts it. Calcarea carbonica represents restrictive and slowed down phenomena as part of its symptom picture. Its use in hypothyroidism becomes obvious. The oyster withdraws from danger and the outer environment by becoming enclosed within its protective shell. It is interesting that hypothyroidism seems to occur most often in persons who are overprotective of themselves and their families and who tend to withdraw from conflict.

The remedy Natrum muriaticum was earlier seen to be symbolically analogous to and therapeutically useful in conditions that are characteristically hyperfunctional and overactive. This is equivalent to the sympathetic nervous system response pattern. Calcarea carbonica, on the other hand, is associated with restriction, passivity and the tendency to withdraw and so is analogous to the parasympathetic nervous system type response.

Case History

Mrs. B is a fifty-year-old woman who developed symptoms of hyperthyroidism, including an enlarged thyroid, fatigue, tremors in the hands, agitated depression, palpitation, weight loss, increased perspiration and hair loss. Although she had felt fatigue for approximately one year prior to the onset of the disease, the hyperthyroidism coincided with severe marital quarreling. She said that she was feeling very incompetent, insecure and continuously feared being abandoned by her second husband, who was four years younger than herself. She had tended to dominate their relationship and tended to "mother" her spouse. When he began to resist this behavior and assert his independence, her symptoms began. It appears that her defense against feelings of insecurity and rejection was to assume a role of controlling her husband's life, since she couldn't control her own life.

This patient related that she had always been dominated by her parents and after spending a week with them she said, "I have to stick up for myself." Never having felt love from her mother, she married at an early age in an attempt to attain security by becoming a mother herself. Because she could never express negative or angry feelings to her mother she felt tightness in her throat. Her excessive passivity towards her mother was transferred to her growing children, whom she smothered in an overcompensating way to give them what she never had. Her children couldn't handle this passive-aggressiveness and eventually left home to avoid further communication.

Specific Treatment of Hyperthyroidism

Nutrition
Hyperthyroidism represents a pitta condition. Holistic treatment for Mrs. B included decreasing stimulating foods such as salt, spices and sweets, as these tend to aggravate an already hyperfunctioning thyroid condition.

Breathing Techniques and Yoga Postures
Mrs. B learned diaphragmatic breathing, alternate nostril breathing and ujjayi to help with gentle relaxation of the throat area. We worked on some gentle neck rolls and neck stretches. Until the hyperactivity of the thyroid was under control, I did not encourage some of the yoga asanas that I teach people with hypothyroidism, including the shoulderstand, the fish and the lion as well as the bridge and the cobra, all of which gently stimulate the thyroid and neck area.

Meditation and Psychotherapy
Spending more time in relaxation and meditation and walking slowly were suggested to help cultivate a quiet state of mind and body. To further promote a calm state, she was instructed to meditate on the thyroid area (fifth chakra) and to visualize the

full moon in a blue sky at this chakra. She used the mantra *Ham*, the sound associated with the fifth chakra, in her daily meditation practice.

Since this patient was not inclined to remember her dreams or take an interest in early childhood experiences, problem solving was employed rather than any kind of intensive analysis. However, during treatment Mrs. B gradually became aware of her immature behavior patterns and underlying fears. She then began to assume a more realistic role as a wife and to let go of her controlling characteristics. She became more independent and actually got a job for the first time in her life. As a consequence, communication with her husband improved and the marriage became relatively harmonious. She came to understand and accept why her children avoided contact with her. In essence, she became a more mature woman.

Homeopathy

Natrum muriaticum, Calcarea iodatum and Medorrhinum were among the more important remedies used. Because the homeopathic remedies were successful, drugs and radiation therapy were not needed. Very occasionally in the past with other patients, I have had to suppress an extremely hyperactive thyroid condition for a short time before beginning homeopathy. I tend to use methimazole, a medication that makes it harder for the body to make thyroid hormone. In the case of an underactive thyroid, I have used thyroid replacement and like to use the natural type such as armour thyroid.

A Holistic Approach to Lower Bowel Disorders

Physiology

Bowel motility (peristaltic movement) is controlled by the parasympathetic system, and under normal situations this process occurs in a precise, gentle and synchronistic way. Diarrhea that is not infectious in causation can occur when parasympathetic overactivation increases bowel motility, rushing food through the small intestine and colon before it can be adequately digested and absorbed. Conversely, when one is in a state of fear, the sympathetic system becomes activated and blood is rechanneled to the organs necessary for immediate survival, such as the muscles and brain.

Activity is inhibited in the other organ systems, such as the urinary and digestive, which are not critical for immediate survival. In order to facilitate the relative slowdown in the function of these two systems, a set of reflexes is triggered that cause the bladder to empty and the bowels to evacuate. The sympathetic system causes the rectal sphincters to relax and the peristaltic and absorbing activities of the bowel to stop. Thus, an underabsorbed, watery stool moves quickly through and out the flaccid large intestine. In acute conditions, fear can cause a child or an animal to defecate or urinate uncontrollably. If a person is in a chronic state of fear or anxiety, a condition of chronic or frequent loose motions will occur. Thus, diarrhea can be due to overactivity of either the parasympathetic or sympathetic nervous systems.

Two common causes of chronic diarrhea are irritable bowel syndrome and ulcerative colitis. Diarrhea associated with spasms of the colon but without observable changes in the colon is called irritable bowel syndrome or spastic colitis. Ulcerative colitis is a more severe form of colitis in which the walls of the colon are covered with tiny ulcers that ooze blood, leading to painful, bloody evacuations. While there are other illnesses associated with chronic diarrhea, such as Crohn's disease and food sensitivities, I will limit our discussion to ulcerative and irritable bowel syndrome.

Causes of Bowel Disorders

Psychosomatic Medicine

Persons with lower bowel disorders are sometimes described as being overly conscientious. At the same time, such persons have a reluctance to exert themself, to engage in systematic work or to fulfill those obligations to which they feel emotionally compelled. This conflict is associated with overactivation of the parasympathetic nervous system. Essentially certain types of chronic diarrhea are the somatic manifestation of a basic lack of self-confidence. The disease is the outward expression of the act of giving to compensate for unconscious feelings of insecurity.

Constipation, another affliction of modern humanity, is a condition in which the stool remains in the colon too long and becomes desiccated and hardened. This creates a wide variety of symptoms, including vague feelings of discomfort or bloating, headache, nausea and vomiting, and in the most extreme cases results in fecal impaction and blockage of the colon. Chronic constipation can often lead to such conditions as diverticulitis (weakening of the colon wall) and hemorrhoids (a condition where the veins around the anus become dilated). In either case, it is the increased pressure created by straining to pass the hardened stool that can lead to the problem.

Some people suffering with chronic constipation often feel rejected and are pessimistic and distrust others. They feel they cannot expect too much from anyone and are afraid to express themselves to others. Thus, they hold back their emotions and the expression of feelings. The retention of feces provides a feeling of well-being or security. It is for this reason that some individuals, despite a high fiber diet and enough water and exercise, may still be troubled with constipation.

Chakra Association

From a yogic perspective, these people exhibit a conflict in the first chakra, which deals physiologically with the act of elimination and psychologically with security and possession. Disturbance in this chakra threatens the instinct for survival and may manifest as constant worry. Weakness of the first chakra can also manifest as chronic diarrhea, a physical manifestation of insecurity on the mental-emotional level.

In both cases, there is a passive response according to psychoanalytic theory, but in constipation the psychological issues are fear of rejection with consequent selfishness (the person tries to possess that which he fears losing). Inability to give of one's self is manifested on the physical level as tightness of the rectum and retention of stool. Chronic diarrhea reflects a more integrated ego where the person feels secure enough at least to attempt to give, even if in an infantile way.

Yoga philosophy calls the energy that is responsible for the process of elimination *apana*. This is analogous to vata in Ayurveda. In healthy individuals the vata or air moves in a downward direction, but occasionally things go awry and the vata begins to move upwards. This condition causes problems that may manifest in a number of ways. Constipation will result, as it is the normal downward force of vata that supplies the energy to move the stool.

Headaches are also a common symptom associated with constipation. No good reason for this relationship has been offered in orthodox medicine. In Ayurveda, it is thought that the obstructed vata moves upwards and fills the head, and the increased "air" pressure causes pain in the cerebral area. In order to correct this situation, an enema may be prescribed to stimulate a reversal of the flow of vata. As vata again begins to flow downwards, the constipation is often relieved and the headache ameliorated. Herbs that counteract vata conditions can also be prescribed.

Flatus (colonic air) is a manifestation of excessive vata, as is diarrhea. The cause may be secondary to diet, such as eating predominantly vatic foods like beans, or to a vatic mental state. Treatment should be designed to rebalance the doshas, using a combination of diet, medicines or meditative exercises.

Holistic Treatment of Bowel Disorders

Nutrition

Although constipation may be due to psychogenic causes, in many instances it may also be due to poor nutrition, lack of exercise and not drinking enough water. It has been noted that the average transit time required for the stool to pass through the large bowel varies tremendously according to the quantity of fiber consumed. African tribesmen, who consume large quantities of fiber, have voluminous stools with a transit time of approximately twelve to twenty-four hours. Europeans and Americans, on the other hand, with their highly refined and processed diets, tend to have smaller stools and a transit time of up to seventy-two hours. In an effort to compensate for the lack of fiber, Americans sometimes substitute large quantities of bran or other bulk agents. However, this is only a symptomatic approach because the basic problem is not a deficiency of bran. What is needed is a more natural diet consisting of foods high in natural fiber, such as fruits and fresh, green leafy vegetables and especially whole grains and legumes. Since these latter two are often absent in the average diet, it should come as no surprise that many people find themselves constipated.

Other dietary measures are also helpful to treat constipation. In Ayurvedic medicine, psyllium seed husks are prescribed to prevent and treat the disorder. These husks have a gelatinous consistency and, unlike bran, are not irritative but have a gentle action. Since they are indigestible, they provide more than adequate quantities of fiber to aid in elimination. Also effective is drinking a glass of hot water with lemon juice, a pinch of salt and honey to taste. This traditional folk remedy is a very effective natural laxative and is very mild. The use of prune juice, coffee, milk of magnesia or other strong laxatives is not generally recommended, since they weaken the body's own ability to eliminate and tend to make the system chronically dependent on their use. Avoiding excess quantities of dairy products, especially cheese, which can be constipating, can also be helpful.

There are many factors that can cause diarrhea. In acute cases it may be due to ingestion of certain foods, microorganisms or toxins that the body rejects and attempts to throw off. Acute diarrhea most commonly occurs in conjunction with acute viral intestinal infection, called the noro virus. Usually in these cases, the process is self-limiting, and a diet of clear liquids or pureed carrot soup will help correct the problem.

The chronic diarrhea of ulcerative or irritable bowel syndrome requires a more complex treatment. Dietary guidelines for treating these conditions have significantly changed over the years. In general, nuts, raw fruits and vegetables, uncooked grains, bran and other foods with heavy roughage should be avoided. Cooked whole grains and cooked vegetables, previously prohibited to patients with chronic diarrhea, are now considered by many physicians to be acceptable and even helpful, the feeling being that the fiber in these foods may act as bulk agents that help to hold the stool together. Yogurt may help provide a favorable environment for repopulation of the microbiome in the colon, as healthy bacteria may have been lost due to the frequent diarrhea. Tofu is an excellent source of nonirritating, easily digestible and high-quality protein. Stewed and peeled apples are helpful since apples contain pectin, which helps form the stool. Cooked whole grains and cooked vegetables are yang and thus can help to balance this condition. Citrus fruit is very yin, according to Chinese medicine, and should be avoided in this yin condition of chronic watery stools.

Exercise and Hatha Yoga

An important factor in preventing constipation is exercise. Joggers don't often complain of constipation because the continuous jostling of the colon stimulates its contraction. Certain hatha yoga exercises such as the stomach lift, plow and knee to chest positions have a gentle massaging effect on the colon and aid in elimination. The biomechanisms of elimination can also be facilitated by squatting. The Western style toilet, although aesthetically appealing, is not very functional. A person familiar with the squatting style of toilet used in the East, or who has defecated in the woods, will attest to the increased efficiency. Squatting is not only an effective way to decrease the amount of straining required, but it can prevent and alleviate hemorrhoids.

Active exercise would be beneficial in the treatment of the chronic diarrhea of spastic or ulcerative colitis. A regular practice of hatha yoga reduces physical tension and promotes calm and relaxation. Hatha postures can be prescribed to promote specific results. For example, in case of diarrhea postures should be held for longer periods to keep the abdominal contents relatively stationary. With constipation, on the other hand, it would be better to repeat the posture in rapid succession to stimulate the sluggish digestive organs. Whereas the abdominal lift might be more beneficial when the bowel movements are loose, agni sara, which is described above in the section on hatha yoga, would help relieve constipation.

Breathing Exercises

The breath is the link between mind and body. That is why breath awareness, diaphragmatic breathing and other breathing exercises that are focused on creating smooth, rhythmic and effortless breath patterns are essential for an individual's total health.

Chest breathing stimulates the sympathetic nervous system (that originates from the back-chest area) to create a state of anxiety. By focusing attention on the solar plexus (third chakra) area while breathing with the diaphragm, greater balance is brought to the sympathetic and parasympathetic nervous systems that innervate this nerve plexus. In addition, diaphragmatic breathing, coupled with a relaxation technique, helps to bring under conscious control emotional responses to psychological conflicts.

Meditation and Psychotherapy

Meditation and/or psychotherapy are of paramount importance in holistic medical therapeutics to prevent or heal lower bowel disorders and ulcers. These practices not only treat the organic dysfunction but also enable the suffering individual to understand the concomitant psychological disturbances that underlie bowel and gastric problems. For example, when bowel movements become irregular, the patient may observe they are feeling particularly selfish or obsessive. Awareness is the first step in problem resolution. Perhaps the person learns by careful scrutiny that wheat, milk or raw foods cause diarrhea, so they avoid them. By practicing breathing exercises they may discover they are primarily doing chest breathing, causing the diaphragm and abdominal muscles to remain frozen. This leads to bowel inactivity and constipation. Such observations need to be followed by taking steps to integrate the knowledge gained with practical methods to eliminate the digestive problems.

Both meditation and psychotherapy can lead to enhanced awareness of how physical habits, personality traits and emotional conflicts lead to disorders of the digestive system. Meditation practices generally involve focusing on simple breath awareness and moving energy up and down the spine. Through the gradual and methodical development of psychological insight, the energy that has been tied up in abnormal physiologic conditions like ulcers and lower bowel disorders can be released and utilized to help better integrate body, mind and spirit.

Homeopathy

The homeopathic remedy Lycopodium (club moss) typifies the symptoms of chronic lower bowel disorders, especially when constipation alternating with loose stools is part of the symptomatology. The abdomen of a person who needs Lycopodium is often distended with trapped gas, and the person may even develop flatus while eating. As is typical of the constipated individual described in psychoanalytic theory, a person who needs Lycopodium is psychologically insecure, lacks confidence and often feels fearful. To compensate for these feelings of inadequacy, they may strive harder in business and tend to overwork because of an insatiable need for power. Such authoritarianism is characterized by the inability to give of oneself. Another important description of a person who needs Lycopodium is haughtiness. The Lycopodium patient tends to become less trustful and fearful that others will usurp his position of power. To cover up their feelings of insecurity they become forceful and aggressive and may even resort to more infantile methods of self-preservation and overprotectiveness. As a consequence, the person's emotional life can suffer; they become hardened, find it difficult to maintain relationships and in general do not take responsibility in intimate relationships. The problem of not being able to give emotionally is reflected on the physical level as retention and inability to give up the stool, resulting in constipation.

Pulsatilla is a remedy suitable to the person with chronic diarrhea. The main characteristics that describe the Pulsatilla personality are emotional unpredictability, changeable and easily suggestible. In general, Pulsatilla is more suitable for women or men who are unafraid of showing their more feminine side. It is useful for people who do not have a strong sense of identity and are easily molded by their environment. All fluids from the body flow easily, including tears whether one is sad or happy, nasal discharge during colds or allergies, and stools. The Pulsatilla personality always wants to please and to give to others. This is very similar to the diarrhea personality as described in the psychosomatic model.

Case History:

LW is a twenty-eight-year-old woman who, six months prior to being seen as a patient, had developed daily episodes of lower abdominal cramping pain, flatulence and diarrhea. These symptoms appeared just as the patient had begun a new job as a store manager. She admitted she had never felt confident about functioning in positions of authority, though she always sought these types of jobs. She tried to push these feelings of inadequacy aside and prove herself capable of this new challenge. However, as her management superiors increased their demands, and as problem solving with the people she was supervising was proving ineffective, the patient's level of anxiety about failing intensified and the above symptoms manifested. Prior to this, similar situations had resulted in anxiety felt in the pit of the stomach and occasional episodes of painless diarrhea. The patient had seen a physician after the cramping pain and diarrhea had persisted for one month. A colonoscopy was performed, and the patient was diagnosed as having irritable bowel syndrome, as there were no obvious pathological changes. A medication to block the overactivity of the parasympathetic nervous system was prescribed, but she experienced only minimal relief of her symptoms. She continued with her job, and her symptoms varied according to the amount of stress she was experiencing in her work.

From the point of view of psychosomatic medicine, this person showed a pattern of symptom development that corresponds with psychological characteristics often seen in colitis patients: an underlying insecurity and lack of basic self-confidence in her ability to adequately perform. When she became stressed beyond her ability to cope, rather than withdrawing by quitting the job, she persevered on a conscious level. But the urge to withdraw was expressed symbolically by activation of the parasympathetic nervous system and the manifestation of the symptoms of colitis.

Specific Treatment Plan

Nutrition

In this case, the approach to therapy focused primarily on a dietary program involving the elimination of coffee, red meat and refined carbohydrates. Fish, poultry and tofu were recommended as high quality and nonirritating protein sources. In addition, fresh cooked vegetables and peeled fruits would provide a healthy source of nonirritating roughage. She also began to take probiotics to enhance her microbiotic health.

Exercise and Hatha Yoga

The patient began a program of regular exercise which consisted of swimming four times per week. This was advised because she liked the sport and a public pool was available. I instructed her to practice yoga postures in a gentle way and modified postures for her such as the spinal twist and the knees to chest posture. As her symptoms improved, I encouraged her to do the inverted postures such as the headstand and shoulderstand. I also taught her agni sara and the abdominal lift.

Breathing Exercises

She was also taught diaphragmatic breathing and relaxation to help balance the overactivity of the parasympathetic nervous system. This also served to provide a tool to discharge the anxiety she felt with the pressures of her job.

Psychotherapy and Meditation

LW decided to enter into weekly psychotherapy, which helped her understand her reluctance to assert herself honestly when she felt she wasn't being heard or acknowledged. We also worked on meditation where she focused her concentration on the first chakra while repeating the mantra *Lam*. She then learned to move her blocked energy up through all the chakras using the mantra associated with each of the chakras. All the above methods and therapies helped her feel much better about herself, to be more efficient and confident at work and less controlling of friends and family.

Homeopathy

As a result of these changes, the patient's colitis improved approximately fifty percent. Once this plateau was reached, she was given the homeopathic remedy Lycopodium because it closely corresponded to her symptoms of constipation alternating with diarrhea, cramping and flatulence. Also, Lycopodium is helpful in conditions where lack of self-confidence is a prominent characteristic. The patient had additional symptoms of always feeling cold and a strong craving for sweets, which are further indications for use of Lycopodium. By the fourth week after taking the remedy, the patient's colitis symptoms were completely resolved, and her anxiety was much reduced, allowing her to healthfully continue her work.

A Holistic Approach to Skin Problems and Acne

Physiology

The skin is the largest organ in the body, weighing over eight pounds in the average male, with an overall area close to eighteen square feet. In the embryo, the skin is derived from a primitive type cell, the ectoderm, which makes up the layer of cells that surrounds the developing embryo. As the embryo grows, most of these cells remain on the outer surface and later develop into the skin. However, a small group of these cells migrate inwards towards the center of the embryo, forming a structure called the neural tube. The neural tube eventually develops into the spinal cord, brain and other nervous tissue.

Since both skin and nervous tissue originate from the same embryonic cell type, there is a close interrelationship between these two organ systems. This intimate connection is demonstrated in the ways in which the skin reflects the emotions or mental states. Blushing with embarrassment, turning white with fear and being purple with rage are all examples of this. Many classic dermatological diseases, such as eczema, psoriasis, acne and neurodermatitis, can be associated with underlying emotional conflicts.

The skin as an organ system performs many essential functions. Primarily, it acts as a barrier to protect the internal environment from the challenges of the external world. Skin is made up of two distinct layers. The deep layer is called the dermis, which is the origin of the nerves, blood vessels and glandular structures like the sweat and oil glands. The more external layer is called the epidermis and contains the cells that make up what is commonly thought of as skin. As the cells at the deepest level of the epidermis divide, the older cells are pushed towards the surface where they eventually die, lose their individual shape, and merge into a single layer of essentially dead tissue. This dead tissue is primarily composed of a protein material called keratin. It is this upper layer of dead cells that gives the skin its tough consistency and provides protection against physical trauma and bacterial invasion.

Located within the skin are special cells called melanocytes. These cells function to produce a darkly colored chemical called melanin. Skin coloring is dependent upon the amount of melanin produced and the number of melanocytes in the skin: the greater their number or activity, the darker the skin. Scandinavians have relatively few melanocytes in their skin as compared to Africans. When exposed to solar irradiation, melanocytes make more melanin to block the irradiation from passing through to the deeper levels of the skin. This serves two functions. First, it protects the skin from being burned, and secondly, it protects the body from overproducing Vitamin D. The production of Vitamin D begins in the deeper layers of the skin. A reaction between the ultraviolet radiation from the sun and a fatty substance found in the skin produces the compound which ultimately becomes Vitamin D. The body needs only a limited amount of Vitamin D every day.

Overproduction of Vitamin D can lead to excessive calcium absorption and possibly kidney stones. Only a small area of skin needs to be exposed to the sun to produce an adequate amount of Vitamin D. In fact, it has been estimated that a fair-skinned individual living in the tropics would only need to expose a postage stamp size area of skin to the sun one hour a day to produce a sufficient amount of Vitamin D. Without the protection provided by melanin, individuals living in the tropics would be in constant danger of overproducing Vitamin D and would suffer from Vitamin D toxicity.

In northern latitudes, where the sun's intensity is diminished, and the weather is cold, people tend to expose less of their bodies to the sun. In the winter the days are short, and so Vitamin D production diminishes. Since Vitamin D is essential for calcium absorption and bone formation, too little Vitamin D can be just as dangerous as too much, leading to deficient calcium absorption and diseases such as rickets. As expected, rickets is more common in urban Blacks than in other groups. This is because their dark pigmentation, along with the other factors listed above, plus the air pollution that blocks the sun's intensity, all predispose them to decreased Vitamin D production. Therefore, dark-skinned people living in northern urban conditions should be careful to obtain an adequate amount of Vitamin D in their diet.

Through the process of sweating, the skin helps to regulate body temperature, water balance and salt balance. The skin also plays an important role in the elimination of wastes and toxins and thus is referred to as a third kidney. For example, during fasting it is common for perspiration to become much more odoriferous, indicating the elimination of certain waste materials. One of the telltale symptoms of kidney failure is the appearance of a whitish discharge on the skin. Urea, a waste product produced by the body as it utilizes protein, is normally eliminated via the kidneys, but when the kidneys fail, the skin tries to compensate and urea is eliminated through perspiration, producing a white discharge called uremic frost.

The skin also acts as a barrier to the evaporation of water that comprises sixty percent of the body's weight. If the skin is injured, as in the case of a serious burn, this mechanism breaks down and large quantities of fluid and salt may exude through the skin. In deep burns the danger of dehydration resulting from fluid loss through the skin is the most immediate cause of fatality.

The importance of the skin as an eliminative organ is emphasized even more in Eastern and other holistic medical systems than in Western medicine. Holistic medicine maintains that physical health is dependent on optimal functioning of the eliminative systems, including the urinary, respiratory and digestive tracts. The liver is also intricately involved in cleansing processes, as it promotes the degradation and metabolism of toxins, drugs and chemicals. If any of these vital body parts is dysfunctional, the skin becomes an alternative organ of elimination of waste products. From this perspective, skin eruptions such as acne or eczema are really a systemic problem representing inner disorder. Skin eruptions are the mind-body's way of throwing off subtler processes that originate in the deeper levels of a person's psyche. If an individual is to be truly cured from a disease process, the process needs to work itself outwards to the surface. Merely treating a skin eruption such as eczema with cortisone cream does not remove the underlying cause or cure the inner disease process. This is evidenced by the return of the symptoms on cessation of the use of the steroid creams.

We have seen that the principle that cure takes place from the inside out is central to many holistic traditions. For example, if a patient is treated by a homeopathic physician, and comes back the next week with the complaint, "Well, since my last visit I feel much better mentally but I have this rash," the homeopath knows that the patient is getting better because the process is moving outwards from the mental to the physical level.

The homeopath also views the commonly ignored eruptions on the skin such as moles and warts as being very significant. According to homeopathy, warts are the external manifestation of an internal imbalance, often related to the sycotic miasm. There is a weakness that allows this virus to grow; when the weakness is corrected, the virus and the warts will be eliminated.

Besides functioning as an instrument of protection and excretion, the skin also serves as an organ of reception and communication. The skin contains hundreds of millions of tiny nerve endings that are sensitive to touch, pressure and temperature. These nerve endings send impulses to the brain where they are interpreted as pain, pleasure, pressure, heat or cold.

More importantly, at least from a psychological perspective, is that the skin allows for the communication of feelings between persons. Physical contact allows a person to "get a feeling" for another individual. A strong, firm handshake transmits a different message from a weak one, and a cold, clammy hand means something different still. A warm embrace conveys quite a different message than a casual hug. Much more can be discerned in a kiss than in the conversation that precedes it. In language, the receptive function of the skin is often used to describe perceptions, for example, "You feel so distant."

The sense of touch is the first to reach maturity in the developing infant. It has been observed that the newborn receives most of its stimulation and communication from the outside world through the skin. It takes several weeks for the eyes and ears to fully develop, but the skin is already a mature sensory organ at birth. For the newborn, the emotions associated with pleasure are fulfilled simply by the security of the mother's embrace.

Bonding between mother and child is extremely important. Many of the psychoneurotic afflictions that are common in Western society may be a result of inadequate or negative sensory stimulation during infancy. Specific modern practices are implicated, such as the early maternal-infant separation that occurs in most nurseries, the practice of bottle feeding as well as general cultural habits such as isolating the child in a crib or carriage as opposed to carrying the infant on one's back or chest. The expressive quality of touch is just as important as the specific message perceived through touch. It is as emotionally fulfilling for the mother to give to her child through loving touch as it is for the baby to receive.

The study of relating surface skin anatomy of the body to internal organ functions is called physiognomy. Through physiognomy a person's health can be ascertained by observing certain features of the skin. It is easy to distinguish a person in glowing health from a terminal patient with sunken features. In fact, the study of the qualities of the skin has always served as an important aspect in the art of medical diagnosis. For example, vitamin B deficiency may manifest as a rash or cracked lip. Zinc deficiency appears as white spots on the nails. Protein deficiency also affects the consistency of the nails, causing horizontal ridging to occur. Diabetes, cancer, gout and most systemic illnesses have demonstrable skin symptoms.

In Western medicine it is recognized that a crease on the earlobe may indicate active or latent heart disease. Coarse facial features are seen in acromegaly (excessive growth hormone effects) and the round moon-shaped face is seen in Cushing's disease (adrenal hyperfunctioning). In traditional medical systems such as Chinese medicine, the study of facial features is highly developed, and the external is considered to be a reflection of the internal. The lines of the face, the shape of the nose and lips and the slant of the eyes are all significant. By observing these characteristics it becomes possible to diagnose liver, kidney and heart problems.

This phenomenon of the external reflecting the internal is most clearly established in the specific acupuncture discipline known as auriculotherapy. *Auriculo* means "ear." Acupuncture describes a point-for-point reflection of every body part on the external ear. Inserting an acupuncture needle in the point on the ear that corresponds to a particular body part will cause numbness in that body part. This is one of the major manipulations used in acupuncture anesthesia. Similarly, in foot reflexology, the organs of the body are considered to correspond to certain areas on the soles of the feet. Pressure on a certain part of the sole may affect the corresponding body part. These two therapies represent specific parts of the body's surface on which the entire anatomy of the body is mapped out in detail. Ayurveda has some similarities to Chinese medicine.

This mirroring of the inner body upon the surface, along with other functions of the skin which have been discussed, such as elimination, protection and communication on emotional and intellectual levels, helps to explain how body massage can influence the person positively through this most sensitive receptor, the skin.

Acne and Other Skin Eruptions

There are many types of skin eruptions, varying in color, texture, type of discharge, degree of inflammation and intensity of pain or itching. Most eruptions, like mild acne, eczema or seborrhea, usually represent a vent for the system's waste products. A small minority of skin problems, like certain skin cancers, severe psoriasis or lupus erythematosis, represent deep systemic disorders that, in a sense, have spilled out onto the skin, or in some cases, the skin is where the disease first manifests.

In this discussion, acne has been chosen as a prototype of a skin eruption because it is perhaps the most common dermatologic problem, and it is also amenable to various types of treatments. It is interesting to compare modern and ancient therapeutics useful in acne. While the major focus will be on acne, skin eruptions in general will be discussed when appropriate.

Causes of Acne

Acne is a condition of recurrent pimple formation that blocks the pores through which the sebaceous glands drain. As a result sebaceous gland oil backs up and seeps into the skin, creating irritation. Secondarily, bacteria may infect this area of inflammation. While most common during adolescence, acne may persist throughout adult life. Several etiologic factors have been incriminated: nutritional deficiencies or excesses, hormonal dysfunction, psychological conflict and infections, but no single agent has been determined to be the definitive cause of acne. Stress is important because it affects the immune system and the secretion of hormones. The male hormones, androgens, are known to cause acne if their levels are too high. According to Eastern and other schools of natural medicine, acne represents the body's way of expelling wastes, and like other chronic diseases, is a manifestation of an underlying imbalance.

Emotional health also has manifestations on the skin. Because the skin and nervous system are closely related, the skin will reflect imbalances of the nervous system. Stress, psychological conflicts and resultant hormonal imbalances are important in the etiology of acne. The human body is a highly resilient and adaptable structure and, if not severely tested, will maintain homeostasis. But if it is continuously overwhelmed by a combination of stresses like poor quality nutrition, lack of exercise and emotional strain, the body's ability to maintain normal physiologic functioning may break down. In this situation, the skin, representing the most external and superficial of the body's organs, can be the area onto which all inner processes are reflected.

From the above discussion, it should be clear that acne is dependent on a variety of factors. It is not due solely to the facial bacteria, too much chocolate or pizza or hormonal problems. Acne can flourish only when the right bacteria begin to grow in a receptive environment prepared by faulty nutrition, an unhealthy psychological matrix and disruptive physiological changes associated with adolescence or the menstrual cycle.

Homeopathic medicine asserts that the depth and degree of illness depends on: (1) inherited predisposition; (2) the intensity of a stressful stimulus, whether environmental, accidental, emotional or microorganism overgrowth; and (3) the nature of the treatment used in terms of strengthening or weakening the defense mechanism. According to homeopathy, when the mind and/or body are disturbed, the natural reaction of the human organism is to attempt to reestablish order and homeostasis. Since the vital force will protect the most vital structures by creating a zone of defense at the most superficial and least harmful levels, symptoms will manifest as far from the more important organs as possible. Thus, the skin, being the most superficial area, is the primary choice for internal disease processes to manifest. From this perspective, skin eruptions are reflections of a defense reaction and are actually protective in nature. Homeopaths consider it to be problematic if the patient displays signs of illness yet does not have the vitality and inner power to throw off the disordered processes onto the skin in the form of heat (fever), rashes, pimples, boils or eczema. In this situation, the internal organs, or even the mind, remain afflicted with the disease process.

Another unfavorable situation can arise when drugs are continuously used to suppress skin manifestations. When this superficial point of defense is removed, a new more internal barrier must be created. Because the original attempt of the system to establish balance was the best possible at that particular moment, the new level occurring after suppression would probably be inferior. If every time psoriasis, eczema or abscesses erupt, their outlet is obstructed by cortisone or coal tar preparations, then the defense mechanism, which was attempting to establish homeostasis by eliminating the disease process on the most peripheral level possible (skin), is inhibited and the vital force is weakened. A secondary defense is established at a less superficial level, which is less effective, more internal and consequently more threatening to the organism. A shock or external stimulus that would normally be neutralized by a strong vital force acting through the defense mechanism, may now overwhelm the weakened vital force. It is in this sense that the disease process is said to have been driven inwards to more vital areas.

The skin is a mirror of health; the color, glow, dryness or oiliness of the skin are reflections of a person's internal condition. Organ dysfunctions manifest themselves on the skin. Likewise, unresolved emotional issues often appear as skin problems. Therefore, a healthy skin often reflects a healthy personality. The approach to an unhealthy skin is not to apply creams, but to work on correcting the internal imbalance by following a good nutritional program and trying to identify and confront psychological problems.

Holistic Treatment

Nutrition

From a holistic medical perspective, nutrition is of utmost importance in preventing acne. It is often helpful to avoid animal fats, refined carbohydrates, chocolate and foods with preservatives. Fresh fruits, green leafy vegetables, whole grains, legumes and lean meats should be emphasized. Zinc and vitamins A, B complex, and C all have a therapeutic effect on acne. Because of its high vitamin A content, carrot juice is helpful.

Exercise and Hatha Yoga

Hatha yoga has a positive effect on skin problems because it enhances relaxation, helps to balance hormone levels and to develop an increased awareness of breathing and psychological difficulties.

Inverted postures are especially helpful because of the shunting of blood to the face and head and the subsequent cleansing effect.

Vigorous active exercise is often helpful in acne and other types of skin eruptions because increased blood circulation to the skin stimulates stagnant areas where sebum and bacteria build up. The induction of perspiration may also help eliminate metabolic and stored environmental waste products. Some people never sweat, and when this function is reestablished, they find their general health improves, because perspiration serves as a natural vent for accumulated waste materials. Thus, sauna baths and steam baths are also advantageous therapy for acne.

Cleansings

Cleanliness is an important preventive in the treatment of acne. Washing helps to reduce surface dirt and oil that may clog skin pores, thus allowing the secretions of the sebaceous glands (sebum) to drain normally. The sebum has antibacterial and antifungal properties and protects and lubricates the skin.

Performing yoga washes (kriyas) such as the upper wash has been advocated, the rationale being that these washes help the body eliminate waste products and mucus from the stomach that would otherwise be discharged through the skin and mucus membranes. Sun exposure, clay, salt packs and other external applications often prove useful. Steaming the face is also recommended. For people with oily skin, the following process can help dry up the skin of the face, clean out blackheads and close off pores. Bring water to a boil, then add rosemary leaves and continue boiling for sixty seconds longer. Turn off the heat and place a towel over the head and steaming vessel so that the vapor with the rosemary essence gently envelopes the face. Keep the face far enough away from the vessel so as not to scald it with the rising steam. Continue for approximately five minutes. Then wash the face with a gentle abrasive soap, such as almond or oatmeal, and warm water. A luffa sponge can also be used to brush off dead scales. A cool water rinse should follow to close the opened pores.

Western Medical Treatment

When cleansing is not sufficient to prevent acne, standard treatment in Western medicine usually consists of antibiotic creams and pills to destroy the bacteria growing on the face, which add to the inflammation by producing secondary infection. Initially this approach might seem beneficial, but its effects are only temporary. The skin improves only so long as the antibiotics are continued. As soon as they are stopped, the acne flares up, often more severely than before. After some time, the bacteria on the skin become resistant to routine antibiotics, and new and often more powerful antibiotics must be used.

Another factor not often associated with the use of antibiotics, is the effect these drugs can have on the intricate relationship between the bacteria living on the skin and the skin itself. Normal skin bacteria are destroyed by the antibiotics and they are replaced by new and often drug-resistant bacteria. Furthermore, it is not only the skin's bacteria that are affected when an antibiotic is taken, but the bacterial population of the throat, colon (microbiome) or vagina may also be altered. When this occurs, the person becomes more susceptible to sore throats, various intestinal difficulties or recurrent vaginitis.

Breathing Exercises

The practice of diaphragmatic breathing and relaxation is essential in the treatment of acne. This simple practice can markedly affect the influence of stress upon the autonomic nervous system and the endocrine (hormone) system. Other breathing exercises are also very beneficial in skin disorders, especially if a slow and gradual increase in capacity is established. Kapalabhati, if vigorously practiced, can exert a cleansing effect on the skin as a fine perspiration is released. Gently rubbing this perspiration is said by advanced practitioners to add a healthy glow to the complexion.

Psychosomatic Medicine

Psychosomatic medicine describes picking of pimples and intense scratching of the skin in general as an expression of hostile, angry impulses that have been deflected from their real target and turned against oneself. Often the reason such a person does not express anger or hostility is because they feel guilty about having such feelings because parents or society mistakenly convey that it is not right to feel or express such feelings. Sexual repression can also lead to inhibited guilt or frustration, which can result in pent-up anger. Picking of pimples as well as scratching so hard that the skin can break serves as an outlet for repressed feelings. And as the person scratches furiously to cause bleeding and scab formation that can result in scarring, the resulting disfigurement can lead to shame and humiliation. This may further cause others to reject them. This helps to promote the attitude that "I am no good anyway," which can serve to ease the feelings of underlying guilt.

Meditation

As the skin is the largest and most ubiquitous organ of the body, meditation through all the chakras is indicated. If someone is interested in Chinese philosophy, I teach the microcosmic orbit meditation, as this helps to circulate energy and chi throughout the energy body.

Homeopathy

Silicea (pure flint) is a homeopathic remedy whose mode of action exemplifies the idea that the system attempts to reestablish homeostasis by expulsion through the skin. The close connection between emotions and personality characteristics and the skin's physical symptomatology also becomes apparent through analysis of this homeopathically prepared mineral. Silicea helps to localize and open abscesses since it promotes suppuration (pus formation). It seems to stimulate a weakened vital force to throw out infectious processes or hardened tissues as well as foreign bodies like splinters. In a constitution that seemingly lacks the necessary strength to establish a strong defense at its periphery (skin), Silicea gives the vital force an extra push to complete the process. Boils or pimples are stimulated to come to a head and then to drain; scar tissue is absorbed and subsequently softens; and, old cracks or fistulous openings on the skin heal. It is interesting to note that the microscopic nature of flint is characterized by very tiny yet extremely sharp points. The essence of Silicea reflects this configuration in that its sharp edge seems to "cut open" the skin so that the disease process can find a vent.

Physical feebleness and lack of reactivity is closely associated with concomitant mental weakness. A person who requires Silicea is typically "yielding, faint-hearted, anxious, sensitive to all impressions, has a lack of vital heat, is cold and chilly and in general has a want of grit, moral or physical."57

Another quote from one of the most brilliant homeopaths of the late nineteenth and early twentieth centuries, James Tyler Kent, MD, eloquently exemplifies the peculiar mental state of the typical patient that responds to Silicea: "The patient lacks stamina. What Silicea is to the stalk of grain in the field, it is to the human mind. Take the glossy, stiff outer covering of a stalk of grain and examine it, and you will realize with what firmness it supports the head of grain until it ripens; there is a gradual deposit of Silicea in it to give it stamina. So, it is with the mind; when the mind needs Silicea it is in a state of weakness, embarrassment and dread, all typical of a state of yielding. If you should listen to the description of this state by a prominent clergyman or a lawyer, or a man in the habit of appearing in public with self-confidence, firmness and fullness of thought and speech, he would tell you he had come to a state where he dreads to appear in public. He feels his own selfhood so that he cannot enter into his subject, he dreads it and fears that he will fail, his mind will not work and he is worn out by prolonged efforts at mental work. But he will say that when he forces himself into the harness he can go on with ease, his usual self-command returns to him and he does well; he does his work with promptness, fullness and accuracy. The peculiar Silicea state is found in the dread of failure. If he has any unusual mental task to perform, he fears he will make a failure of it, yet he does it well. This is the early state; of course, there comes a time when he cannot perform the work with accuracy and he may need Silicea."58

The homeopathic remedy Sulphur offers another interesting study of mind-body-skin interrelatedness. Mentally, a person needing Sulphur is irritable, volatile, angry and emotionally eruptive. They tend to argue vehemently about all sorts of meaningless issues and thus deserve the label "the ragged philosopher." As J T Kent says: "He has long, uncut hair and a dirty face; his study is uncleanly, it is untidy; books and leaves of books are piled up indiscriminately; there is no order. It seems that Sulphur produces this state of disorder, a state of untidiness, a state of uncleanliness, a state of "I don't care how things go" and a state of selfishness. He becomes a false philosopher and the more he goes on in this state the more he is disappointed because the world does not consider him the greatest man on earth."59

The Sulphur anger and hostility are either expressed in volatile outbursts or are repressed and sublimated into other areas like study or philosophical dissertation. This work, however, is disorderly and disorganized as the misdirected and dissipated focus of attention makes the quality of the work poor. The repressed anger is also expressed as uncleanliness or extreme itching that eventually causes the skin to become raw, red and ugly. Both situations act as a mechanism to keep other people away or to cause rejection by others. Thus, the guilt that arose from hostile impulses is expiated.

The Sulphur skin is characterized by a similar eruptive nature. All sorts of eruptions occur: vesicular, pustular, scaly, herpetic or eczematous. Like its corresponding hot-tempered personality, the Sulphur discharges are hot, corrosive and burning. As the Sulphur patient is unclean and odoriferous generally, the discharges are also foul-smelling.

Another prominent skin symptom of the Sulphur type illness is that intense itching accompanies most problems. This is particularly aggravated by wool, warm rooms or beds, and baths (the Sulphur patient despises bathing), and is generally worse at night. Relief often is afforded through voluptuous scratching until the skin becomes raw and begins to burn.

Case History

Miss T is a twenty-eight-year-old woman with a history of several skin disorders, including cystic acne since adolescence and chronic recurring eczema since childhood. Both dermatologic problems would aggravate during times of high emotional stress. Arguments with her parents and siblings particularly exacerbated her symptoms. Instead of expressing her opinion, she either sulked or exploded in rage. In either case, she was ill at ease expressing angry feelings. As a consequence, inner frustration and built up anger manifested in an outbreak of eczema, which she scratched until the skin bled as though she were attacking herself.

Her mother had given her subtle messages that she was incompetent to make her own decisions, and she slowly developed feelings of inadequacy and in general, lacked self-confidence. Her disfiguring eczema reconfirmed her negative self-image. To compound the problem, her father constantly offered her money for vacations and luxuries. Despite earning a good salary, she felt obliged to accept these monetary gifts so that her father would not be upset. As a result, she felt even more dependent, which further decreased her feelings of self-worth and self-esteem and worsened her acne condition.

Specific Treatment

Nutrition

Treatment for Miss T was multifaceted. Nutritionally, she was taken off all animal fats including beef, pork and eggs. Lighter vegetable oils such as cold pressed sesame, sunflower seed and olive oils were allowed. Dairy products were restricted, not only because the fat seemed to make her acne worse, but also because she proved to be allergic to milk protein, which exacerbated her eczema.

Specific supplements that were helpful for the acne included vitamins A and C and zinc as well as the herbs goldenseal and Echinacea. For the eczema, vitamin B was added. She was advised to keep areas of eczema dry and exposed to sunlight, and to apply topically a combination of oil of Calendula (marigold), vitamin E and sesame oil. A facial sauna and herbal clay packs were prescribed for her facial acne.

Breathing Exercises

She was advised to practice the cleansing breathing techniques, kapalabhati and bhramari, daily. Relaxation techniques and diaphragmatic breathing helped her realize how tight her muscles were. I recommended she take a yoga class and do the entire sequence of twelve postures she had been learning. She also took a tai chi course and was able to do both a hatha yoga practice three days weekly and alternate this with four days of a chen tai chi practice. This helped her manage the stress in her life.

Psychotherapy

Slowly through psychotherapy and meditation, she began to recognize her anger and learned to confront her parents more directly when they discouraged her efforts to assert herself. She began to refuse her father's money and moved into her own apartment. She generally assumed a more honest and mature relationship with her parents. Simultaneously, the intensity of her eczema reactions diminished, and her acne greatly improved.

Homeopathy

Several homeopathic remedies were used, the most important being Graphites (Graphite) when her eczema oozed a sticky substance and she was depressed and constipated, Sepia (ink of the female cuttlefish) when she was withdrawn and her acne and eczema erupted during the premenstrual period, Silicea to help open cysts and Sulphur when her anger was self-directed and she scratched her eczema until it bled.

In Retrospect

As I am in my seventy-second year in this life's journey, patients, family and friends have been asking me when I plan to retire from my medical practice. I too have pondered this question. The truth is the practice of holistic medicine and caring for people is part job and part spiritual practice for me. While I help take care of people who are suffering, I also get to discuss the benefits of eating natural healthy foods, exercise, hatha yoga and meditation. In fact, my spiritual life is so intertwined with my medical practice that they have become one and the same.

The doctor's black bag I carry with me contains not only the instruments for diagnosis such as a stethoscope and otoscope, scalpels, syringes and suture material to mend a person's body, but also homeopathic remedies, a summary of yoga postures and breathing techniques, and ideas about what meditation practices would be best used during times of illness, stress or anxiety. These are useful as I show my patients which yoga postures could be used therapeutically for such conditions as an underactive thyroid or low back pain. I also teach breathing exercises for patients who are suffering from asthma, anxiety or depression.

In a sense, I practice the different types of yoga, including karma yoga when I serve people and their health needs as selflessly as possible. I practice bhakti yoga by caring deeply about my patient's overall well-being with as much compassion and empathy as possible. Through my study and teachings, I practice jnana yoga, and ultimately the practice of raja yoga gathers it all together. I help others see how ethical and simple living can combine with healthy physical and dietary habits and the practice of meditation, to become the best person they can be.

When I look back on my career, I am so grateful to have practiced preventive medicine on multiple levels. I have been privileged to treat four generations in the same family and to see how patterns of behavior and health are passed on through the ages, what homeopaths call miasms. Besides my public health work with its community and global implications, my private family practice is preventive in its focus with an emphasis on good nutrition, exercise, natural medicines when possible and holistic practices. As a physician whose practice encompasses many of the subjects discussed in this book, I can without hesitation state that my experiences have been very rewarding and fulfilling. I feel I have been very blessed to have had the opportunity to care for patients and to guide them on the path of holistic and healthful living.

Endnotes

1. Frawley, David. *Yoga and Ayurveda.* Delhi, India: Motilal Banarsidas Publishers, 1999. 87-104.
2. Chernin, Dennis and Greg Manteuffel. *Health: A Holistic Approach.* Wheaton, Illinois: Quest Books,1984. 84-99.
3. Rama, Swami, Rudolph Ballentine, and Alan Hymes. *The Science of Breath.* Honesdale, PA: Himalayan Institute Press, 1998. 72-112. And Avalon, Arthur. *The Serpent Power: The Secret of Tantric and Shaktic Yoga.* New York: Dover Publications, 1974. 257-498.
4. Trugman, Avraham. *Shema Yisrael.* Israel: Ohr Chadash, 2016. 66-67.
5. Koch, Christof. *Consciousness: Confessions of a Romantic Reductionist.* Cambridge: MIT Press, 2012. 124.
6. Ibid, Koch. 80.
7. Rama, Swami. *Emotions to Enlightenment.* Honesdale, PA: Himalayan Institute Press, 1987. Whole Book.
8. Vishnudevananda. *Mantra and Meditation.* Delhi, India: Motilal Banarsidas, 2003. 148-151.
9. Ajaya, Swami. *Yoga Psychology: A Practical Guide to Meditation.* Honesdale, PA: Himalayan Institute Press, 1976. 16-18.
10. Rama, Swami. *Path of Fire and Light.* Honesdale, PA: Himalayan Institute Press, 1986. 114-116. And Ajaya. *Yoga Psychology.* 80-86.
11. Chernin. *Health: A Holistic Approach.* 99-118.
12. Suzuki, Shunryu. *Zen Mind, Beginner's Mind.* New York: Weatherhill, 1974. 21-22.
13. Gia-Fu Feng and Jane English. *Lao Tzu and the Tao Te Ching.* Toronto, Canada: Vintage Books, 1972. 36.

14. Wong, C.henchen "Effect of tai chi versus aerobic exercise for fibromyalgia: comparative effectiveness randomized controlled trial." BMJ 2018. 360.K851.

15. Huston, Patricia and Bruce McFarlane. "Health Benefits of Tai Chi : What is the Evidence." *Canadian Family Physician (Le Medecin de famille canadien)* 62 (2016): 881-890.

16. 16. Mookerjee, Ajit. *Kundalini.* Rochester, VT: Destiny Books, 1986. 71-83.

17. Pandit, MP. *Kundalini Yoga.* Pomona, CA: Auromere Publications, 1979. 50-60. And Swami Vishnu Tirtha. *Devatma Shakti.* Delhi, India: Swami Shivan Tirth Publications, 1962. 76-78. And Rama. *Path of Fire and Light.* 134-144.

18. Johari, Harish. *Chakras.* Rochester, VT: Destiny Books, 1987. 47-84. And S. Goswami. *Layayoga: The Definitive Guide to the Chakras and Kundalini.* Rochester, VT: Inner Traditions, 1999. 143-286. And MP Pandit. *Kundalini Yoga.* 50-60.

19. Glick, Yoel Rabbi. *Walking the Path of the Jewish Mystic.* Woodstock, VT: Jewish Life Publishing, 2015. 3-15.

20. Yang, JM. *Qigong Meditation: Small Circulation.* Boston, MA: YMAA Publication: 1st Edition. 2016. Whole book.

21. Vishnudevananda. *Mantra and Meditation.* 148-151.

22. *World Book Science Annual 1974, The 1973 Encyclopedia Britannica Yearbook of Science. The Time-Life 1973 Nature Science Annual.*

23. Kaplan, Aryeh. *Jewish Meditation.* New York: Schocken Books, 1985. 35-36.

24. Khanna, Madhu. *Yantra: The Tantric Symbol of Cosmic Unity.* London, England: Thames and Hudson, 1994. 109-130.

25. Maher, E. *The Mind Gut Connection.* NY: Harper Collins Publisher, 2016. 12.

26. Melville, Nancy. "Gut Bacteria, Diet Significant in Multiple Sclerosis." Medscape.com. Consortium of Multiple Sclerosis Centers Annual Meetings. June 05, 2018.

27. Sabate, Joan. "Unscrambling the Relations of Egg and Meat Consumption with Type 2 Diabetes Risk." *The American Journal of Clinical Nutrition.* 108, Issue 5 (2018): 1121-1128.

28. Environmental Working Group. April 2016, www.ewg.org.

29. Vishnudevanada Swami. *Sivananda Yoga Teacher Training Manual.* Val Marin Quebec, Canada: International Sivananda Vedanta Centre Headquarters. 2018. Whole Manual.

30. Coulter, David. *Anatomy of Hatha Yoga.* Marlboro, VT: Body and Breath Inc. 2017. Whole Book.

31. Kaminoff, Leslie and Amy Matthews. *Yoga Anatomy.* Champaign, IL: Human Kinetics. 2015. Whole Book.

32. Chernin. *Health: A Holistic Approach.* 99-118.

33. Rama, *Path of Fire and Light,* 16-21. And A. Van Lysbeth. *Pranayama.* London, England: Mandala Books, 1979. 140-178. And Swami Sivananda. *The Science of Pranayama.* Garhwal, India: The Divine Life Society, 1971. 74-84.

34. *World Book Science Annual 1974, the 1973 Encyclopedia Britannica Yearbook of Science, the Time-Life 1973 Nature Science Annual.*

35. Walsh, Nancy. "Can Yoga Tame OCD." *Patient Care* 34, Issue 7 (2000): 14.

36. Chernin. *Health: A Holistic Approach.* 99-118.

37. Ibid 99-118.

38. Austin, James. *Zen and the Brain.* Cambridge, MA: MIT Press, 1998. 57-148. And Lynda Freeman and G F Lawlis. *Complementary & Alternative Medicine.* St. Louis, MO: Mosby, 2001. 166-196.

39. Cahn, B Rael et al. "Yoga, Meditation and Mind-Body Health: Increased BDNF, Cortisol Awakening Response." *Frontiers in Human Neuroscience* 11 (2017): 315.

40. Mahajan, Aarti Sood. "Role of Yoga in Hormonal Homeostasis." *International Journal of Clinical and experimental Physiology* 1, Issue 3 (2014): 173-178.

41. <u>Masoumeh, Shohani et al.</u> "The Effect of Yoga on Stress, Anxiety and Depression in Women." *International Journal of Preventive Medicine* 9(21) (2018): 242-255.

42. Cabral, <u>Patricia,</u> B.A., <u>Hilary B. Meyer,</u> B.A., and <u>Donna Ames,</u> M. "Effectiveness of Yoga Therapy as a Complementary Treatment for Major Psychiatric Disorders: A Meta-Analysis." *Primary Care Companion,* CNS Disorders 2011: 13.

43. Arora, Sarika and Jayashree Bhattacharjee. "Modulation of Immune Responses in Stress by Yoga." *International Journal of Yoga* 2 (2008): 45-55.

44. Mohandas, E "Neurobiology of Spirituality." *Mens Sana Monographs* 6(1) (2008): 63-80.

45. Lagouge, Marie et al. "Resveratrol Improves Mitochondrial Function and Protects against Metabolic Disease by Activating SIRT1 and PGC-1alpha." *Cell* 127(6) (2006): 1091-1093.

46. McMackin, Craig and Michael Widlansky. "Effect of Combined treatment with Alpha Lipoic Acid and Acetyl-L-carnitine on Vascular Function and Blood Pressures in Coronary Artery Disease." *Journal of Clinical Hypertension* 9(4) (2007): 249-255.

47. Bhasin, Manoj K et al. "Relaxation Response Induces Temporal Transcriptome Changes in Energy Metabolism, Insulin Secretion and Inflammatory Pathways." *Plos One.* 12(2) (2017): 12.

48. Waltham, Clare, Chuang Tzu. *Genius of the Absurd.* NY, NY. Ace Books. 1971 (Chuang Tzu, "The Butterfly as Companion: Meditations on the First Three Chapters of the Chuang Tzu)."

49. Clarke, Nicholas. *Paracelsus: Essential Readings.* Berkeley, CA. North Atlantic Books 1999. Whole Book.

50. Ullman, Dana. *The Consumer's Guide to Homeopathy.* Berkeley, CA: Homeopathic Education Services. 1984. 14.

51. Kunzli, Jost et al. *Hahnemann, Samuel. The Organon of Medicine.* Blain, Washington: Cooper Publishing, 1996. 1-218.

52. Ullman, Dana. "Principles of Homeopathy." *Co-Evolution Quarterly* 1981. 66.

53. Bridgman, Percy Williams. *The Physics of High Pressure.* London, England. G. Bell and Sons, 1931. Whole Book.

54. Ibid. Kunzil. Section 1, paragraph 9.

55. Fitch, KD et al. "Effects of Swimming Training on Children with Asthma." *Archives of Disease in Childhood* 51. 1976): 190-194.

56. Alexander, Franz. *Psychosomatic Medicine.* NY, NY: W. W. Norton. 1950. 104.

57. Boericke, William. *Material Medica with Repertory.* New Delhi: Jain Publishing Co. 1976. 891.

58. Kent, James Tyler. *Lectures on Homeopathic Materia Medica.* Chicago, IL: B. Jain Publishers, 1923. 925-9.

59. Ibid. 952.

Bibliography

Ajaya, Swami. *Yoga Psychology: A Practical Guide to Meditation.* Honesdale, PA: Himalayan Institute Press, 1976.

—. *Psychotherapy East and West.* Honesdale, PA.: Himalayan Institute Press, 1983.

Alexander, Franz. *Psychosomatic Medicine.* NY, NY: W. W. Norton, 1950.

Austin, James. *Zen and the Brain: Towards an Understanding of Meditation and Consciousness.* Cambridge, MA: MIT, 1998.

Avalon, Arthur. *The Serpent Power: The Secret of Tantric and Shaktic Yoga.* New York: Dover Publications, 1974.

Besserman, Perle. *Kabbalah and Jewish Mysticism.* Boston, MA: Shambhala, 1997.

Boericke, W. *Materia Medica with Repertory.* New Delhi: Jain Publishing Co., 1976.

Chernin, Dennis, and Greg Manteuffel. *Health: A Holistic Approach.* Wheaton, IL.: Quest Books, 1984.

Chernin, Dennis. *How to Meditate Using Chakras, Mantras and Breath.* Ann Arbor, MI: Think Publishing, 2006.

—. *The Complete Homeopathic Resource for Common Illnesses,* Berkeley, CA: North Atlantic Books and Homeopathic Educational Services. 2006.

Clarke, NG. *Paracelsus: Essential Readings.* Selected Works of, Berkeley, CA, 1999.

Cooper, David. *God is a Verb: Kabbalah.* NY, NY. Riverhead Books, 1997.

Coulter, David. *Anatomy of Hatha Yoga.* Albany, CA, 2015.

Digambayi, Swami. *Hathapradipika.* Dehli, India: Kaivalya-dhama,1970.

Eliade, Mircea. *Yoga: Immortality and Freedom.* Princeton, N.J.: Princeton University Press, 1969.

Epstein, Perle. Kabbalah: *The Way of the Jewish Mystic.* NY, NY: Samuel Weiser, 1978.

Feurerstein, Greg. *Tantra: The Path of Ecstasy.* Boston, MA: Shambhala, 1998.

Frawley, David. *Yoga and Ayurveda.* Lotus Press, Twin Lakes, WI USA, www.lotuspress.com.

Freeman, L. and G.F. Lawlis. *Complementary & Alternative Medicine.* St. Louis, MO: Mosby, 2001.

Gia-Fu Feng and Jane English. *Lao Tzu and The Tao Te Ching.* Toronto, Canada: Vintage Books, 1972.

Glick, Yoel Rabbi. *Walking the Path of the Jewish Mystic.* Woodstock, VT: Jewish Life Publishing, 2015.

Goldstein, J., and Jack Kornfield. *Seeking the Heart of Wisdom: The Path of Insight Meditation.* Boston, MA: Shambhala, 1987.

Goswami, S. Layayoga: *The Definitive Guide to the Chakras and Kundalini.* Rochester, VT: Inner Traditions, 1999.

Govinda, Lama. *Foundations of Tibetan Mysticism.* York Beach, ME: Samuel Weiser, 1969.

Iyengar, B. K. S. *Light on Yoga.* New York: Schocken Books, 1975.

Johari, Harish. *Chakras.* Rochester, VT: Destiny Books, 1987.

Judith, Anadea. *Eastern Body Western Mind: Psychology and the Chakra System.* Berkeley, CA.: Celestial Arts, 1996.

Kabat-Zinn, Jon. *Wherever You Go There You Are.* New York: Hyperion, 1994.

Kaplan, Aryeh. *Jewish Meditation.* New York: Schoken Books, 1985.

Kaminoff. Leslie and Amy Matthews. *Yoga Anatomy.* Champaign Il. Human Kinetics, 2015.

Kent, *Lectures on Homeopathic Materia Medica.*

Khalsa, D. et al. "Randomized Controlled Trial of Yogic Meditation Techniques for Patients with Obsessive-Compulsive Disorder." *CNS Spectrums* 4.4 (1999): 34-47.

Khanna, Madhu. *Yantra: The Tantric Symbol of Cosmic Unity.* London: Thames and Hudson, 1994.

Koch, Christof. *Consciousness: Confessions of a Romantic Reductionist.* Cambridge: MIT Press, 2012.

Kornfield, Jack. *After the Ecstasy, the Laundry.* NY, NY: Bantam Books, 2000.

LeShan, Lawrence. *How to Meditate.* Boston, MA.: Back Bay Books, 1999.

Maher, E. *The Mind Gut Connection.* NY, NY: Harper Collins Publisher, 2016.

Mookerjee, Ajit. *Kundalini.* Rochester, VT: Destiny Books, 1986.

Pandit, M. P. *Kundalini Yoga.* Pomona, CA: Auromere Publications, 1979.

Prabhavananda, S., and C. Isherwood. *How to Know God: The Yoga Aphorisms of Patanjali.* New York: Mentor Books, 1969.

Rama, Swami. *Choosing a Path.* Honesdale, PA.: Himalayan Institute Press, 1988.

—. *Lectures on Yoga.* Honesdale, PA: Himalayan Institute Press, 1976.

—. *Path of Fire and Light: Advanced Practices of Yoga.* Honesdale, PA: Himalayan Institute Press, 1986.

—. *Emotions to Enlightenment.* Honesdale, PA: Himalayan Institute Press, 1987.

Rama, S., R. Ballentine., and S. Ajaya. *Yoga and Psychotherapy.* Glenview, IL: Himalayan Institute Press, 1976.

Rama, S., R. Ballentine., and A. Hymes. *The Science of Breath.* Honesdale, PA.: Himalayan Institute Press, 1998.

Saraswati, Swami. *Asana Pranayama Mudra Bandha.* Bihar, India: Bihar School of Yoga, 1977.

Sivananda, Swami. *The Science of Pranayama.* Garhwal, India: The Divine Life Society, 1971.

Suzuki, Shunryu. *Zen Mind, Beginner's Mind.* New York: Weatherhill, 1974.

Tigunat, Rajmani. *The Path of Mantra and the Mystery of Initiation.* Honesdale, PA: Himalayan Institute Press, 1996.

Tirtha, Swami Vishnu. *Devatma Shakti.* Delhi, India: Swami Shivan Tirth Publications, 1962.

Trugman, Avraham. *Shema Yisrael.* Israel: Ohr Chadash, 2016.

Ullman, Dana. *The Consumer's Guide to Homeopathy.* Berkeley, CA, 1995.

Van Lysbeth, A. *Pranayama*. London, England: Mandala Books, 1979.

Vishnudevanada, Swami. *Sivananda Yoga Teachers Training Manual*, International Sivananda Vedanta Centre Headquarters. 673 8th Avenue, Val Marin Quebec, J0T 2 R0 Canada.

Vishnudevananda, Swami. *Mantra and Meditation*. New Delhi, India.: Jain Printing, 2013.

Waltham, Clare. Chuang Tsu: *Genuis of the Absurd*. NY, NY. Ace Books, 1971. "Chuang Tzu, *The Butterfly as companion: Meditations on the first Three Chapters of the Chuang Tzu.*"

White, John. *The Highest State of Consciousness*. New York: Doubleday, 1972.

About the Author

Dennis K. Chernin, MD, MPH received his BA and the Phi Beta Kappa honorary from Northwestern University and his MD and MPH from the University of Michigan. He did residencies in psychiatry and preventive medicine and is board certified in preventive medicine.

Even before he had completed his medical education he began to explore meditation and the spiritual dimensions of life. His personal experience with meditation and spirituality has led him to further explore many different avenues to expand his never-ending quest for further knowledge. Although he has never completely left his Western medical training, he is dedicated to providing holistic care to his patients and teaching them to take responsibility for their own health. He currently practices holistic and family medicine in Ann Arbor, Michigan using nutrition, yoga, exercise, breathing exercises, meditation therapies and homeopathy.

Dr. Chernin has actively practiced and taught meditation and breathing techniques worldwide for over forty years based upon the ancient teachings of Tantra, Vedanta and Samkhya philosophies. He is also a certified yoga teacher.

He is also the medical director of two county health departments and lectures at the University of Michigan Medical School. He continues to work with the underprivileged and rural population of Michigan to improve their life circumstances and health care.

In addition, Dr. Chernin teaches and studies Chinese martial arts, including the Yang and Chen forms of tai chi and Yin style bagua. He is a lead singer, harmonium player and co-founder of a kirtan group, Ann Arbor Kirtan.

He is the author of several books, the most recent being *The Complete Homeopathic Resource for Common Illnesses* and *How to Meditate Using Chakras, Mantras and Breath* (with audio CD of guided meditation).

Dr. Chernin has a big and loving family, including his life partner, Ruma Banerjee, PhD, his three children, Abe, Ethan and Ari and their spouses, Sarah, Leah and Michael. He is crazy about his nine grandchildren.

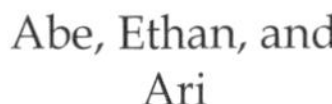

Abe, Ethan, and Ari

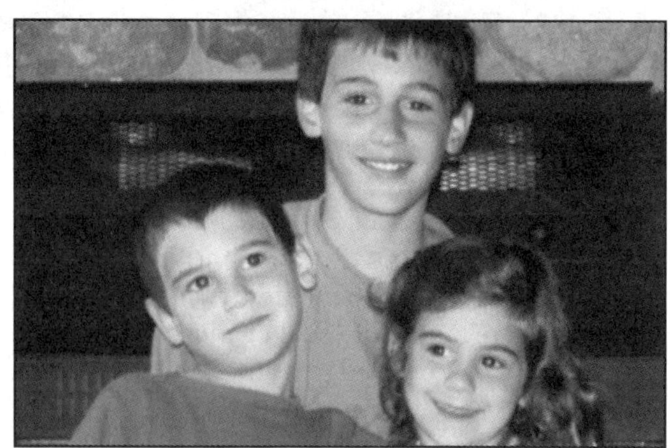

The family now (below)

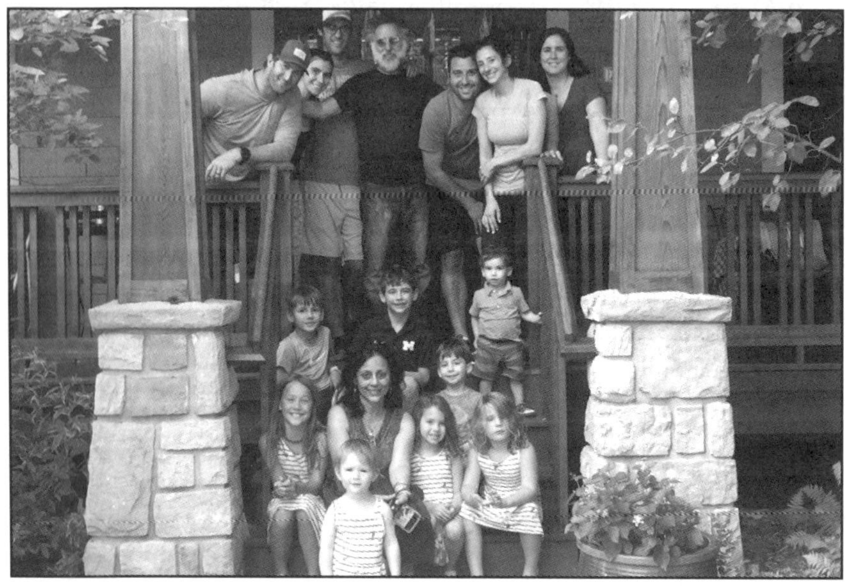

Himalayan Institute Hospital Trust

The Himalayan Institute Hospital Trust (HIHT) was conceived, designed and orchestrated by Dr. Swami Rama, a yogi, scientist, researcher, writer and humanitarian. The mission of HIHT is to develop integrated and cost-effective approaches to health care and development for the country as a whole, and for underserved populations worldwide.

Swamiji started this project in 1989 with an outpatient clinic of only two rooms. The hospital at HIHT currently has a thousand beds and is serving approximately 10 million people of Garhwal, Kumaon and adjoining areas. The hospital includes a Reference Laboratory, Emergency Wing, Operation Theaters, Blood Bank, Eye Bank, Dialysis Unit, I.C.U., C.C.U., Cath Lab., and a state-of-the-art Radiology Department. The Cancer Research Institute at HIHT is providing radiation therapy in addition to chemotherapy and surgical oncology.

The Rural Development Institute is providing health care, education, income generation opportunities, water and sanitation programs, adolescent awareness programs and other quality of life improvement programs in the villages of Uttarakhand and adjoining rural areas.

The Himalayan Institute of Medical Sciences has become Swami Rama Himalayan University, a state university promoted by the Himalayan Institute Hospital Trust, and established by the Govt. of Uttarakhand under section 2(f) of UGC Act vide Act no. 12 of 2013. The University runs undergraduate (MBBS) and postgraduate courses (MD/MS and Diploma) in 15 disciplines. The medical faculty also conducts paramedical degree courses in Medical Laboratory Technology, Radiology & Imaging Technology, and Physiotherapy. This University includes the Himalayan College of Nursing, the Himalayan School of Engineering and Technology, and the Himalayan School of Management Studies.

The College of Nursing offers a three-year GNM diploma program, a four-year BSc program, a two-year Post Basic BSc program and a two-year MSc program. The uniqueness of these nursing programs is that nursing students are provided hands-on training, both in the community and with the rural population.

Two new departments have been added to the Faculty of Medicine: the Dept. of Biosciences and the Dept. of Yoga Sciences and Holistic Health. The Dept. of Biosciences offers undergraduate and postgraduate degree programs in Biochemistry, Microbiology and Biotechnology. The Dept. of Yoga Sciences and Holistic Health currently offers a bachelor's degree program and plans to add a diploma program in the future.

In keeping with Swamiji's mission of integration, the hospital runs outpatient Ayurveda and Homeopathy clinics, and the Ayurveda Center provides a residential panchakarma therapy program for detoxification, rejuvenation and treatment of chronic ailments.

For information contact:

Himalayan Institute Hospital Trust
Swami Ram Nagar
P.O. Jolly Grant, Dehradun 248016
Uttarakhand, India
91-135-247-1200
pb@hihtindia.org
www.hihtindia.org

Swami Rama Society, Inc.

The Swami Rama Society is a registered nonprofit, tax-exempt organization committed to Swami Rama's vision of bridging the gap between Western science and Eastern wisdom. The Society was established to provide financial assistance and technical support to institutions and individuals who are ready to implement this vision in the USA and abroad.

For information contact:Swami Rama Society, Inc., 5000 W. Vliet St, Milwaukee, WI 53208 U.S.A. 414-454-0500, info@swamiramasociety.org, www.swamiramasociety.org.

Samadhi the Highest State of Wisdom

Yoga the Sacred Science, vol. one
Swami Rama

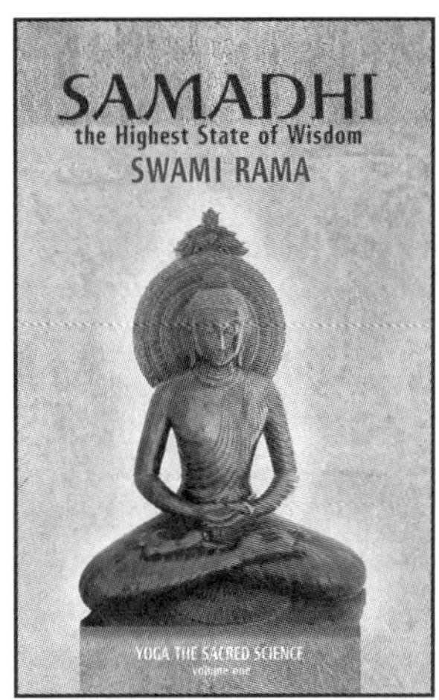

"A clear and relevant guide to the deeper practices of Yoga for those who are looking for more than mere asanas. Swami Rama addresses Patanjali's Yoga up to its highest state of samadhi and makes it accessible and understandable for the contemporary student."
David Frawley, author,
Yoga and Ayurveda, Tantric Yoga

ISBN 978-81-88157-01-3, $14.95, paperback, 256 pages

Sadhana the Path to Enlightenment

Yoga the Sacred Science, vol. two
Swami Rama

"All sadhana is meant to purify the mind and make the mind one-pointed and inward so it can be directed toward the center of consciousness within the inner chamber of your being. Physical growth is in the hands of nature; mental growth and spiritual growth are in your hands. The second chapter of the Yoga Sutras is completely devoted to sadhana and is replete with methods of practice to help you improve yourself by learning to control your mind and its modifications. Then, you can attain a state of samadhi and realize the Self within."   *Swami Rama*

ISBN 978-81-88157-68-6, $18.98, paperback, 310 pages

Distributed by Lotus Press, P.O. Box 325, Twin Lakes, WI 53181 U.S.A., www.lotuspress.com, 1-262-889-8561, lotuspress@lotuspress.com.

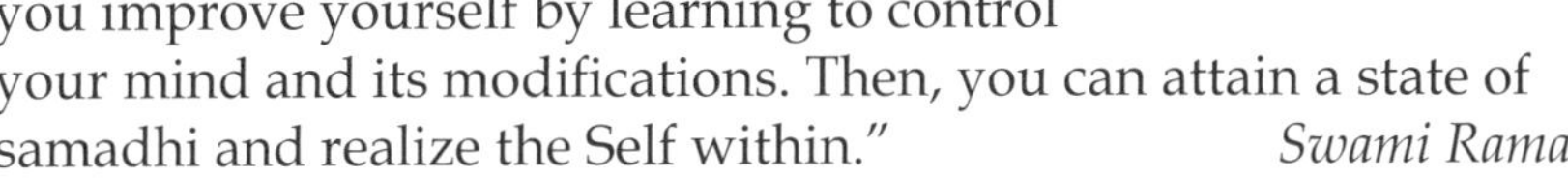

Sacred Journey
Living Purposefully and Dying Gracefully
Swami Rama

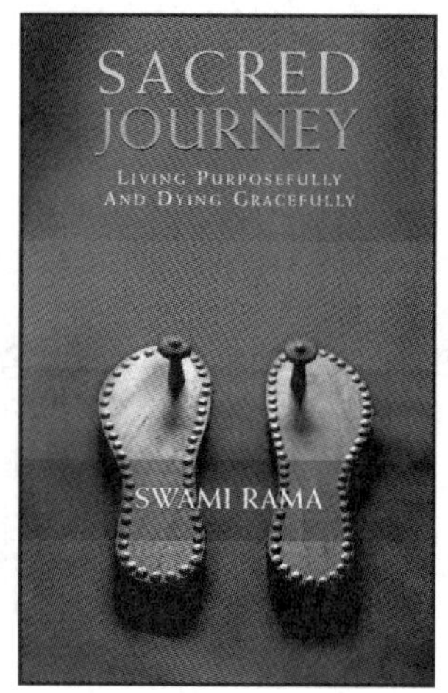

"People today spend more time preparing for a vacation than for death. Swami Rama unveils the mysteries of the afterlife, well known to the yoga masters of the Himalayas, and teaches us how to live—and die—with serenity and full awareness."
Linda Johnsen, author, *The Living Goddess*

ISBN 978-81-88157-00-6, $12.95, paperback, 136 pages

Let the Bud of Life Bloom
A Guide to Raising Happy and Healthy Children
Swami Rama

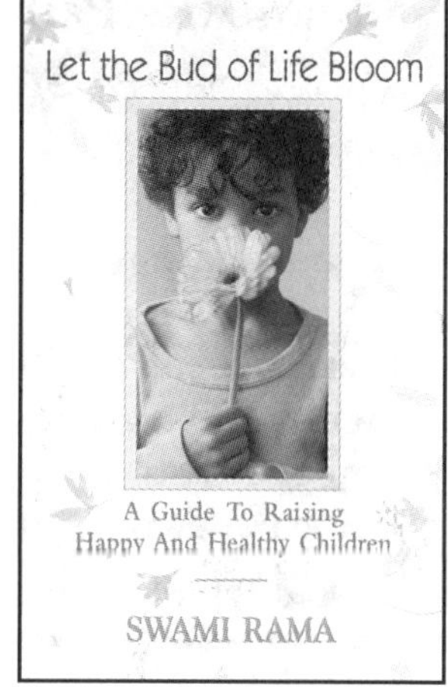

"Raising healthy, well balanced children may be one of the greatest challenges most people ever face. Swami Rama has some amazingly practical, loving and insightful advice for those of us navigating the choppy waters of parenthood."

Linda Johnsen, contributing editor, *Yoga International*

ISBN 978-188157-04-4, $12.95, paperback, 102 pages

Distributed by Lotus Press, P.O. Box 325, Twin Lakes, WI 53181 U.S.A., www.lotuspress.com, 1-262-889-8561, lotuspress@lotuspress.com.

Holistic Living Manual
The Teachings of Swami Rama of the Himalayas
Presented by
Prakash Keshaviah, Ph.D.

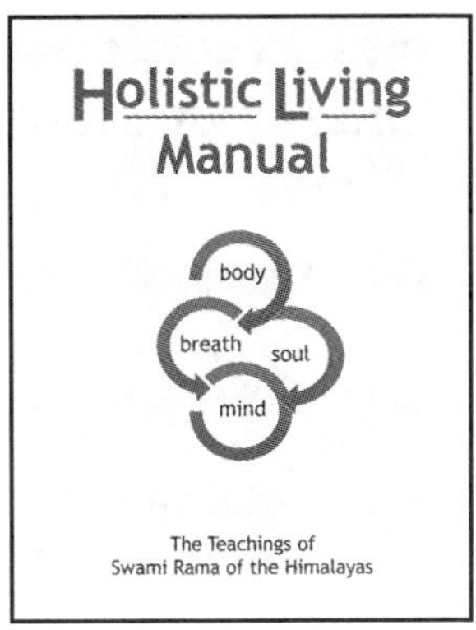

"Preventive medicine is an important part of modern life. Why should we be sick? We should be aware of health, we should be aware of diet and nutrition, we should be aware of good living, of how to eat right."   Swami Rama

The word "holistic" comes from the Greek root "holos," which means whole, total, entire. Holistic means to understand the entire human being. In holistic health, the entire human being is considered, paying attention to the interaction and integration of the biological and physiological (body and breath), psychological (conscious and unconscious mind) and philosophical (soul) dimensions. The emphasis is on treating the whole patient and not just the symptoms of disease.

Man has to realize that he is not a body alone. He is a breathing being and a thinking being with complex emotions, appetites and desires.

The purpose of life is to be happy and free from pains, fears and miseries. This can be achieved by practicing a self-training program as set forth in this manual.

ISBN 978-81-88157-71-6, 128 pages, $18.95

Distributed by Lotus Press, P.O. Box 325, Twin Lakes, WI 53181 U.S.A., www.lotuspress.com, 1-262-889-8561, lotuspress@lotuspress.com.

Yogic Practcices of the Himalayan Tradition
as Taught by H.H. Swami Rama
by Prakash Keshaviah, Ph.D.

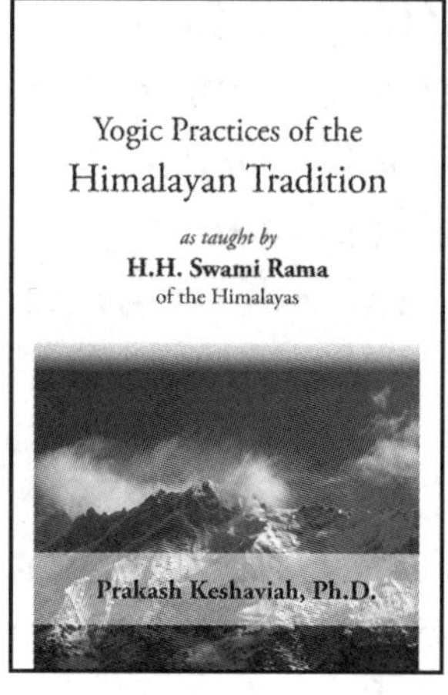

As H.H. Swami Rama always reminded his students, the purpose of human life is to attain a state that confers true happiness, bereft of all pains, miseries and bondages.

The purpose in compiling this book is to create for spiritual aspirants a ready reference of the many kriyas (yogic practices, derived from the Sanskrit kri, to act) of the Himalayan tradition that H.H. Swami Rama taught his students during the more than two decades that he spent in the United States. The vast majority of these kriyas was taught by Swamiji during seminars, workshops and lectures and have found their way into the books authored by Swamiji. However, they are scattered through many books and there is no ready reference wherein all of these kriyas are compiled and presented. It is hoped that this volume will serve that purpose. Fortunately, many of the kriyas were personally taught to the compiler of this volume during small group sessions, seminars and workshops and the writings have been compiled from his notes.

This book may be considered a progression in sadhana from the beginning practices included in the *Holistic Living Manual*. The 2-audio CD set, "Basic Practices of the Himalayan Tradition" provide complementary audio guidance for some of the practices in this volume.

ISBN 978-81-88157-97-6, paperback, 136 pages, $15.95

Distributed by Lotus Press, P.O. Box 325, Twin Lakes, WI 53181 U.S.A., www.lotuspress.com, 1-262-889-8561, lotuspress@lotuspress.com.